Orofacial Pain
From Basic Science to Clinical Management
Second Edition

Orofacial Pain

From Basic Science to Clinical Management

The Transfer of Knowledge in Pain Research to Education

Second Edition

Edited by

Barry J. Sessle, MDS, PhD, DSc(hc), FRSC, FCAHS

Gilles J. Lavigne, DMD, FRCD(C), PhD

James P. Lund, BDS, PhD, FCAHS

Ronald Dubner, DDS, PhD

Quintessence Publishing Co, Inc

Chicago, Berlin, Tokyo, London, Paris, Milan, Barcelona, Istanbul, São Paulo, Mumbai, Moscow, Prague, and Warsaw

Library of Congress Cataloging-in-Publication Data

Orofacial pain : from basic science to clinical management : the transfer of
knowledge in pain research to education / Barry J. Sessle ... [et al.]. --
2nd ed.
        p. ; cm.
  Includes bibliographical references and index.
  ISBN 978-0-86715-458-0 (hardcover)
  1. Orofacial pain. 2. Temporomandibular joint--Diseases. I. Sessle,
Barry J., 1941-
  [DNLM: 1. Facial Pain. 2. Facial Pain--therapy. 3. Temporomandibular
Joint Disorders. WE 705 O742 2008]
  RK322.O765 2008
  617.5'206--dc22
                                    2008016356

© 2008 Quintessence Publishing Co, Inc

Quintessence Publishing Co, Inc
4350 Chandler Drive
Hanover Park, IL 60133
www.quintpub.com

Editor: Bryn Goates
Design: Dawn Hartman
Production: Sue Robinson

Printed in Canada

Table of Contents

Preface to the Second Edition

Some of the most common pains occur in the orofacial region. Because this region of the body has special importance in eating, drinking, speech, and the expression of our feelings, pain occurring in this region has particular significance to the orofacial pain patient. The effect of chronic orofacial pain on a patient is particularly serious because it can be associated with emotional, psychologic, and social disturbances that compromise the patient's quality of life and well-being. Furthermore, changing population demographics will likely increase their bearing on dental practice in most countries over the coming decades as more people become middle-aged or elderly—the age range when chronic orofacial pain conditions are most prevalent.

Thus, there is a rapidly growing interest in the field of orofacial pain. In the 8 years since the first edition of this book was published, new approaches have been developed in the diagnosis and management of orofacial pain conditions, and our knowledge of the neurobiologic, molecular, and genetic processes involved in orofacial pain has advanced. However, the decision to publish a second edition was based on a need not only to update the basic science and clinical information, but also to expand the book's reach by including new topics related to pain genetics, pain and motor control and dysfunction, and management of headaches and pain-related movement disorders. We accomplished these goals by providing updated information in the relevant chapters and by adding four new chapters. New cases have also been added to illustrate how orofacial pain conditions may be differentially diagnosed and managed (see chapter 27).

The philosophy of this second edition remains true to that of its predecessor, namely to provide a comprehensive, integrated, concise, and evidence-based synthesis of the topic of orofacial pain through a translational bridging from molecules and cellular mechanisms to diagnostic and management approaches. The main target audience of the book is still dental students and clinicians; in addition, it will undoubtedly prove a valuable source of information for neuroscience graduate students and medical residents who want to learn more about orofacial pain processes and their clinical correlates, and for those scientists and clinicians interested in translational research using pain models.

We are grateful to Fong Yuen (University of Toronto Faculty of Dentistry) for her excellent work as editorial assistant for this second edition of the book and to the staff at Quintessence Publishing for their dedication and help in bringing it to fruition. We also thank the authors of the chapters, who have worked with the editors to ensure that each chapter provides an up-to-date and evidence-based overview of its topic.

Preface to the First Edition

The model for this book is the *Studies in Physiology Series* published by the British Physiological Society (Cody FWJ [ed]; Portland Press, London, 1995). The purpose of these publications is to present a summary of current knowledge in a particular field to teachers of physiology. Contributing authors are asked to keep their papers short and simple, so that they are readily accessible to undergraduate students. They are also told to use summary figures and diagrams rather than complex reports of data, to keep the number of references small, and to cite reviews rather than research reports whenever possible.

Drs James Lund and Gilles Lavigne saw that this approach would be useful for teachers of oral biology, oral medicine, and facial pain; for students in faculties of dentistry and medicine; and for clinicians who want to be better informed. While scientists and graduate students use original reports and sophisticated literature reviews of the type published in *Critical Reviews in Oral Biology and Medicine* for their research and coursework, there is a paucity of material on dental and orofacial research suitable for the nonexpert. This problem is of growing importance because, as many dental faculties heed the call to improve the teaching of basic and applied science and in particular to integrate emerging scientific evidence into patient care, appropriate materials are not available to their students. Drs Lund and Lavigne recognized that there was a particular need for concise summaries of knowledge about orofacial pain and asked two of the pre-eminent experts in the field to join them as coeditors: Dr Ronald Dubner, chief editor of the journal *Pain*, and Dr Barry Sessle, editor-in-chief of the *Journal of Orofacial Pain* and president of the International Association for the Study of Pain.

Some of you may ask, why another volume on orofacial pain? Aren't there enough published reviews and textbooks on the subject already? It is true that much has been written, particularly about temporomandibular disorders (TMDs), but the best of the newer publications are written for the researcher and graduate student. Most of those books that are written for the dental student and clinician are heavy on opinion but light on evidence. In preparing this book, we have tried to include the major topics that would be found in an undergraduate curriculum. In partic-ular, we made sure that acute pain and chronic pain states other than TMDs are covered. We asked each of the authors, who were chosen for their expertise in the field, to distinguish between data and anecdote; if they could find no good evidence for or against current practice, they were asked to state so. Each of us took responsibility for one of the four sections (Section I, The Clinical Problem and Epidemiology; Section II, Neurobiology of Pain; Section III, Pain and Behavior; and Section IV, Management of Orofacial Pain) and worked with the contributing authors to ensure a uniformity of expression and continuity of content within and between the sections. We have tried to make sure that the book provides a comprehensive, integrated synthesis of the topic and that it is not just a series of loosely connected chapters.

Most of the chapters in this book were first presented as papers at a symposium for teachers of orofacial pain held in Vancouver on March 10, 1999, in conjunction with the American and Canadian Associations of Dental Schools and the International Association for Dental Research. We wish to thank Dean Edward Yen of the Faculty of Dentistry of the University of British Columbia for facilitating the organization of the conference and Mmes Christiane Manzini and Francine Guitard for their assistance in Vancouver. Mme Lucille Gendron was our editorial assistant and coordinated the arrangements for the conference.

We also acknowledge the financial support of the Canadian Medical Research Council, Block Drug Company Inc, the Quebec Oral Health Network of the Fonds de Recherche en Santé du Québec, the Association of Canadian Faculties of Dentistry, the International Association for Dental Research—Neuroscience Group, the Canadian Association for Dental Research, the American Academy of Orofacial Pain, the Association of University Teachers of Orofacial Pain Programs, and the Oral Physiology Commission of the International Union of Physiological Sciences.

We owe special thanks to the authors, who had to put up with more interference than usual from the editors, and finally to Quintessence for their help with the production of the book, which we hope is only the first in a series. We have already begun to plan the next on normal and abnormal movements of the orofacial region and upper aerodigestive tract.

Contributors

Pierre Blanchet, MD, FRCP(C), PhD
Associate Professor
Department of Stomatology
Faculty of Dental Medicine
Université de Montréal
Neurologist
Université de Montréal Hospital Centre
Montreal, Quebec, Canada

M. Catherine Bushnell, PhD
Harold Griffith Professor of Anesthesia
Director, Alan Edwards Centre for Research
  on Pain
Department of Anesthesia and Faculty of Dentistry
McGill University
Montreal, Quebec, Canada

Thuan T.T. Dao, DMD, MSc, PhD, FRCD(C)
Associate Professor
Faculty of Dentistry
University of Toronto
Toronto, Ontario, Canada

Antoon De Laat, LDS, GHO
Professor
Department of Oral and Maxillofacial Surgery
School of Dentistry
Catholic University of Leuven
Leuven, Belgium

Raymond A. Dionne, DDS, PhD
Scientific Director
National Institute of Nursing Research
National Institutes of Health
Bethesda, Maryland, USA

Mark Drangsholt, DDS, PhD
Assistant Professor
Departments of Oral Medicine and Dental Public
  Health Science
School of Dentistry
University of Washington
Seattle, Washington, USA

Ronald Dubner, DDS, PhD
Professor and Chair
Department of Biomedical Sciences
University of Maryland Dental School
Baltimore, Maryland, USA

Samuel F. Dworkin, DDS, PhD
  (Hon: DSci, DrOdont)
Professor Emeritus
Department of Oral Medicine
School of Dentistry
Department of Psychiatry and Behavioral Sciences
School of Medicine
University of Washington
Seattle, Washington, USA

Eli Eliav, DMD, PhD
Professor and Director of the Division of Orofacial
  Pain
Robert and Susan Carmel Endowed Chair in
  Algesiology
Department of Diagnostic Sciences
New Jersey Dental School
The University of Medicine and Dentistry of New
  Jersey
Newark, New Jersey, USA

Jocelyne S. Feine, DDS, HDR
Professor and Director of Graduate Studies in
  Oral Health Sciences
Faculty of Dentistry
Department of Epidemiology and Biostatistics
Department of Oncology
Faculty of Medicine
McGill University
Montreal, Quebec, Canada

James R. Fricton, DDS, MS
Professor
Department of Diagnostic and Biological Sciences
School of Dentistry
University of Minnesota
Minneapolis, Minnesota, USA

Sharon M. Gordon, DDS, MPH, PhD
Associate Professor
Biomedical Sciences Director of Curriculum
University of Maryland Dental School
Baltimore, Maryland, USA

Jean-Paul Goulet, DDS, MSD, FRCD(C)
Professor
Department of Stomatology
Faculty of Dental Medicine
Université Laval
Quebec, Quebec, Canada

Charles S. Greene, BS, DDS
Clinical Professor and Director of Orofacial Pain
    Studies
Department of Oral Medicine and Diagnostic
    Sciences
College of Dentistry
University of Illinois at Chicago
Chicago, Illinois, USA

Kenneth M. Hargreaves, DDS, PhD
Professor and Chair
Department of Endodontics
University of Texas Health Science Center at
    San Antonio
San Antonio, Texas, USA

G. Rex Holland, BSc, BDS, PhD
Professor
Department of Cariology, Restorative Sciences,
    and Endodontics
School of Dentistry
University of Michigan
Ann Arbor, Michigan, USA

Yoshiki Imamura, DDS, PhD
Professor
Department of Oral Diagnosis
School of Dentistry
Nihon University
Tokyo, Japan

Koichi Iwata, DDS, PhD
Professor and Chairman
Department of Physiology
School of Dentistry
Nihon University
Tokyo, Japan

Takafumi Kato, DDS, PhD
Associate Professor
Division of Oral and Maxillofacial Biology
Institute for Oral Science
Matsumoto Dental University
Shiojiri, Japan

Asma A. Khan, BDS, PhD
Assistant Professor
Department of Endodontics
University of Texas Health Science Center at
    San Antonio
San Antonio, Texas, USA

Gilles J. Lavigne, DMD, FRCD(C), PhD
Professor and Canada Research Chair
    in Pain, Sleep and Trauma
Department of Oral Health
Faculty of Dental Medicine
Université de Montréal
Montreal, Quebec, Canada

Linda LeResche, ScD
Professor
Department of Oral Medicine
School of Dentistry
University of Washington
Seattle, Washington, USA

Frank Lobbezoo, DDS, PhD
Professor
Department of Oral Function
Academic Centre for Dentistry Amsterdam
University of Amsterdam
Amsterdam, The Netherlands

Marco L. Loggia
McGill Centre for Research on Pain
Department of Neurology and Neurosurgery
McGill University
Montreal, Quebec, Canada

James P. Lund, BDS, PhD, FCAHS
Professor
Alan Edwards Centre for Research on Pain
Faculty of Dentistry
McGill University
Montreal, Quebec, Canada

William Maixner, DDS, PhD
Professor and Director
Center for Neurosensory Disorders
Departments of Endodontics and Pharmacology
School of Dentistry
University of North Carolina
Chapel Hill, North Carolina, USA

Bruce Matthews, BDS, PhD
Professor
Department of Physiology and Pharmacology
School of Medical Sciences
University of Bristol
Bristol, United Kingdom

Mitchell B. Max, MD
Visiting Professor of Anesthesiology and Medicine
Director of Molecular Epidemiology of Pain Program
Center for Pain Research
University of Pittsburgh
Pittsburgh, Pennsylvania, USA

Pierre Mayer, MD, FRCP(C)
Associate Professor
Faculty of Medicine
Director, Sleep Laboratory
Centre Hospitalier de l'Université de Montréal
Montreal, Quebec, Canada

Charles McNeill, DDS
Professor Emeritus and Director
UCSF Center for Orofacial Pain
University of California, San Francisco
San Francisco, California, USA

Jeffrey S. Mogil, PhD
E.P. Taylor Professor of Pain Studies
Canada Research Chair in the Genetics of Pain
Department of Psychology and Alan Edwards
  Centre for Research on Pain
McGill University
Montreal, Quebec, Canada

Greg Murray, BDS, MDS, PhD, FRACDS
Professor of Dentistry
Jaw Function and Orofacial Pain Research Unit
Faculty of Dentistry
University of Sydney
Sydney, New South Wales, Australia

Jeffrey P. Okeson, DMD
Professor and Chair
Department of Oral Health Science
Director of Orofacial Pain Program
College of Dentistry
University of Kentucky
Lexington, Kentucky, USA

Sandro Palla, Dr Med Dent
Professor and Chair
Department of Masticatory Disorders, Removable
  Prosthodontics and Special Care Dentistry
Center for Dental and Oral Medicine and
  Cranio-Maxillofacial Surgery
University of Zurich
Zurich, Switzerland

Pierre Rainville, PhD
Associate Professor
Department of Stomatology
Faculty of Dental Medicine
Université de Montréal
Montreal, Quebec, Canada

Ke Ren, MD, PhD
Professor
Department of Biomedical Sciences
University of Maryland Dental School
Baltimore, Maryland, USA

Michael W. Salter, MD, PhD, FRSC
Professor and Canada Research Chair in
    Neuroplasticity and Pain
Faculties of Dentistry and Medicine
Director of University of Toronto Centre for
    the Study of Pain
University of Toronto
Senior Scientist and Head
Program in Neurosciences & Mental Health
Hospital for Sick Children
Toronto, Ontario, Canada

Eric L. Schiffman, DDS, MS
Associate Professor
Department of Diagnostic and Biological Sciences
University of Minnesota
School of Dentistry
Minneapolis, Minnesota, USA

Petra Schweinhardt, MD, PhD
Assistant Professor
Alan Edwards Centre for Research on Pain
Faculty of Dentistry
McGill University
Montreal, Quebec, Canada

Ze'ev Seltzer, BMS, Dr Med Dent
Professor and Canada Research Chair in
    Comparative Pain Genetics
Faculties of Dentistry and Medicine
University of Toronto
Toronto, Ontario, Canada

Barry J. Sessle, MDS, PhD, DSc(hc), FRSC,
    FCAHS
Professor and Canada Research Chair in
    Craniofacial Pain and Sensorimotor Function
Faculties of Dentistry and Medicine
University of Toronto
Toronto, Ontario, Canada

José Tadeu Tesseroli de Siqueira, DDS, PhD
Orofacial Pain Clinic
Dentistry Division and Neurology Department
Hospital das Clinicas
School of Medicine
University of Sao Paulo
Sao Paulo, Brazil

Christian S. Stohler, DDS, Dr Med Dent
Professor and Dean
Baltimore College of Dental Surgery
University of Maryland Dental School
Baltimore, Maryland, USA

Peter Svensson, DDS, PhD, Dr Odont
Professor and Chair
Department of Clinical Oral Physiology
School of Dentistry
Faculty of Health Sciences
University of Aarhus
Aarhus, Denmark

Edmond Truelove, DDS, MSD
Professor and Chair
Department of Oral Medicine
University of Washington
Seattle, Washington, USA

Chantal Villemure, PhD
Research Associate
Alan Edwards Centre for Research on Pain
McGill University
Montreal, Quebec, Canada

Charles G. Widmer, DDS, MS
Associate Professor
Department of Orthodontics
University of Florida
Gainesville, Florida, USA

Alain Woda, DDS, PhD
Professor
Laboratory DIDO
Faculty of Dentistry
Université d'Auvergne
Clermont-Ferrand, France

Section I

Orofacial Pain: Classification, Epidemiology, and Beliefs

What Is Pain and How Do We Classify Orofacial Pain?

Charles McNeill
Ronald Dubner
Alain Woda

Pain is one of the most common symptoms for which patients seek treatment, and management of pain and relief of suffering should be at the core of the health care provider's commitment to patients. However, most curricula devote little time to pain biology, and pain management is often neglected. We know that proper management of pain is essential, not only to bring relief of the primary symptom, but also to prevent the consequences of unrelieved pain. It is now recognized that unrelieved pain can delay healing and depress the immune system. Unrelieved pain can also cause stress, autonomic symptoms, and alterations in the peripheral nervous system (PNS) and central nervous system (CNS) that may result in persistent pain or chronic pain syndromes.

There is every medical and ethical reason to treat pain aggressively using all the evidence-based resources that are likely to benefit patients. This chapter defines pain and different terms used to discuss its features, and outlines how pain, including orofacial pain, can be classified. The first goal of definition and classification is to minimize, as much as possible, the confusion caused by using either different terms to name the same symptoms and conditions or, even worse, the same word to name different pain symptoms or conditions. By using

the same terminology, clinicians and researchers can understand each other better, and consequently, the exchange of information is much improved. Standardization also helps to address a second goal: to constitute groups of subjects for clinical research studies whose outcomes can be compared worldwide.

What Is Pain?

The definition of pain

Pain is defined as an unpleasant sensory and emotional experience associated with actual or potential tissue damage or described in terms of such damage.[1] Although we often refer to pain as a *sensation*, it is probably better described as a multidimensional or multifactorial experience encompassing sensory, affective (emotional), motivational, and cognitive dimensions. While there are certain sensory qualities of somatic sensations that are almost exclusively associated with pain, such as stinging, pricking, burning, and aching, pain is also an unpleasant emotional experience. It is because of this emotional dimension that the adjective *painful* is sometimes applied to other emotional experiences in the absence of sensory stimulation. Pain also has a strong motivational component, evoking both withdrawal reflexes and highly organized avoidance and escape behavior. The motivational aspect of pain is a primary function, and without it the organism will not survive. The cognitive component of pain refers to its meaning to the individual. For example, if the pain is believed to be due to a malignant tumor, its effect on the individual will be much greater than if the pain is believed to result from minor trauma due to a fall.

Theories of pain

Various theories of pain have been proposed. One of the oldest that still has some salience is that a noxious stimulus evokes a specific sensation (pain), which is basically similar to vision and touch, with hardwired lines from specific "pain receptors" to regions in the CNS that process only pain-related signals (specificity theory). Another group of theories proposes instead that noxious stimulation activates several different types of receptors, including tactile receptors, and that summation of the signals in the CNS leads to pain (intensive or summation theory). A third theory proposes that the pattern of signals produced by the noxious stimulus would be important for the recognition of pain and its distinction from other sensations (pattern theory).

     More recently, evidence was produced that a large amount of interactions exist between nociceptive and non-nociceptive inputs to the CNS. A theory was formulated based on the potential for inhibition of nociceptive transmission in the CNS by low-threshold mechanosensitive afferent inputs to the CNS. This theory explains, for example, why rubbing an acutely injured body part can often, at least temporarily, produce some pain relief. A few years later, research demonstrated that the "gating" of nociceptive transmission in the spinal cord and brainstem could also be provoked by controls descending from brain centers located higher in the CNS and involved in stress, emotion, cognition, distraction, etc. While not all elements of this so-called gate control theory as originally proposed have held up to detailed scientific scrutiny, this theory has had a huge impact on the understanding of pain by provoking an intense research interest over the past 40 years. The resulting advances in understanding pain from anatomic, physiologic, pharmacologic, neurochemical, molecular, and behavioral research have pointed to the high level of neural integration and the multiple factors involved in pain.

Acute, persistent, and chronic pain

We have all experienced the pain of touching a hot kettle. The pain is sharp but soon subsides. We call this *acute* (or *transient*) pain, and it is protective; it warns us of impending tissue damage. A stimulus that is damaging or potentially damaging to tissues is considered noxious. Pain that lasts for a few days or a few weeks can follow athletic injuries of the elbow, knee, or elsewhere. We call this *persistent* pain; it can also be protective since it forces us to rest the injured part and avoid further damage. In some clinical conditions, however, pain persists long after an injury has apparently healed, possibly for months or years, resulting in *chronic pain*. This type of pain can be nonprotective. In this book, the terms *persistent pain* and *chronic pain* will be used interchangeably. In clinical terms, pain that lasts for at least 3 to 6 months is considered *chronic*. In contrast, *persistent* pain can refer to pain that lasts for just hours or days.

Pain terms

A number of terms are used to describe various features of pain. Box 1-1 is a glossary of terms customarily used to describe common aspects of acute, chronic, or persistent pain.

Box 1-1 Pain glossary[2]

Algesia	Any pain experience following a stimulus
Allodynia	Pain or a painful sensation due to a stimulus that does not normally provoke pain or which is innocuous (eg, skin touch after a sunburn)
Causalgia	Pain after a trauma to a nerve that may be associated with vasomotor dysfunction
Habituation	A decrease or loss of response in nerve terminals or neurons following repetitive stimulations
Hyperalgesia	An increased pain response to a noxious stimulus in an affected area versus a control area
Hypoalgesia	A diminished pain response to a noxious stimulus in an affected area versus a control area
Hypoesthesia	A decreased sensitivity to stimulation that feels similar to the effect of local anesthesia
Neuroma	A mass of peripheral neurons formed by a healing scar at a damaged nerve that can cause hyperexcitability of neurons or spontaneous discharge (also termed *ectopic discharge*)
Neuropathic pain	Aberrant pain induced by an injury to a sensory nerve or neuron; may be evoked by thermal, mechanical, or chemical stimuli or may be secondary to a disease (eg, diabetes mellitus, postherpetic neuralgia); may also be central in origin; may occur spontaneously
Nociception	The reception and transmission of nociceptive messages
Pain	An unpleasant sensory, emotional, and motivational experience, associated with actual or potential tissue damage, that requires consciousness
Pain threshold	The lowest level of stimulation perceived as painful by a subject (> 50% of the time)
Pain tolerance	The highest level of pain a subject is prepared (able) to tolerate
Paresthesia/dysesthesia	An abnormal sensation that is termed *dysesthesia* when it becomes unpleasant
Sensitization	The increased excitability of nerve terminals or neurons produced by trauma or inflammation of peripheral tissues; can be peripheral or central or both
Sprouting	The extensive spread of regenerated nerve endings into surrounding tissue following nerve damage

Methods Used in Classification

To properly manage orofacial pain, the clinician must be able to appreciate the underlying pain mechanisms. This includes a working knowledge of functional neuroanatomy, PNS and CNS pathways, descending pain modulating systems, changes that take place in the CNS that may underlie persistent pain, and the affective or emotional aspects of pain. The clinician must have knowledge of the various categories of persistent pain of the head, neck, and face. For this reason, a number of different methods of classifying pain have been developed.

Medical taxonomy is a pragmatic affair. It needs, however, to be based as much as possible on a scientific approach. There are three methodologies that can be used to classify orofacial pain. Historically, the first to appear was expert opinion (or other authority-based consensus), followed by diagnostic criteria and then cluster analysis. Curiously, in a logical approach, they should be used in exactly the reverse order. First, cluster analysis should be used to identify the different possible entities among a whole population of patients. Then, in a second step based on diagnostic criteria, a small group of signs and symptoms should be selected to characterize each of the previously determined entities; and finally in a third step, a group of experts should be gathered to organize the experimental data obtained during the first two steps and to decide how to answer the questions that the two previous methods have not been able to address. The following discussion addresses each of these three approaches.

Cluster analysis approach

The first problem encountered by scientists trying to classify orofacial pain entities is deciding which groups of patients constitute a homogenous entity. It is clear that irreversible acute pulpitis constitutes a single entity, but how many entities can be identified among temporomandibular disorders (TMDs)? Cluster analysis can be used to solve this type of problem. The method relies on signs and symptoms recorded from a large sample of patients with a large array of pain conditions. At the end of the analysis, the whole sample is seen as a "cloud" of points that may or may not constitute several clusters of patients. Finally, each cluster is considered as a separate entity whose name depends on the diagnostics that have been made for the majority of patients forming the cluster.

Cluster analysis has been used to define subdivisions in ill-defined chronic pain entities (such as so-called complex regional pain syndrome and irritable bowel syndrome) and in pain studies to determine prognosis and treatment orientations, largely based on psychopathologic measurements. Its use in orofacial pain has been mostly limited to the impact of psychologic and sociobehavioral factors. This methodology was recently applied to the entire group of chronic orofacial pains in a prospective multicenter study.[3] The expectation was that

the clustering of the signs and symptoms used as variables might reflect pathophysiologic mechanisms and clinical significance. The outcome of this experiment is represented in Fig 1-1. It must be considered as a general framework that needs to be detailed through other classification methods.

Diagnostic criteria

In the diagnostic criteria approach, groups of patients are defined on the basis of an a priori set of inclusion criteria used to select a group of patients representing a given pain entity. These inclusion criteria are generally defined by a group of experts or from a preceding classification. Then, signs and symptoms observed in the selected patients are recorded, and a small set of signs and symptoms is selected to characterize the entity. The choice of these diagnostic criteria is made according to their discriminating properties (sensitivity, specificity; see chapter 18). There is clear circular reasoning in this approach since the entity is already defined by the initial inclusion criteria. Therefore, it cannot be used to identify entities. In other words, the diagnostic criteria method does not say whether a group of cases belongs to a single disease or lies on a continuum of overlapping cases. This approach is, however, of great value in forming homogenous groups of patients for research purposes. The scientific methodology used to determine these diagnostic criteria makes it possible to draw up consensus definitions that can be adopted worldwide by different groups of researchers. Another advantage is that relatively small numbers of subjects can be used to characterize a new disease. This is particularly helpful for infrequent diseases.

As pioneers of the method, Dworkin and LeResche published the TMD research diagnostic criteria (RDC) in 1992.[5] The TMD RDC articular and masticatory muscle conditions have been reduced to the subsets listed in Box 1-2. Dworkin and LeResche used the primary signs and symptoms (pain, tenderness) to place patients into one of

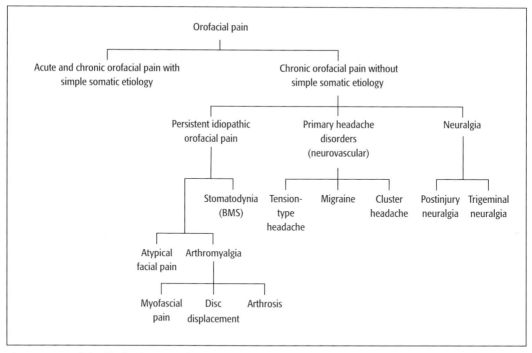

Fig 1-1 Proposed classification for orofacial pain after multidimensional analyses. The term *arthromyalgia* is intended to exclude TMDs and masticatory muscle disorders with well-identified causes or mechanisms, which were not considered in the analyses. Persistent idiopathic orofacial pain includes stomatodynia (ie, burning mouth syndrome [BMS]), arthromyalgia and atypical facial pain. Atypical facial pain includes atypical odontalgia. Atypical facial pain and arthromyalgia are located lower than stomatodynia in the classification tree because they could be separated only by topographic signs and symptoms. Adapted with permission from Woda.[4]

Box 1-2 Research diagnostic criteria, Axis I: Clinical TMD conditions

Group I: Muscle disorders
- Myofascial pain
- Myofascial pain with limited opening

Group II: Disc displacements
- Disc displacement with reduction
- Disc displacement without reduction, with limited opening
- Disc displacement without reduction, without limited opening

Group III: Arthralgia, arthritis, arthrosis

Table 1-1   Main characteristics of two basic methods used for building classification systems*

Method for classification	What it can do	Limitations	Flaws	Advantages
Cluster analysis	Determine what entities really exist	Needs large sample Cannot define entities with very small prevalence	Observed groups must be labeled from a preexisting classification Circular reasoning	Probably closer to mechanisms
Diagnostic criteria	Characterize an already selected group	A large fraction of the cases are left unclassified	Diagnostic criteria must be extracted from a group of patients chosen with preexisting inclusion criteria Circular reasoning	Allows standardization of inclusions in clinical studies

*Reprinted with permission from Woda.[4]

three groups—muscle (group I), disc displacement (group II), and joint (group III) disorders—and then subdivided groups I and II depending on range of motion. To the traditional clinical measures based on somatic signs (Axis I), they added Axis II pain-related measures, which cover pain severity, psychologic status, and pain-related disability. It is important to note that the RDC deals only with TMDs and does not include other important clinical conditions.

Authority-based consensus

The main characteristics of the above two approaches are displayed in Table 1-1. Their flaws can be summarized by the following statement: cluster analyses implicate very large samples but can not identify entities with low prevalence, whereas the diagnostic criteria approach may characterize non-existing entities. Therefore, these two methods should be combined while leaving room for a more subjective approach in which expert opinion plays a role.

In the last few decades, groups of experts have been gathered by scientific societies and institutions to establish various classification systems. These organizations sought to control for "individual leadership subjectivity." However, scientific societies and institutions themselves can be subjective, as shown by the large differences observed between the resulting classification systems. Despite the limitations, these classification systems have proven over time to be invaluable in providing a common worldwide language for clinical researchers. Actually, two leading scientific societies, the International Headache Society (IHS) and the International Association for the Study of Pain (IASP), have published comprehensive and detailed classification systems.[1,6] The American Academy of Orofacial Pain (AAOP) expanded the first IHS classification[7] to include all head, face, and neck conditions that could be associated with orofacial pain.[8,9] This led to a classification (Box 1-3) that must be considered as a work in progress since updated editions will be published as new research data appear.

Box 1-3 Classification of all head, face, and neck conditions that could be associated with orofacial pain*

Orofacial pain: Diagnostic range

Intracranial pain disorders
- Neoplasm, aneurysm, abscess, stroke, multiple sclerosis

Primary headache disorders (neurovascular disorders)
- Migraine, migraine variants, cluster headache, paroxysmal hemicrania, SUNCT, tension-type headache

Secondary headache related to disease/substances

Neurogenic/neuropathic pain disorders
- Paroxysmal neuralgias (trigeminal, glossopharyngeal, occipital)
- Continuous pain disorders (deafferentation pain: peripheral neuritis, postherpetic neuralgia, postinjury neuralgia)
- Sympathetically maintained pain

Extracranial pain disorders
- Eye, ear, nose, paranasal sinuses, lymph nodes, throat, salivary glands, neck

Intraoral pain disorders
- Dental pulp, periodontium, mucogingival tissues, tongue

Persistent idiopathic orofacial pain
- TMD conditions (see Box 1-2), atypical facial pain, stomatodynia (eg, BMS)

Mental disorders
- Somatoform disorders, pain syndromes of psychogenic origin

SUNCT=Short-lasting unilateral neuralgiform headache attacks with conjunctival injection and tearing; BMS=burning mouth syndrome.
*Adapted with permission from Okeson.[9]

Entities That May Cause Pain in the Orofacial Area

Many head and neck conditions present as orofacial pain. Therefore, it is critical for all health care providers, regardless of disciplinary boundaries, to have an extensive knowledge of the array of disorders that may be responsible for the symptoms. Because different disease entities present with similar pain patterns in the head, face, and neck, clinicians must consider diseases unrelated to the masticatory system in their differential diagnoses.

It can be daunting to correctly identify all of the possible sources of a patient's orofacial pain complaints, so it is essential to have a systematic approach. The scope of practice for the oral health care provider includes: (1) intraoral pain conditions, (2) musculoskeletal pain conditions affecting the mandible and associated structures, and (3) related medical conditions that either directly cause pain, refer pain to the region, or masquerade as orofacial pain.

Intraoral pain conditions

Intraoral pain includes odontogenic pain (see chapter 20) and pain associated with the mucogingival tissues, tongue, and salivary glands (see chapter 23). *Odontogenic pain* is defined as pain associated with the teeth and periodontium. Tooth pain includes reversible and irreversible pulpitis and pulpal necrosis. The pain is often referred to other teeth as well as to distant areas in the head, neck, and mandible. Pain conditions associated with the supporting tissues of the teeth include acute apical periodontitis, acute apical abscess, and acute periodontal abscess.

Mucogingival and tongue pain disorders may be localized or generalized throughout the mouth. Localized pain conditions include acute necrotizing ulcerative gingivitis, recurrent aphthous stomatitis, herpes simplex, candidiasis, and injury from trauma. Pain disorders associated with salivary disease or dysfunction can result from trauma, neoplasia, infection (eg, mumps), inflammation (eg, acute suppurative and chronic recurrent sialadentitis), and sialolithiasis (salivary calculi or "stones"). Systemic disorders and their treatments also can contribute to orofacial pain (eg, HIV, chemotherapy, radiation therapy).

Musculoskeletal pain disorders

Musculoskeletal conditions are the major cause of nonodontogenic pain in the orofacial region. They include cervical spine disorders and TMDs (see chapters 19 and 22). TMDs, as classified by the AAOP, include a disparate group of articular and nonarticular conditions that often have similar signs and symptoms. The temporomandibular joint (TMJ) disorders include developmental or acquired articular disorders, articular disc disorders, inflammatory-immune disorders, infection, osteoarthritis, condylar dislocation, ankylosis, and fracture. Develomental disorders of the condyle include agenesis, aplasia (faulty development), hypoplasia (incomplete or underdevelopment), and hyperplasia (non-neoplastic overdevelopment). Acquired disorders include benign, malignant, or metastatic neoplasms. TMJ disc disorders involve disc displacement with reduction and without reduction as well as disc adhesion. Inflammation can occur in the synovium (synovitis)

and/or capsule (capsulitis), and it can be related to a systemic polyarthritic or collagen disease (eg, rheumatoid arthritis, lupus, reactive arthritis). Osteoarthritis is a degenerative condition of the TMJ that can be active or stable (osteoarthrosis). Condylar subluxation or dislocation occurs when the condyle becomes positioned anterior and superior to the articular eminence and is unable to return to a seated position in the fossa. Fracture of the condyle usually results from direct trauma to the mandible but can be idiopathic, iatrogenic, or secondary to another pathologic process (see chapter 22). Masticatory muscle disorders include myofascial pain, myositis, myospasm or trismus, local myalgia (unspecified, eg, postexercise myalgia), contracture, and neoplasia (see chapter 22).

Related medical conditions masquerading as orofacial pain disorders

Medical conditions that are associated with orofacial pain can masquerade as orofacial pain conditions; these include intracranial disorders, neurovascular disorders (primary headache), neuropathic disorders, and extracranial disorders. The site of pain in the head, neck, and orofacial region is often not the primary source of the pain, making differential diagnosis extremely difficult. Referral of pain from one structure to another is common and is explained in part by the convergence of noxious input in the trigeminal spinal tract nucleus (see chapter 5).

Usually, disorders of the intracranial structures (such as neoplasia, aneurysm, hemorrhage, or hematoma) can be easily differentiated from orofacial pain conditions. They should be considered first in the diagnostic process because they can be life threatening and require immediate attention.

Neuro-vascular disorders associated with orofacial pain include migraine headaches, migraine-variant headaches, cluster headaches, chronic paroxysmal hemicrania, and tension-type headaches (see chapter 25). Migraine headache is divided into migraine with aura (*classic migraine*) and migraine without aura (*common migraine*). Tension-type headaches are believed to be a type of chronic or episodic migraine-like headache and may be associated with pericranial muscle tenderness.

Neuropathic pain is defined as pain initiated or caused by a primary lesion or dysfunction in the PNS (see chapters 7 and 24). Neuropathic pain disorders can be divided into either *paroxysmal conditions* or *continuous painful* conditions. The paroxysmal conditions associated with orofacial pain include trigeminal neuralgia and glossopharyngeal neuralgia (see chapter 24). The continuous neuropathic pain disorders associated with orofacial pain are syndromes characterized by compression or distortion, demyelination, infarction, or inflammation of the cranial nerves. Atypical facial pain and/or atypical odontalgia (phantom tooth pain, stomatodynia, or burning mouth syndrome [BMS]), acute herpes zoster, chronic postherpetic neuralgia, and neuromas are some examples of continuous pain conditions.

Extracranial pain disorders associated with orofacial pain include pain related to the eyes, ears, nose, sinuses, and throat. They can also be associated with cervical spine dysfunction involving the muscles, ligaments, joints, bones, and/or neural tissues of the neck. This can be explained by the convergence of noxious input from the upper cervical nerves with the trigeminal nerve, resulting in referred pain to the orofacial region (see chapter 5).

Summary

This chapter first considered the definition of pain and the main theories that have been proposed to explain the physiologic mechanism of pain, and also provided a glossary of pain terms. Methods used in classification were described in the second part. As noted in this introductory chapter, classification is the result of a dynamic process based on experimental evidence as well as consensual opinions of experts. This means that definitions and classifications will never be definitively fixed; on the contrary, they will always be changing with the flow of new information. The third part of the chapter extended far beyond orofacial pain conditions in the stricter sense by outlining all the medical conditions that may cause pain in the orofacial area.

References

1. Merskey H, Bogduk N (eds). Classification of Chronic Pain: Descriptions of Chronic Pain Syndromes and Definitions of Pain Terms. Seattle: IASP Press, 1994:59–76.
2. Lavigne G, Woda A, Truelove E, Ship JA, Dao T, Goulet JP. Mechanisms associated with unusual orofacial pain. J Orofac Pain 2005;19:9–21.
3. Woda A, Tubert-Jeannin S, Bouhassira D, et al. Towards a new taxonomy of idiopathic orofacial pain. Pain 2005; 116:396–406.
4. Woda A. A rationale for the classification of orofacial pain. In: Türp JC, Sommer C, Hugger A (eds). The Puzzle of Orofacial Pain. Integrating Research into Clinical Management. Vol 15: Pain and Headache. Basel: Karger, 2007:209–222.
5. Dworkin SF, LeResche L. Research diagnostic criteria for temporomandibular disorders: Review, criteria, examinations and specification, critique. J Craniomandib Disord 1992;6:301–355.
6. Headache Classification Subcommittee of the International Headache Society. The international classification of headache disorders, ed 2. Cephalalgia 2004;24(suppl 1):9–160.
7. Olesen J. Classification and diagnostic criteria for headache disorders, cranial neuralgias and facial pain. Cephalalgia 1988;8(suppl 7):1–96.
8. McNeill C (ed). Temporomandibular Disorders: Guidelines for Classification, Assessment, and Management. The American Academy of Orofacial Pain, ed 2. Chicago: Quintessence, 1993.
9. Okeson JP (ed). Orofacial Pain: Guidelines for Assessment, Diagnosis, and Management. Chicago: Quintessence, 1996:45–52.

Epidemiology of Orofacial Pain: Prevalence, Incidence, and Risk Factors

Linda LeResche
Mark Drangsholt

This chapter introduces important epidemiologic concepts and reviews what is known about the epidemiology of specific orofacial pain conditions. The aim is to provide an understanding of how epidemiologic data can contribute to clinical practice as well as to provide information on the rates of and risk factors for specific orofacial pain problems.

What Is Epidemiology?

Epidemiology is the study of the distribution, determinants, and natural history of disease in populations.[1] Although epidemiology has traditionally focused on well-defined diseases, epidemiologic methods are increasingly employed to study symptoms such as pain and other conditions for which patients are defined based on self-report or a combination of self-report and clinical findings. Morris[2] has identified seven uses of epidemiology. For the clinician, the most important of these are the following: The use of epidemiologic data *(1)* in predicting an individual's risk of having or developing a particular disease or disorder; *(2)* in completing the clinical picture, that is, in understanding where in the spectrum of disease an individual patient's condition falls; and *(3)* in the clues it may provide about causes of a disease and, therefore, possible approaches to its treatment. Knowing the rates with which specific pain conditions occur in the population as a whole, as well as their rates in specific age and sex groups, can aid the clinician in thinking about the most probable diagnosis in a particular patient. Of course, a thorough history, examination, and appropriate diagnostic tests are warranted in any patient before making a definitive diagnosis.

Inherent in the definition of epidemiology are three important perspectives[3]: *(1)* the *population perspective*, which implies that, to understand the full spectrum of pain problems, pain conditions must be studied in entire populations, not only in persons seeking treatment; *(2)* the *developmental perspective*, which suggests that understanding pain across the life cycle is essential because factors influencing a specific pain condition may vary with age; and *(3)* the *ecologic perspective*, in which disease agents, characteristics of the host, and characteristics of the environment are all important in determining whether or how a condition manifests itself in a given person. This is similar to the *biopsychosocial perspective* on pain, which views pain as the result of the dynamic interaction of biologic, psychologic, and social factors.

Epidemiologic Measures

Most of the epidemiologic data on chronic orofacial pain are prevalence data. *Prevalence* is simply the proportion of the population with a condition at a given time. Prevalence differs from *incidence*, which is the rate of onset of new cases of a condition over a specific period, usually a year. Incidence and prevalence are related such that:

Prevalence = Incidence × Mean Duration

It makes sense that the number of cases in the population at any given time is a function not only of the rate at which new cases occur but also of how long the condition typically lasts. (If the rate of onset of two conditions is the same, but one lasts 1 year and the other lasts 2 years, twice as many cases of the second condition will be found at any given time.) Although pain arising from caries and periodontal disease is generally acute if treatment is provided, most other orofacial pain conditions in the population follow a chronic-recurrent course.

In the epidemiologic sense, *risk* is the likelihood that people without a disease who are exposed to certain factors (called *risk factors*) will acquire the disease. It is useful to think about two kinds of risk factors: those that we can change, like smoking, are known as *modifiable risk factors*; and those that we cannot control, like age and sex, are sometimes called *risk indicators*.

Orofacial Pain Conditions

Toothache, periodontal pain, and oral soft tissue pain

Because caries is the most common cause of pain in the teeth, the prevalence of toothache in a population depends on the rate of caries and the factors that influence that rate, such as diet, social class, and levels of fluoride in the water supply. One US national study[4] found an overall preva-lence of 12.2% among adults for toothache in the preceding 6 months, with little difference in preva-lence rates for men and women. Rates decreased with age from 16.9% in 18- to 34-year-olds to 3.4% among those aged 75 years or older. A slightly higher prevalence was found in a survey of Toronto residents,[5] where 14.1% of adults reported experiencing toothache in the previous 4 weeks. Toothache is likely the most common cause of oro-facial pain among children; for example, a study of Australian schoolchildren found that about 12% had experienced at least one toothache before their fifth birthday, and almost one-third (31.8%) had experienced toothache by the age of 12 years.[6]

Few epidemiologic investigations of pain in the periodontal and oral soft tissues have been con-ducted. Population-based studies of herpes simplex and aphthous stomatitis, common oral lesions that typically cause acute, self-limiting pain, have found point prevalences of 1.6% and 0.9%, respectively.[7] *Pericoronitis*, an acute infection around erupting third molars, commonly causes acute pain and trismus among persons in their late teens or early twenties, although no population-based prevalence data have been reported.

Temporomandibular disorder pain

Temporomandibular disorders (TMDs) are muscu-loskeletal conditions characterized by pain in the temporomandibular joint (TMJ) and/or the associ-ated muscles of mastication (see chapters 17, 18, and 22). TMD pain is by far the most common chronic orofacial pain condition, and it is similar to back pain in its intensity, persistence, and psycho-logic impact.[8] TMD pain is rare in children prior to puberty.[9] Table 2-1 lists several studies that in-quired into the presence of ongoing pain in the temporomandibular region in adult populations (for review, see Drangsholt and LeResche.[9]). Rates range from 9% to 15% for women and from 3% to 10% for men. Considering the differences in defini-tions and in populations examined in the different

Table 2-1 Prevalence of pain in the temporomandibular region in adult populations

Authors	Prevalence (%)		F:M ratio	Peak age
	Women	Men		
Locker and Slade[10]	9.5	5.0	1.9	< 45
Von Korff et al[8]	15.0	8.0	1.9	25–44
Goulet et al[11]	9.0	5.0	1.8	35–54
Helkimo[12]	14.0	10.0	1.4	35–44
Matsuka et al[13]	11.7	9.9	1.2	20–39

studies, these rates are remarkably consistent. Interestingly, TMD pain appears to be 1.5 to 2 times as common in women than in men in nearly every study. Also, in all studies where there was a clear pattern for age-specific prevalence, the peak age was around 35 to 45 years.

Although standardized research diagnostic criteria for TMDs are now available,[14] few studies have yet used these criteria to examine the prevalence of *myalgia* (pain in the masticatory muscles) and/or *arthralgia* (pain in the TMJ) in nonpatient populations.

The few studies of onset rates of TMD pain that have been conducted (Table 2-2) indicate that incidence rates of TMD pain are approximately 2% to 3% per year. This fairly low incidence suggests that the high prevalence of TMD pain in the population is because of its relatively long duration, rather than high rates of onset.

Recent epidemiologic research has investigated risk factors for TMD pain. Both age and sex appear to strongly influence TMD prevalence, suggesting that some factor in women of reproductive age may be a risk factor (see also chapter 13). Preliminary studies[19,20] indicate that estrogen may contribute to the development of these disorders. Two well-designed studies found that persons with pain in other body sites (eg, back pain, abdominal

pain) were at increased risk for developing TMD pain.[14,17,21] As with other chronic pain conditions, depression and psychosocial distress are likely important risk factors. The etiology of TMDs also appears to include genetic factors.[22] Other hypothesized risk factors such as physical trauma, bruxism, dental extractions, antidepressant medications, and dental occlusal variables have insufficient evidence to support or refute their involvement as risk factors for TMDs at this time.

Headaches

There is a large amount of epidemiologic literature on headaches and on migraine headache in particular (see chapter 25 for diagnosis and treatment).[23] Migraine headache is more prevalent in women than in men, and prevalence varies with age, peaking between age 35 and 45 for both genders. In this age group, prevalence averages about 20% for women and 7% for men. Nonmigrainous headaches (primarily tension-type headaches) are very common conditions experienced by 60% to 80% of adults. The prevalence of nonmigrainous headache is higher in women than in men, but the gender difference is much smaller than for migraine.

Table 2-2 TMD pain incidence studies

Authors	Population	Incidence rate (per 100 person-years)
Von Korff et al[15]	1,062 US adult HMO enrollees	2.2
Kitai et al[16]	361 Japanese adolescent girls	2.4 to 3.9
Heikinheimo[17]	167 Finnish adolescents	1.8
Nilsson et al[18]	2,255 Swedish adolescents	2.9
LeResche et al[19]	1,674 US 11- to 14-year-olds	2.3

Neuralgias

Trigeminal neuralgia is head or face pain characterized by sudden, brief paroxysmal stabbing pain along one or more distributions of the trigeminal nerve (see chapters 1 and 24). Rare types of facial neuralgia, including glossopharyngeal neuralgia and postherpetic neuralgia, will not be reviewed here. Because neuralgia is much less common than TMDs, population-based prevalence studies to determine the number of cases would require investigating a huge number of people. However, because people with trigeminal neuralgia nearly always seek treatment for their pain problem, the number of people seeking treatment for the first time in a defined geographic region can serve as a fairly good measure of its incidence. Annual incidence rates for trigeminal neuralgia from two studies[24,25] are based on records of treated cases over long periods of time in defined populations. Overall incidence rates are approximately 3 to 5 onsets per year per 100,000 people (ie, about 1/1,000 the rate of onset of TMD pain). The incidence rate rises with age in both studies; but one study shows a large sex difference, with higher rates in women, while the other shows a smaller difference. A recent UK study reports higher incidence rates for trigeminal neuralgia, about 27 per 100,000 person-years, also showing an increase with age and in women, but this study may include all types of trigeminal neuropathic pains.[26]

In addition to increased age and female gender, other possible risk factors for acquiring trigeminal neuralgia are multiple sclerosis, hypertension, and abstinence from alcohol and tobacco.

Other orofacial pain conditions

A few population-based studies exist for dysesthesias characterized by burning pain or discomfort in the oral soft tissues, eg, burning mouth syndrome (BMS) (see chapters 1 and 23 for diagnosis and treatment). Lipton et al[4] found that less than 1% of the US population reported "a prolonged unexplained burning sensation in [the] tongue or any other part of [the] mouth." Rates were somewhat higher in women than in men. Two other studies using broader case definitions reported rates of 4.5%[4] and almost 15%[27]; the especially high rate in the latter study might be due in part to the older age of its population. Women and the very elderly seem to be at an increased risk for burning mouth pain. Loss of hormones with menopause may increase the risk, but the research on this subject is far from clear. The risk may also be much higher for persons of Asian or American Indian ancestry than for whites or African Americans.[4] Many studies have found higher rates of psychologic disorders in persons seeking care for BMS than in control groups. However, no prospective population-based studies are available to assess whether the pain or psychologic distress occurred first, which limits the interpretation of these observations.

Two conditions of great interest to clinicians are *atypical odontalgia*, which is localized, usually throbbing pain in a tooth or tooth site without identifiable pathology, and *atypical facial pain*, which is continuous, nagging, deep, diffuse pain in the absence of other pain diagnoses or identifiable pathology (see chapters 1, 20, and 24). There is increasing evidence that a majority of these conditions are neuropathic, although no population-based data exist. Two studies have reported that 3% of patients[28] and 12% of patients[29] still had persistent tooth pain 1 month and 1 year, respectively, after endodontic treatment was completed, although some of the subjects in the latter study may have had persistent pain at the start of the study, which explains the high prevalence. This latter study also showed that being female, having previous chronic pain conditions, or reporting preexisting tooth pain were strong risk factors for persistent pain after a year or more.

Other clinical studies also indicate that women are much more likely than men to seek care for atypical odontalgia and atypical facial pain, and that the mean age of persons seeking care is around 40 to 55 years. High rates of psychologic disturbance also seem to occur in clinical populations of these patients, but again, it is unclear whether these disturbances precede or follow the unremitting pain, and whether they are associated with having the pain problem or with seeking care.

The impact of orofacial pain

Pain can disrupt a number of aspects of everyday life, including work, social and recreational activities, and sleep. A study of residents of Toronto[30] found that the most common impact of pain was worrying about one's health, which was experienced by over 70% of persons reporting pain. Forty-four percent of those with pain consulted a doctor or dentist; about 29% took medication; 14% reported sleep disturbance; and 4% to 8% reported taking time off from work, staying in bed, or avoiding family and friends. The more severe the pain, the more likely people were to report significant impacts. Many TMD patients experienced substantial psychologic impact and disruption of social and recreational activities.[8]

Summary

Epidemiologic research can help clinicians understand the frequency, etiology, diagnosis, prognosis, treatment, and prevention of orofacial pain disorders. This chapter has noted the limited epidemiologic research on types of orofacial pain other than TMDs; more research is likely to provide large gains in our knowledge. Toothache is the most prevalent acute orofacial pain condition in children and adults, while TMDs are rare in children but cause the most prevalent chronic orofacial pain in adults. BMS and atypical odontalgia/atypical facial pain are less common, while trigeminal neuralgia is rare. Risk factors for TMDs include female gender, having preexisting pain conditions, and depression. Risk factors for other chronic orofacial pains are less well known but are likely similar. The impact of orofacial pain is often substantial and should not be underestimated.

References

1. Lilienfeld AM, Lilienfeld DE. Foundations of Epidemiology, ed 2. New York: Oxford Univ Press, 1980.
2. Morris JN. Uses of Epidemiology, ed 3. Edinburgh: Churchill Livingstone, 1975.
3. Dworkin SF, Von Korff MR, LeResche L. Epidemiologic studies of chronic pain: A dynamic-ecologic perspective. Ann Behav Med 1992;14:3–11.
4. Lipton JA, Ship JA, Larach-Robinson D. Estimated prevalence and distribution of reported orofacial pain in the United States. J Am Dent Assoc 1993;124:115–121.
5. Locker D, Grushka M. Prevalence of oral and facial pain and discomfort: Preliminary results of a mail survey. Community Dent Oral Epidemiol 1987;15:169–172.
6. Slade GD, Spencer AJ, Davies MJ, Burrow D. Intraoral distribution and impact of caries experience among South Australian school children. Aust Dent J 1996;41:343–350.
7. Schulman JD, Beach MM, Rivera-Hidalgo F. The prevalence of oral mucosal lesions in U.S. adults: Data from the Third National Health and Nutrition Examination Survey, 1988-1994. J Am Dent Asso 2004;135:1279–1286.
8. Von Korff M, Dworkin SF, LeResche L, Kruger A. An epidemiologic comparison of pain complaints. Pain 1988;32:173–183.
9. Drangsholt M, LeResche L. Temporomandibular disorder pain. In: Crombie IK, Croft PR, Linton SJ, LeResche L, Von Korff M (eds). Epidemiology of Pain: A Report of the Task Force on Epidemiology of the International Association for the Study of Pain. Seattle: IASP Press, 1999:203–233.
10. Locker D, Slade G. Prevalence of symptoms associated with temporomandibular disorders in a Canadian Population. Community Dent Oral Epidemiol 1988;16:310–313.
11. Goulet JP, Lavigne GJ, Lund JP. Jaw pain prevalence among French-speaking Canadians in Quebec and related symptoms of temporomandibular disorders. J Dent Res 1995;74:1738–1744.
12. Helkimo M. Studies on function and dysfunction of the masticatory system. IV. Age and sex distribution of symptoms of dysfunction of the masticatory system in Lapps in the north of Finland. Acta Odontol Scand 1974; 32:255–267.
13. Matsuka Y, Yatani H, Kuboki T, Yamashita A. Temporomandibular disorders in the adult population of Okayama City, Japan. Cranio 1996;14:158–162.
14. Dworkin SF, LeResche L. Research diagnostic criteria for temporomandibular disorders: Review, criteria, examinations and specifications, critique. J Craniomandib Disord 1992;6:301–355.
15. Von Korff M, LeResche L, Dworkin SF. First onset of common pain symptoms: A prospective study of depression as a risk factor. Pain 1993;55:251–258.
16. Kitai N, Takada K, Yasuda Y, Verdonck A, Carels C. Pain and other cardinal TMJ dysfunction symptoms: A Longitudinal survey of Japanese female adolescents. J Oral Rehabil 1997;24:741–748.
17. Heikinheimo K, Salmi K, Myllarniemi S, Kirveskari P. Symptoms of craniomandibular disorder in a sample of Finnish adolescents at the ages of 12 and 15 years. Eur J Orthod 1989;11:325–331.
18. Nilsson IM, List T, Drangsholt M. Incidence and temporal patterns of temporomandibular disorder pain among Swedish adolescents. J Orofac Pain 2007;21:127–132.
19. LeResche L, Mancl L, Sherman JJ, Gandara B, Dworkin SF. Changes in temporomandibular pain and other symptoms across the menstrual cycle. Pain 2003;106:253–261.
20. LeResche L, Sherman JJ, Huggins KH, et al. Musculoskeletal orofacial pain and other signs and symptoms of temporomandibular disorders during pregnancy: A prospective study. J Orofac Pain 2005;19:193–201.
21. LeResche L, Mancl LA, Drangsholt M, Huang G, Von Korff M. Predictors of onset of facial pain and temporomandibular disorders in early adolescence. Pain 2007; 129:269–278.
22. Diatchenko L, Slade GD, Nackley AG, et al. Genetic basis for individual variations in pain perception and the development of a chronic pain condition. Hum Mol Genet 2005;14:135–143.
23. Scher AI, Stewart WF, Lipton RB. Migraine and headache: A meta-analytic approach. In: Crombie IK, Croft PR, Linton SJ, LeResche L, Von Korff M (eds). Epidemiology of Pain: A Report of the Task Force on Epidemiology of the International Association for the Study of Pain. Seattle: IASP Press, 1999:159–170.
24. Rothman KJ, Monson RR. Epidemiology of trigeminal neuralgia. J Chronic Dis 1973;26:3–12.
25. Katusic S, Beard CM, Bergstralh E, Kurland LT. Incidence and clinical features of trigeminal neuralgia, Rochester, Minnesota, 1945-1984. Ann Neurol 1990;27:89–95.
26. Hall GC, Carroll D, Parry D, McQuay HJ. Epidemiology and treatment of neuropathic pain: The UK primary care perspective. Pain 2006;122:156–162.
27. Tammiala-Salonen T, Hiidenkari T, Parvinen T. Burning mouth in a Finnish adult population. Community Dent Oral Epidemiol 1993;21:67–71.
28. Marbach JJ, Hulbrock J, Hohn C, Segal AG. Incidence of phantom tooth pain: An atypical facial neuralgia. Oral Surg Oral Med Oral Pathol 1982;53:190–193.
29. Polycarpou N, Ng YL, Canavan D, Moles DR, Gulabivala K. Prevalence of persistent pain after endodontic treatment and factors affecting its occurrence in cases with complete radiographic healing. Int Endod J 2005;38:169–178.
30. Locker D, Grushka M. The impact of dental and facial pain. J Dent Res 1987;66:1414–1417.

3

Current Beliefs and Educational Guidelines

Charles G. Widmer

The patient with orofacial pain is a challenge to health care providers because of the complexity of presenting signs and symptoms and the diversity of conditions that may elicit pain in this region. To accurately diagnose the cause of orofacial pain, a practitioner must have knowledge of a wide variety of disciplines including the basic biomedical sciences, epidemiology of orofacial pain conditions, validity and reliability associated with parameters used in diagnosis and treatment, pathologies that may present as pain in the orofacial region, and the psychosocial impact of pain on the individual.

The purpose of this chapter is to examine the current beliefs in the field of orofacial pain and to review an educational framework that has been proposed for orofacial pain curricula in dental schools.

Overview of Current Beliefs

Current beliefs regarding orofacial pain are quite diverse. Although the number of well-controlled randomized clinical trials is growing, most beliefs are still based on philosophic interpretations of clinical observations, rather than evidence-based practice (see chapter 18). The local dogma in each dental program will vary according to the philoso-

phy of the department or the practitioner teaching about orofacial conditions. This general overview of the most important orofacial pain conditions emphasizes musculoskeletal pain, since this has traditionally generated the most controversy.

Intraoral pain conditions

Odontalgia

Examples of orofacial pain conditions that have a well-understood etiology include odontalgia associated with either an irreversible pulpitis secondary to a caries infection, or a reversible pulpitis associated with trauma (see chapter 20). However, not all people who present with tooth pain have pulpitis. Some have atypical odontalgia, which has no clear etiology. This condition has been linked to several possible pathologies, including osteomyelitis and neuralgias. One variant of this condition, phantom tooth pain, occurs after an extraction of a tooth or group of teeth. Although the true etiologies of these persistent pain conditions have not been established, there is a tendency to group them with neuropathic pains (see chapters 7 and 24).

Mucosal and gingival pain associated with inflammation

Another orofacial pain that has a well-understood etiology is that associated with fungal infections (candidiasis) or viral infections (herpes simplex) of the oral mucosa. These infections respond to antifungal and antiviral agents, respectively. Acute necrotizing ulcerative gingivitis is associated with an acute gingival infection, whereas desquamative gingivitis is associated with abnormal hormonal levels or allergic reactions involving the gingival tissues, such as reactions to components of crowns or partial denture frameworks. These pains decline in a predictable fashion as the infections clear and the tissues repair. Chronic periodontal disease causes pain in only 6% of patients with the condition,[1] which may be one of the reasons for its high prevalence in many population groups and the primary reason that it remains untreated in many patients (see chapters 2 and 23).

Temporomandibular disorders

Until recently, most authors did not separate myalgia and arthralgia because they believed that both disorders had a common cause (see chapters 19 and 22). Some of the most common etiologic theories are listed below.

Dental and occlusal etiologies

Costen,[2] an otolaryngologist, proposed that tooth loss was the cause of impaired hearing, stuffy ears, tinnitus, dull muscle and joint pain, dizziness, sinus symptoms, and headaches. He stated that correction of an overbite or replacement of lost molar support would remove the pressure that the displaced condyle was exerting on adjacent structures, including the dura mater and middle ear. In dentistry, this belief led to a major emphasis for five decades on occlusal-based treatment approaches and diagnostic devices for temporomandibular disorders (TMDs). Currently, this explanation is not generally accepted, although some practitioners still persist in occlusally based diagnostic and therapeutic approaches. Some evidence suggests that loss of posterior support, such as missing molars, may be linked to a higher incidence and severity of arthritis in the temporomandibular joint (TMJ),[3] but these data must be interpreted with caution because of the possible link to a third variable—age.

Occlusal discrepancies, particularly centric occlusion interferences and balancing interferences, have also been cited as a cause of musculoskeletal pain. These concepts were based on the clinical observations of musculoskeletal pain improvement after elimination of nonideal contacts. However, epidemiologists have determined that a significant proportion of the population has these occlusal discrepancies without experiencing musculoskeletal pain.[4] Others have placed experimental occlusal or placebo interferences in normal subjects, but these devices were not found to be associated with the development of TMD-like symptoms.[5]

Skeletal abnormalities

One theory of masticatory and cervical musculoskeletal pain is that poor body alignment, including cervical posture (eg, forward head posture), pelvic tilt, and uneven leg lengths, can initiate and propagate the pain condition. To prove that poor body alignment is an etiologic factor, a practitioner would need to show that it predisposed the patient to musculoskeletal pain, but this has not been done. In fact, the prevalence of one of the misalignments that has frequently been invoked as a cause of TMDs, the so-called forward head posture, has been found to be as high as 93% in teenaged girls, suggesting that it is biologically very normal.[6] Other postural or skeletal deviations from a philosophic ideal are probably just as high. For example, one concept states that the mandibular condyle should occupy a central position within the fossa. However, studies using tomography to examine the condylar position in asymptomatic participants and TMD patients found that variation from the ideal position was equally high in both samples.[7,8]

Another theory links orofacial pain with misalignment of the cranial bones coupled with stress along the sutures. The basis for this concept is the impression of improvement in musculoskeletal pain after cranial bone manipulation. To date, there is no evidence that the cranial bones are mobile in the adult, and no randomized clinical trials have been carried out to test the efficacy of manipulation.

Psychologic disturbances

The belief that patients with chronic pain are psychologically or emotionally disturbed is rather widespread. When no evidence of local pathology is found, the default diagnosis for some practitioners is a psychosomatic disorder. Although depression is a frequent symptom in patients with chronic orofacial pain, as it is in any chronic pain group, there is no evidence that depression, or indeed any psychologic trait or disorder, is a cause of TMDs or related conditions. Depression is likely to be secondary to the pain (see chapter 12).

Psychophysiologic theory of muscle pain

The psychophysiologic theory was proposed by Laskin[9] to describe the relationship between stress, increased muscle activation patterns, and muscle and TMJ pain. As a group, patients with chronic pain show relatively high levels of stress[10,11]; however, most experimental studies of induced stress have not shown parallel changes in muscle activity and pain levels. Although a small increase of masticatory muscle electromyographic (EMG) activity (2 to 4 μV) during high relevant stress has been reported in a study[12] using imagery or reaction times, this is not evidence that stress-induced hyperactivity causes TMD pain. In fact, this EMG activity may be caused by low-level activation of the facial muscles rather than the jaw muscles. A

number of treatment techniques that aim to reduce stress, such as biofeedback, relaxation therapies, and counseling, apparently lead to a reduction in muscle pain. However, it is important to understand that most studies of the efficacy of these techniques have been, at best, loosely controlled, which precludes the drawing of causal relationships.

Bruxism and other parafunctional behavior

The presence of bruxism in TMD patients has been reported to be very high in some studies, but the criteria used to identify bruxers were very loose (see chapters 16 and 26). Although chronic clenching or grinding of the teeth involves the excessive activation of the masticatory muscles that sometimes leads to pain, there are many people who qualify as bruxers who do not have a history of masticatory muscle pain. These conflicting data cloud the picture.

Related medical conditions

Neuropathic pains

Several neuropathic pain conditions affect the orofacial region (see chapter 24). These include trigeminal neuralgia, postherpetic neuralgia, burning mouth syndrome (BMS), and complex regional pain syndrome (CRPS). For these conditions, etiologies are difficult to identify. This difficulty has resulted in various viewpoints regarding the possible etiology and management of each condition. Most of these viewpoints are not based on evidence and often lead to ineffective and sometimes deleterious treatment approaches. For example, trigeminal neuralgia has been traditionally associated with vascular compression of the trigeminal nerve by an adjacent artery, but vascular decompression does not provide relief of pain in all these patients. Postherpetic neuralgia has an identified etiology (herpes virus), but the mechanism of pain during flareups is poorly understood at best. BMS, sometimes called *stomatodynia*, occurs most frequently in postmenopausal women and has been linked to hormonal changes. However, this syndrome has been difficult to diagnose due to the lack of diagnostic indicators, and it has been incorrectly labeled by many practitioners as psychosomatic in origin. CRPS presents with signs or symptoms of edema, color changes, or sweating; it appears to reflect abnormal regional activity of the sympathetic nervous system. However, these regional changes can also be observed in other categories of neuropathic pain. The current consensus regarding these neuropathies is that they are associated with neuroplastic changes at one or several levels in the nervous system (see chapter 7).

Headaches

There are many different varieties of headaches, but the most common are tension-type, migraine, and cluster (see chapter 25). Tension-type headache was originally called *tension headache* or *muscle-contraction headache* and was attributed to the excessive contraction of the muscles of the scalp (frontalis, temporalis, and occipital muscles). Treatments to reduce the "spasm" of muscles were pursued without evidence of tonic muscle contraction. However, in 1988 the International Headache Society[13] changed the name to *tension-type headache* to recognize the fact that muscle contraction was unlikely to be the cause of the pain (see also chapters 15 and 17). Treatment has traditionally consisted of mild analgesics such as nonsteroidal anti-inflammatory drugs (NSAIDs).

Migraine headache and the throbbing characteristic of its pain has been attributed to vasodilatation of cranial blood vessels such as the middle meningeal artery. However, magnetic resonance imaging (MRI) evidence suggests that the meninges are inflamed in a subset of migraine patients during an attack.[14] This finding has prompted the testing of ibuprofen and other NSAIDs along with vasoconstriction medications or serotonin antago-

nists such as triptans. One therapy that has not been shown to be effective for migraine or tension-type headaches in randomized, double-blind clinical trials is botulinum toxin A.[15] These findings are contrary to open-label studies using this toxin. This lack of efficacy of a popular toxin for pain management reinforces the need to follow evidence-based techniques (see chapter 18).

Cluster headache is more common in middle-aged men and is associated with autonomic signs on the side ipsilateral to the periorbital headache. Currently, the etiology is unknown, although evidence suggests a neuroendocrine etiology.[16] Treatment for cluster headache is empiric, but serotonin agonists such as sumatriptan have been used with good results.[17]

The Need for Knowledge in the Basic Sciences

Dentistry has traditionally approached orofacial pain problems such as TMDs with a narrow vision. Dentists deal with teeth, and therefore it has been easy for many to accept that these pains must be tooth related. Although there are some practitioners who still believe that generalized musculoskeletal pain can be caused by abnormal occlusal contacts, the more astute clinicians ponder the larger picture. What causes some conditions associated with pain to become chronic (see chapters 5 and 7)? Why do most chronic pain conditions have a female predominance (see chapter 13)? Why are many chronic pain conditions exacerbated by stress and the immune system (see chapter 6)? Is there a genetic tendency for experiencing pain (see chapter 9)? These are just some examples of the challenging questions facing the pain field, and progress will be gained through a better understanding of the physiology of pain and the impact of other systems on the initiation, persistence, and modulation of pain transmission and perception. An integrated approach to the teaching of basic,

---

Box 3-1 Educational guidelines for orofacial pain*

Pain as a public health problem
- Pain as an obstacle to optimum care
- Epidemiology
- Economics of pain
- Medicolegal and ethical issues

Definition of pain
- Acute, recurrent, and persistent pain
- Terminology of pain
- Philosophic issues associated with pain
- Historic perspectives of pain studies
- Biologic significance of acute and chronic pain

Neurobiology of pain
- Theories of pain
- Peripheral neuroanatomy/receptors/mechanisms
- Central nociceptive pathways
- Neurochemicals associated with pain
- Affective, cognitive, behavioral, and developmental aspects
- Interpersonal and psychosocial issues associated with pain

Pain assessment
- Measurement of pain and disability, distress, and suffering
- Assessment of pain relief

Management of pain
- Preoperative and operative pain management
- Managing postoperative pain

Acute and chronic orofacial pain
- Orofacial pain taxonomy
- Assessment of orofacial pain
- Diagnostic features, etiology, mechanisms, and management

*Adapted from the International Association for the Study of Pain, Internet communication, 1993.

---

behavioral, and clinical sciences must form a part of the training in dental schools. Without this foundation, it will be difficult for the practitioner to adequately evaluate and treat patients with orofacial pain as newer concepts emerge. Unfortunately, many dental schools provide limited curricular time and little exposure for the dental student to pain mechanisms, diagnosis, and management, despite orofacial pain being so common and despite educational guidelines being available.

Current educational guidelines

The current educational guidelines have evolved from workshops conducted in the early 1990s and 2002[18] and from the International Association for

the Study of Pain Proposed Outline Curriculum on Pain for Dental Schools (Internet communication, 1993). These guidelines serve as a basis for a standardized and integrated curriculum to prepare the student to meet standards of dentistry excellence today and for the next 40 years of an evolving dental practice (Box 3-1).

The guidelines cover six topics beginning with general concepts about pain and progressing to the specifics of orofacial pain. The first section covers pain as a public health problem, including prevalence of pain in the general population. The second section covers definitions and includes a discussion of the philosophic, historic, and biologic significance of the pain experience. It prepares the student for a broadened appreciation of the effect pain has in our daily lives. The next topic reviews the neurobiology of pain as it travels from the site of injury in the periphery to the central nervous system; the modulation of this pain by various processes; and the theories of pain resulting from injury, inflammation, and neuropathic changes. The basic principles of neuroanatomy; receptors and mechanisms of pain initiation, transmission, and maintenance; and the interpersonal and psychosocial factors associated with pain are included in this third section. The integration of these topics reflects the interdependence of the physical and psychosocial axes. The fourth section describes the methods used to measure pain, relief, and suffering. This topic is followed by a fifth section on pain management. The last topic focuses on orofacial pain and a review of taxonomy, diagnostic techniques and features, and management approaches specific to this group of pain disorders.

Summary

This chapter has noted that the etiology of most acute pain conditions of the teeth and oral mucosa is well understood, and the management of these pains is usually uncomplicated. In contrast, the origin of most chronic pain of the orofacial region is uncertain, and for some diseases, no specific treatments have been found. In general, the most popular etiologic hypotheses are not well supported by data.

Students of dentistry need to understand current knowledge about pain and pain conditions, and they need to be trained to find and incorporate new knowledge into their future practices.

References

1. Brunsvold MA, Nair P, Oates TW Jr. Chief complaints of patients seeking treatment for periodontitis. J Am Dent Assoc 1999;130(3):359–364.

2. Costen JB. A syndrome of ear and sinus symptoms dependent upon disturbed function of the temporomandibular joint. 1934. Ann Otol Rhinol Laryngol 1997;106(10 Pt 1):805–819.

3. Seligman DA, Pullinger AG. The role of intercuspal occlusal relationships in temporomandibular disorders: A review. J Craniomandib Disord 1991;5:96–106.

4. Seligman DA, Pullinger AG. The role of functional occlusal relationships in temporomandibular disorders: A review. J Craniomandib Disord 1991;5:265–279.

5. Magnusson T, Enbom L. Signs and symptoms of mandibular dysfunction after introduction of experimental balancing-side interferences. Acta Odontol Scand 1984; 42:129–135.

6. Alderman M. An Investigation of the Need for Posture Education Among High School Girls and a Suggested Plan of Instruction to Meet These Needs [thesis]. Univ of Texas, 1966.

7. Blaschke DD, Blaschke TJ. Normal TMJ bony relationships in centric occlusion. J Dent Res 1981;60:98–104.

8. Katzberg RW, Keith DA, Ten Eick WR, Guralnick WC. Internal derangements of the temporomandibular joint: An assessment of condylar position in centric occlusion. J Prosthet Dent 1983;49:250–254.

9. Laskin DM. Etiology of the pain-dysfunction syndrome. J Am Dent Assoc 1969;79:147–153.

10. Carlson CR, Reid KI, Curran SL, et al. Psychological and physiological parameters of masticatory muscle pain. Pain 1998;76:297–307.

11. Wolfe F, Hawley DJ. Psychosocial factors and the fibromyalgia syndrome. Z Rheumatol 1998;57(suppl 2):88–91.

12. Ohrbach R, Blascovich J, Gale EN, McCall WD Jr, Dworkin SF. Psychophysiological assessment of stress in chronic pain: Comparisons of stressful stimuli and of response systems. J Dent Res 1998;77:1840–1850.

13. Classification and diagnostic criteria for headache disorders, cranial neuralgias and facial pain. Headache Classification Committee of the International Headache Society. Cephalalgia 1988;8(suppl 7):1–96.

14. Cao Y, Welch KM, Aurora S, Vikingstad EM. Functional MRI-BOLD of visually triggered headache in patients with migraine. Arch Neurol 1999;56:548–554.

15. Evers S, Olesen J. Botulinum toxin in headache treatment: The end of the road? Cephalalgia 2006;26:769–771.

16. May A, Bahra A, Buchel C, Frackowiak RS, Goadsby PJ. Hypothalamic activation in cluster headache attacks. Lancet 1998;352:275–278.

17. Hardebo JE, Dahlof C. Sumatriptan nasal spray (20 mg/dose) in the acute treatment of cluster headache. Cephalalgia 1998;18:487–489.

18. Mohl ND, Attanasio R. The third educational conferenceto develop the curriculum in temporomandibular disorders and orofacial pain: Introduction. J Orofac Pain 2002;16:173–175.

Section II

Neurobiology of Pain

Peripheral Mechanisms of Orofacial Pain

Bruce Matthews
Barry J. Sessle

In general, the peripheral mechanisms of pain in the tissues innervated by the trigeminal (V) nerve are much the same as those in other parts of the body. However, the sensory receptors associated with pain in pulp and dentin appear to have rather different properties from other nociceptors; these differences may be more a result of the different environments provided by the tissues in which they are located than of fundamental differences in the receptors themselves. The pulp and dentin are also unusual in that virtually all the afferents that innervate these tissues seem to be capable of producing pain. Because of their particular clinical relevance to dentistry, this chapter will focus on nociceptive mechanisms in the dentin and pulp, but nociceptors in other orofacial tissues will also be mentioned because pain associated with them is also encountered in clinical practice.

General Features of Receptors Including Nociceptors

Those nerve cells with axons (ie, fibers) innervating peripheral tissues are termed *primary afferent* (sensory) *neurons* and can be divided into groups on the basis of their axonal diameter and degree of myelination, both of which influence axonal conduction velocity. Large-diameter axons conducting impulses (action potentials) in the 70 to 120 m/s and the 30 to 70 m/s ranges are called A-α and A-β *afferent fibers*, respectively. The smaller, finely myelinated axons are termed A-δ *afferent fibers* and conduct impulses at approximately 3 to 30 m/s, whereas unmyelinated axons, called *C-fiber afferents*, conduct impulses at 0.5 to 3.0 m/s. Many A-β afferents terminating peripherally in specialized sense organs (ie, receptors) are excited by light tactile stimuli applied to the peripheral tissues that they innervate and are termed *low-threshold mechanoreceptors*. In contrast, many of the A-δ and C-fiber afferents terminate in the peripheral tissues as free nerve endings that provide the peripheral basis for pain. They act as nociceptors; that is, they are the sense organs that are activated by noxious stimulation of peripheral tissues, and their activation may result in the production of action potentials in the small-diameter (A-δ or C) afferent fibers with which they are associated. The action potentials are then conducted along the fibers into the central nervous system (CNS), where they are processed so that the quality, intensity, duration, and location of the noxious stimulus can be perceived. The frequency of the impulses and the duration of the series of impulses in the nociceptive afferent fiber provide the peripheral basis for coding the intensity and duration of the noxious stimulus. The peripheral feature of importance for stimulus localization is the *receptive field* (RF) of the fiber: the area of skin, mucosa, or deep tissue from which an afferent fiber, or central neuron, and its associated receptors can be excited by a threshold stimulus. In the case of a nociceptive afferent fiber, the threshold for its excitation from its RF is extremely high and in the noxious range; the RF area is usually less than 1 mm^2.

Nociceptive endings can be activated by a wide range of noxious stimuli, but their sensitivity may increase following mild injury (eg, when the threshold of the nociceptors is lowered by chemical agents or repeated noxious stimuli). This increased responsiveness, called *nociceptor* or *peripheral sensitization*, appears to be a major factor in the production of hyperalgesia and allodynia (see chapters 1 and 6). Biomechanical factors, such as tissue compliance, may also influence the responsiveness of nociceptive afferents. Sometimes after peripheral injury, afferent fibers may also fire spontaneously. A number of chemicals are involved in peripheral sensitization of these peripheral endings and their activation by noxious stimuli (see chapter 6), and some mechanically insensitive nociceptors (*silent nociceptors*) may be responsive only to chemical stimuli. The increased nociceptor activity inevitably leads to an increased afferent barrage into the CNS, followed by functional changes known as *central sensitization* (see chapter 5).

Pulp and Dentin

Dental pulp is a highly vascular and richly innervated connective tissue that forms the soft tissue core of a tooth. In many respects the pulp of a fully formed tooth has physiologic properties similar to those of loose connective tissue elsewhere in the body, but it is different in at least two important

respects: *(1)* it is exquisitely sensitive, so much so that just touching exposed pulp with a wisp of cotton wool can cause severe pain; and *(2)* in a fully formed, intact tooth, it has a very low compliance. This low compliance is because of the surrounding calcified dentin, which prevents any significant volume change when the pressures within the tissue change. Because of this low compliance, the equilibrium between the various factors that affect blood flow and the circulation of tissue fluid in pulp is different from that in most other tissues. In contrast, dentin is an avascular tissue. Nevertheless, it can be highly sensitive despite its sparse innervation. While there is considerable evidence that stimulation of these tissues evokes only the experience of pain, there is some evidence that nonpainful sensations may be elicited under certain conditions.[1-5]

The innervation of pulp and dentin

The nerve fibers that innervate the pulp arborize extensively, especially in the coronal part of the tooth, and form a subodontoblastic plexus (Fig 4-1). The branches of the V nerve that innervate teeth contain both afferent and postganglionic sympathetic efferent axons.[6,7] The V primary afferents have their cell bodies in the V ganglion and are primarily sensory in function, although some—when stimulated—produce vasodilatation, a component of neurogenic inflammation (see chapter 6). The sympathetic efferents supply pulp vessels (see Fig 4-1) and are vasoconstrictive. Their cell bodies are in the superior cervical ganglion, from which the axons pass to the V ganglion and then on to the tooth in the branches of the V nerve. Unlike the lip and some other orofacial tissues, there is no conclusive evidence that the pulp receives a parasympathetic vasodilator innervation.

Classes of nerve fibers that innervate the pulp

The pulp is innervated by myelinated A-β and A-δ fibers and nonmyelinated C-fibers. About 50% of

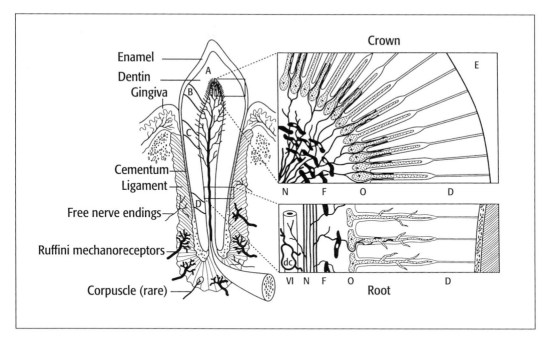

Fig 4-1 Schematic of a mature erupted tooth and its rich dentinal, pulpal, and periodontal innervation, with various structures indicated. More than 40% of dentinal tubules are innervated at the tip of the pulp horn (zone A), with decreasing percentages of innervated tubules in zones B (4.1% to 8.3%), C (0.2% to 1.0%), and D (0.02% to 0.2%). The higher-magnification panels show differences in intradentinal nerve (N) incidence, pulpal fibroblasts (F), odontoblast morphology (O), dentin (D), and enamel (E) for the crown and root. Perivascular dendritic cells (dc) and vascular innervation (VI) are shown in the root diagram. Reprinted with permission from Byers and Närhi.[2]

the myelinated axons are A-β, which is surprising for a tissue whose afferent innervation appears to support only pain sensation. Histologically, the pulp appears to contain large numbers of small myelinated and nonmyelinated axons. However, this picture is distorted by the fact that the terminals of the axons in the pulp are smaller in diameter than their more central parent axons, as well as by the fact that axons myelinated in the nerve trunk outside the tooth may have unmyelinated terminals within the pulp. The number of nerve terminals in the pulp is also much greater than the number of sensory neurons that innervate the tissue because each neuron may have many terminal branches.

The innervation of dentin and the contents of dentinal tubules

The dentinal tubules taper from a diameter of about 2 μm at their pulpal ends to 0.5 μm or less at their periphery. Each tubule contains the process of an odontoblast whose cell body is situated at the pulpal end of the tubule.[8] Adjacent cell bodies are functionally limited by gap junctions.[9] The odontoblast processes extend no more than half the length of the tubules, and under the tip of the cusp, they are much shorter. There is no evidence that vital cellular elements are present in the tubules past the ends of the odontoblast processes, although the luminal contents have a granular appearance,[10,11] indicating that they contain something in addition to simple extracellular fluid. As noted in Fig 4-1, some dentinal tubules also contain one or more fine nerve terminals. Quantitative data mainly from the permanent canine teeth of cats[12] reveal that these nerve terminals are unmyelinated (diameter approximately 0.1 μm) and penetrate up to 100 μm into the dentinal tubules. Innervation density is highest under the tip of the cusp where almost every tubule contains a nerve terminal, but the density decreases rapidly below this level (see Fig 4-1).

There are no myelinated axons in the odontoblast cell layer. It is not clear whether the nerve endings there and in the dentinal tubules are the nonmyelinated terminals of myelinated or of nonmyelinated pulpal axons, although some evidence suggests that there might be a differential distribution of endings from unmyelinated and small-diameter myelinated afferents in the pulp versus the dentin.[2,5,6] Some of the dental nerve endings contain neuropeptides, including substance P and calcitonin gene-related peptide (CGRP). Indeed, several neurochemicals have been found in neural elements (eg, substance P, CGRP, nerve growth factor) and in non-neural tissues (eg, histamine, serotonin [5-HT], opioids) of the pulp, and have been implicated in the responses of pulp afferent fibers to noxious stimuli, injury, and inflammation, as well as in processes related to regeneration and repair[2,6] (see chapter 6). The pulp innervation is thus in a dynamic state, and injury or aging, for example, can be associated with changes in the neurochemicals within pulp afferents as well as in the type, structure, and distribution of these afferents. For example, dentin cavity preparations can induce increased production of pulpal nerve growth factor and sprouting of CGRP-containing nerve fibers.

Sensory mechanisms of dentin

The dentin is normally well protected from the environment, although this may change because of dental caries, attrition, or tooth fracture. Heat, cold, mechanical stimulation, drying, large changes in hydrostatic pressure, and solutions of high osmotic pressure excite intradental nerves and can cause pain in human dentin.[1–5] With the exception of the thermal stimuli, these must be applied to an exposed dentin surface to produce pain, and they are most effective when the ends of the dentinal tubules are patent. Despite the lack of vital cellular elements in the outer ends of the dentinal tubules, this area of the dentin is sensitive to stimulation, and very gentle mechanical probing of the dentoenamel junction will evoke a discharge of impulses in intradental nerves if the smear layer left by drilling has been removed. So where are the receptors that respond to the pain-producing stimuli, and how are they excited?

Several theories have been proposed, and the three most significant are illustrated in Fig 4-2. Experimental data over the last two to three decades have not lent much support to the so-called neural theory and odontoblast transduction theory; most evidence supports the hydrodynamic theory.[1–3,5,10,14] From simple physical principles, it would be expected that all the different forms of stimulation capable of causing pain from dentin are also capable of producing movement of the contents of the underlying dentinal tubules; this expectation has been confirmed experimentally in extracted teeth. It seems that the dentinal tubules act as passive hydraulic links between the site of stimulation and nerve endings sensitive to pressure changes or deformation located more deeply, either at the pulpal ends of the tubules or in the underlying pulp.

In addition, the latencies of sensory responses to cold stimuli in humans and of neural responses in the cat, which are less than a second, are too short to be accounted for by a mechanism that involves a temperature change in the pulp or at the pulp-dentin interface where the nerves are known to terminate. Movement of fluid in the tubules can account for this short latency because the move-

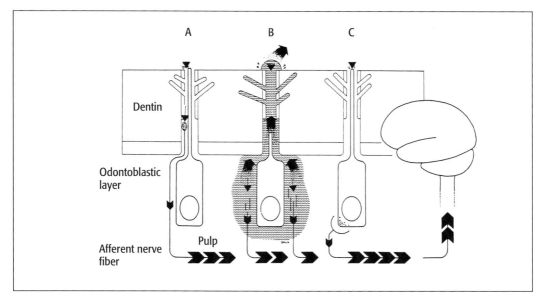

Fig 4-2 Three major theories for activation of dental nerve fibers by stimuli applied to enamel or dentin. Stimuli are indicated by arrowheads. The *neural theory* (A) attributes activation to an initial excitation (*arrow*) of those nerves ending within the dentinal tubules that generates nerve impulses, which are then conducted along the parent primary afferent nerve fibers in the pulp into the dental nerve branches and then into the brain. The *hydrodynamic theory* (B) proposes that the stimuli cause a displacement of the fluid within the dentinal tubules in either an outward direction (as shown) or an inward direction (not shown); this mechanical disturbance is thought to activate the nerve endings in the dentin or pulp. The *odontoblastic transduction theory* (C) proposes that the stimuli initially excite the odontoblast process or body, the membrane of which may come into close junctional apposition with that of the nerve endings in the pulp (as shown) or in the dentinal tubule (not shown), and that the odontoblast transmits this excitation to these associated nerve endings. Adapted with permission from Nanci and Ten Cate.[13]

ment begins at the moment the stimulus is applied and a temperature gradient is set up in the tooth. Further support is provided by the observation that removing the smear layer from exposed dentin increases the neural response evoked by nonthermal stimuli such as probing, drying, and changes in hydrostatic pressure. But probably the most conclusive evidence is the finding that many afferents each respond to many of the different stimuli that cause pain; this suggests that these afferents may operate through a common transduction system, although it is not known how the displacement of tubule contents generates impulses in nerve endings in the dentinal tubules or in the adjacent pulp. In addition, not all intradental afferents are excited by such a hydrodynamic mechanism; pulpal C-fibers and some of the slowest A-δ fibers appear to respond directly to thermal and chemical stimuli. Indeed, there is some evidence for specific cold receptors in teeth: etching dentin in humans increases the intensity of the pain produced by cold stimuli, but at the same time decreases the fluid flow through the tubules,[15] indicating that a hydrodynamic mechanism was not responsible for the pain caused by the cold stimuli. There is also evidence that heat as well as cold-sensitive transient receptor potential (TRP) ion channels (see chapter 6) are expressed in neurons that innervate the pulp.[16,17]

Other Orofacial Tissues

Periodontal ligament and oral mucous membrane

In addition to a dense innervation by low-threshold mechanoreceptors, the periodontal ligament contains free nerve endings (see Fig 4-1). These are associated with A-δ and C-fiber nociceptive afferents that may respond to mechanical, thermal, and/or chemical stimuli.[3] The different classes are, in general, similar to nociceptors in other tissues. Some periodontal nociceptive afferents branch to innervate the pulp of an adjacent tooth.

Limited data are available on the properties of nociceptors in the oral mucosa, but it is known that A-δ and C-fiber nociceptors exist, that they are sensitive to a variety of noxious stimuli, and that their responsiveness may be influenced by biomechanical factors in the tissues.[18]

Cornea

In the cornea, nerve terminals penetrate into the epithelium, and the sensory receptors are highly exposed to changes in the external environment. When stimuli of different types are applied to the corneal surface, the most prominent sensations evoked are of pain and irritation, but careful sensory testing has established that a cooling sensation can also be perceived. These observations correlate well with recordings from corneal afferent nerves in experimental animals, in which it has been shown that the cornea contains mechano-nociceptors, polymodal nociceptors, and low-threshold cold receptors.[19]

Facial skin

The cutaneous tissues of the orofacial region have a dense innervation, especially in the perioral region. Three major classes of nociceptive afferent fibers have been described[3,18]: *(1)* A-δ mechano-thermal nociceptive afferents that respond to intense thermal and mechanical stimuli; *(2)* C-polymodal nociceptive afferents that are excited by strong mechanical, thermal, and chemical stimuli; and *(3)* high-threshold mechanoreceptive afferents that respond best to intense mechanical stimuli (most of these conduct in the A-δ range, although some may have conduction velocities in the A-β and C-fiber ranges).

Temporomandibular joint and masticatory muscles

The endings of many of the small-diameter afferents innervating the temporomandibular joints (TMJs) and masticatory muscles may respond to a wide range of peripheral stimuli that cause pain in humans[3,18,20] (eg, heavy pressure, algesic chemicals, and inflammatory agents). Ischemia also is an effective stimulus of small-diameter muscle afferents if it is prolonged and associated with muscle contractions. There is also evidence that differences may exist in some of these responses between males and females.[20]

Cranial vessels and meninges

Small-diameter afferent fibers supply cranial vessels, and many can be activated by noxious stimuli.[18,21] Their activation may also be associated with the subsequent development of vasodilatation related to so-called neurogenic inflammation (see chapter 6). Their activation and their modulation by peripheral neurochemical processes (eg, 5-HT) appear to be important factors in the initiation and control of certain headaches such as migraine.

Connections of V nociceptive afferents in the brain stem

In the brain stem, V primary afferent fibers project to a column of nuclei consisting of the V main sensory nucleus and the V spinal tract nucleus, the latter of which is subdivided into three sub-nuclei: oralis, interpolaris, and caudalis. Nociceptive afferents from many different orofacial tissues project ipsilaterally and make synaptic connections predominantly with neurons in the subnucleus caudalis (see chapter 5).

Summary

This chapter has provided a general description of the properties of nociceptors and then has focused on the physiologic mechanisms underlying nociception in the pulp and dentin. It is pointed out that the dentinal tubules as well as the pulp are innervated, and that the afferents can respond to a wide variety of stimuli that predominantly, if not exclusively, produce pain. There are a large number of small-diameter myelinated and unmyelinated afferents innervating the teeth, but some large A-β intradental afferents also exist. Evidence currently favors a hydrodynamic mechanism for activation of intradental afferent fibers. Small-diameter nociceptive afferents have also been described in other orofacial tissues, and their discharges to several forms of stimulation are conducted into the brain stem, where the central neural events leading to the experience of pain are initiated.

References

1. Anderson DJ, Hannam AG, Mathews B. Sensory mechanisms in mammalian teeth and their supporting structures. Physiol Rev 1970;50:171–195.
2. Byers MR, Närhi MV. Dental injury models: Experimental tools for understanding neuroinflammatory interactions and polymodal nociceptor functions. Crit Rev Oral Biol Med 1999;10:4–39.
3. Dubner R, Sessle BJ, Storey AT. The Neural Basis of Oral and Facial Function. New York: Plenum Press, 1978.
4. Matthews B. Peripheral and central aspects of trigeminal nociceptive systems. Philos Trans R Soc Lond B Biol Sci 1985;308:313–324.
5. Närhi M, Yamamoto H, Ngassapa D, Hirvonen T. The neurophysiological basis and the role of inflammatory reactions in dentine hypersensitivity. Arch Oral Biol 1994;39:(suppl) 23S–30S.
6. Hildebrand C, Fried K, Tuisku F, Johansson CS. Teeth and tooth nerves. Prog Neurobiol 1995;45:165–222.
7. Matthews B, Robinson PP. The course of post-ganglionic sympathetic fibres distributed with the trigeminal nerve in the cat. J Physiol (Lond) 1980;303:391–401.
8. Holland GR. The odontoblast process: Form and function. J Dent Res 1985;64(special issue):499–514.
9. Ushiyama J. Gap junctions between odontoblasts revealed by transjunctional flux of fluorescent tracers. Cell Tissue Res 1989;258:611–616.
10. Matthews B, Hughes SH. The ultrastructure and receptor transduction mechanisms of dentine. Prog Brain Res1988;74:69–76.
11. Yoshiba K, Yoshiba N, Ejiri S, Iwaku M, Ozawa H. Odontoblast processes in human dentin revealed by fluorescence labeling and transmission electron microscopy. Histochem Cell Biol 2002;118:205–212.
12. Holland GR, Matthews B, Robinson PP. An electrophysiological and morphological study of the innervation and reinnervation of cat dentine. J Physiol (Lond) 1987;386:31–43.
13. Nanci A, Ten Cate AR. Ten Cate's Oral Histology: Development, Structure and Function, ed 6. St Louis: Mosby, 2003:235.
14. Andrew D, Matthews B. Displacement of the contents of dentinal tubules and sensory transduction in intradental nerves in the cat. J Physiol (Lond) 2000;529(pt 3):791–802.
15. Chidchuangchai W, Vongsavan N, Matthews B. Sensory transduction mechanisms responsible for pain caused by cold stimulation of dentine in man. Arch Oral Biol 2007;52:154–160.
16. Morgan CR, Rodd HD, Clayton N, Davis JB, Boissonade FM. Vanilloid receptor 1 expression in human tooth pulp in relation to caries and pain. J Orofac Pain 2005;19: 248–260.
17. Park CK, Kim MS, Fang Z, et al. Functional expression of thermo-transient receptor potential channels in dental primary afferent neurons: Implication for tooth pain. J Biol Chem 2006;281:17304–17311.
18. Sessle BJ. Mechanisms of trigeminal and occipital pain. Pain Rev 1996;3:91–116.
19. Acosta MC, Belmonte C, Gallar J. Sensory experiences in humans and single-unit activity in cats evoked by polymodal stimulation of the cornea. J Physiol (Lond) 2001; 534(pt 2):511–525.
20. Lam DK, Sessle BJ, Cairns BE, Hu JW. Neural mechanisms of temporomandibular joint and masticatory muscle pain: A possible role for peripheral glutamate receptor mechanisms. Pain Res Manag 2005;10:145–152.
21. Strassman AM, Levy D. Response properties of dural nociceptors in relation to headache. J Neurophysiol 2006; 95:1298–1306.

5

Central Nociceptive Pathways

Barry J. Sessle
Koichi Iwata
Ronald Dubner

This chapter focuses on central trigeminal (V) pathways and mechanisms that underlie nociceptive transmission. It describes the afferent inputs and organization of the brain stem elements, then outlines how nociceptive information is transmitted or modulated and relayed to other brain centers, and concludes with an outline of processes at some higher levels of the central nervous system (CNS).

Afferent Inputs and Brain Stem Organization

Most V primary afferents that innervate cutaneous, intraoral, deep tissues (eg, joints, muscle, cranial vessels) have their cell bodies in the V ganglion and project to the V brain stem sensory nuclear complex (VBSNC). Most axons travel in the V spinal tract and give off collaterals that activate second-order neurons within or adjacent to the VBSNC. The VBSNC can be subdivided into two major components: the main or principal sensory nucleus and the spinal tract nucleus, which contains three subnuclei: oralis (Vo), interpolaris (Vi), and caudalis (Vc) (Fig 5-1). The Vc is a laminated structure re-

sembling the spinal cord dorsal horn; it extends into and merges with the cervical spinal cord.[1–6] It also receives afferent inputs from other cranial nerves and cervical nerves, as well as from other brain stem or higher CNS centers that provide part of the substrate for modulation of V neurons (see chapter 8).

The neurons in the VBSNC are somatotopically arranged (an exception is the Vi/Vc transition zone). Most dorsal neurons in each component have inputs from the mandibular branch of the V nerve as well as receptive fields (RFs) within its territory (an RF is that portion of the body which, when stimulated at threshold, excites the neuron). The ventral neurons have an ophthalmic RF; neurons having a maxillary RF occur between the dorsal and ventral parts of each component. However, in Vc the pattern of representation of the face and mouth may shift such that RFs in the perioral region are found in the rostral part of the subnucleus and RFs in the more lateral regions of the face are located more caudally; this particular somatotopic pattern in Vc has sometimes been referred to as an "onion-skin" arrangement.[1,2,3,6]

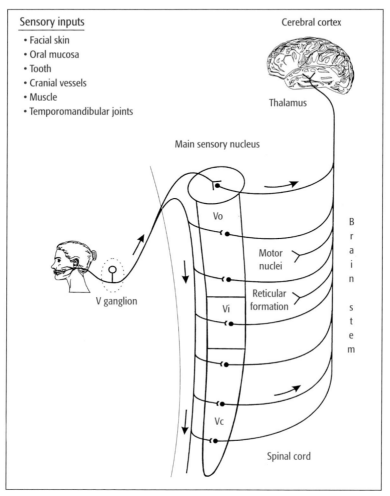

Fig 5-1 Major somatosensory pathway from the mouth and face. Trigeminal (V) primary afferents have their cell bodies in the V ganglion and project to second-order neurons in the VBSNC. These neurons may project to neurons in higher levels of the brain (eg, in the thalamus) or in brain stem regions such as the cranial nerve motor nuclei or the reticular formation. Not shown are the projections of some cervical nerve and cranial nerve VII, IX, X, and XII afferents to the VBSNC and the projection of many V, VII, IX, and X afferents to the solitary tract nucleus. Reprinted with permission from Sessle.[1]

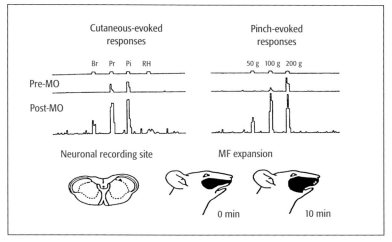

Fig 5-2 Example of a Vc NS neuron showing changes in spontaneous activity and mechanoreceptive field (MF) properties after application of the inflammatory irritant, mustard oil (MO), to the maxillary right molar pulp. The top series of traces on the left show the neuronal responses to brush (Br), pressure (Pr), pinch (Pi), and radiant heat (RH) applied to the RF in control conditions prior to MO application (ie, Pre-MO). Bottom traces show the neuronal responses to the same stimuli 20 minutes after MO application (ie, Post-MO). On the right are the neuronal responses to 3-second graded mechanical stimuli (50, 100, and 200 g). Note that after MO application to the tooth pulp, this NS neuron became responsive to Br and RH of the cutaneous RF and more strongly responsive to graded Pi stimuli; these changes reflect a central sensitization. The lower part of the figure shows the neuronal recording site in Vc and the MF expansion 10 minutes after MO application. Modified with permission from Chiang et al.[7]

Brain Stem Nociceptive Transmission

Involvement of Vc

Most evidence indicates that Vc is the principal first relay site of V nociceptive information. By virtue of its close functional and structural similarity to the spinal dorsal horn, which is the essential region of the spinal cord for pain, Vc is now often termed the *medullary dorsal horn*. The small-diameter (A-δ and C-fiber) afferents carrying nociceptive information (see chapter 4) predominantly terminate in laminae I, II, V, and VI of Vc; in contrast, the large A-fibers conducting low-threshold mechanosensi-

tive (tactile) information terminate primarily in the more rostral components of the VBSNC and in laminae III to VI of Vc. Transection of the V spinal tract (*V tractotomy*) at the level of Vc produces a marked reduction in pain perception, especially in the face, and has been used to relieve the excruciating pain of V neuralgia (see chapter 24).[1,3] Similar lesions in animals reduce behavioral, muscle, and autonomic responses to facial noxious stimuli.[1]

Additional evidence of a crucial role for Vc in craniofacial pain comes from microelectrode recordings of the activity of its neurons. These show that many Vc neurons are activated by cutaneous nociceptive inputs. The neurons have been categorized as either nociceptive-specific (NS) or wide dynamic range (WDR) (Fig 5-2) and are predominantly located in the superficial (I/II) and deep (V/VI) laminae of Vc. NS neurons respond only to noxious stimuli (eg, pinch, heat) applied to a small RF and receive inputs from A-δ and/or C-fiber nociceptors, whereas WDR neurons also receive A-fiber inputs that transmit non-noxious (eg, tactile) information. WDR neurons have a large RF with low-threshold and high-threshold areas. Both NS and WDR neurons increase their firing frequency as the intensity of noxious stimulation is increased or as more of the RF is stimulated. These RF and response properties of Vc nociceptive neurons determine our ability to localize, detect, and discriminate cutaneous noxious stimuli,[1,3,8,9] although some neurons may receive other convergent afferent inputs and are involved in deep pain. In addition, all nuclei and subnuclei of the VBSNC contain low-threshold mechanoreceptive (LTM) neurons that are responsive to light tactile stimulation of a localized RF in the facial skin or mouth, but not noxious stimuli, and provide the brain stem substrate for the localization, detection, and discrimination of touch. Some VBSNC neurons respond to non-noxious mechanical stimulation of deep tissues.

Further evidence indicates that, like the spinal dorsal horn, the central endings of nociceptive primary afferents transmit the nociceptive signals to the second-order V NS and WDR neurons by releasing excitatory amino acids (eg, glutamate) and neuropeptides (eg, substance P, calcitonin gene-related peptide [CGRP])[1,10,11] (Fig 5-3). Glutamate activates the nociceptive neurons via metabotropic glutamate receptors and two ionotropic receptors: N-methyl-D-aspartate (NMDA) and non-NMDA receptors (eg, α-amino-3-hydroxy-5-methyl-4-isoxazole-propionic acid [AMPA]) (see Fig 5-3). Activation of the AMPA receptor is rapid and short-lived, whereas the NMDA receptor has a longer period of activation; this is one reason the NMDA receptor is thought to be important in the processes

called *wind-up* and *central sensitization*. Among the neuropeptides involved in nociceptive transmission, the neurokinin substance P is particularly important. It is concentrated in afferent endings in the superficial and deep Vc laminae, where the nociceptive neurons predominate. Furthermore, noxious craniofacial stimulation causes release of substance P within Vc, where it acts through neurokinin receptors to produce sustained excitation of the nociceptive neurons (see Fig 5-3).

Also like the spinal dorsal horn, the nociceptive Vc neurons have receptors for inhibitory neurotransmitters that modulate the nociceptive transmission process (see Fig 5-3). These include, in lamina II, the *substantia gelatinosa* (SG); the axons of most SG neurons arborize locally within the VBSNC and release neuromodulatory substances such as enkephalin or γ-aminobutyric acid (GABA).[1,4,5] The SG receives a mix of inputs from other areas in the brain, as well as from craniofacial afferent inputs, and is one of the main sites by which peripheral afferents and CNS centers modulate somatosensory transmission (see chapter 8).

The Vi/Vc transition zone

A distinctive feature of Vc is that its most rostral part, the Vi/Vc transition zone, has properties different from the more caudal Vc. Whereas the latter has a somatotopic organization (see above), neurons in Vi/Vc receive converging input from all tissues in all V dermatomes, and its ventral portion has bilateral inputs. It has been proposed that Vi/Vc has a purpose beyond discriminative sensory function. This view is supported by findings that somatovisceral and somatoautonomic inputs caused by injury to masticatory muscles and the temporomandibular joint (TMJ) are bilaterally integrated in this zone[13,14] and that its ventral portion plays a significant role in responses to deep tissue injury.[13–15]

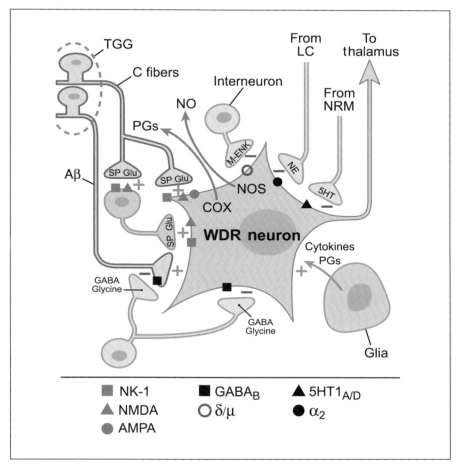

Fig 5-3 Neurochemical processes related to nociceptive transmission in Vc. In this example, activation of nociceptive fibers leads to the release of glutamate (Glu) and substance P (SP), which are conveyed across a synapse to a WDR neuron which projects to the thalamus. Glutamate binds and activates either NMDA or AMPA receptors, while SP binds and activates the neurokinin 1 (NK-1) receptors. The afferent fibers can activate the WDR neuron directly, or indirectly via contacts onto excitatory interneurons. Several intracellular signal transduction pathways have been implicated in modulating the responsiveness of the nociceptive neurons, including the protein kinase A (PKA) and protein kinase C (PKC) pathways. The neurons can themselves modulate nearby cells by synthesis and release of prostaglandins (PGs) via cyclooxygenase (COX) and nitric oxide (NO) via nitric oxide synthase (NOS). Glia can modulate nociceptive processing by release of substances such as cytokines and prostaglandins. Descending terminals of fibers originating in CNS regions such as the nucleus raphe magnus (NRM) or locus coeruleus (LC) can release serotonin (5-HT) or norepinephrine (NE). In addition, note receptors on the neuron for substances released from other neurons (interneurons) within Vc: met-enkephalin (M-ENK), glycine, and γ-aminobutyric acid (GABA). The major proposed receptors for these neurotransmitters are also depicted. Drugs that alter these receptors or neurotransmitters have potential as analgesics. TGG = trigeminal ganglion. Reprinted with permission from Hargreaves and Goodis.[12]

Involvement of other components of the VBSNC

The more rostral subnuclei, Vi and Vo, have also been implicated in nociception. Lesions of Vi and Vo disrupt some orofacial pain behaviors, and they contain NS and WDR neurons, with cutaneous RFs that are usually localized to intraoral or perioral areas. Many of these neurons can be activated by tooth pulp stimulation.[1] These and other findings suggest that rostral nociceptive neurons, particularly those in Vo, are principally involved in intraoral and perioral nociceptive processing.

Convergence, neuroplasticity, and central sensitization

Most NS and WDR neurons can be excited not only by cutaneous afferents but also by peripheral afferents from other tissues, eg, tooth pulp, cranial blood vessels, TMJ, or muscle.[1,9] The extensive convergent afferent input patterns are a particular characteristic of NS and WDR neurons in Vc. This may explain the poor localization of deep pain, in addition to the spread and referral of pain typical of most toothaches, headaches, and temporomandibular disorders.

Several chemicals released from the peripheral tissues (including primary afferent nerve endings) by injury or inflammation can increase the excitability of nociceptors (so-called nociceptor or peripheral sensitization; see chapters 1, 4, and 6). This produces a barrage of action potentials conducted along the nociceptive primary afferents to the CNS. Peripheral nerve damage or lesions can also increase nociceptive input (see chapter 7). This nociceptive afferent barrage can lead to prolonged functional alterations that have been termed *central sensitization* (see Fig 5-2). For example, activity caused by damage or inflammation of tooth pulp, TMJ, or muscle induces spontaneous activity, RF expansion, lowering of the RF threshold, and enhancement of responses of Vc NS and WDR neurons that may include a gradually augmenting response to a series of repeated noxious stimuli (ie, wind-up).

These alterations indicate that the afferent inputs and brain stem circuitry are not "hard-wired" but are plastic; that is, they reflect activity-dependent neuroplastic changes in the RF and response properties of the nociceptive neurons. The neurons' responses to their convergent afferent inputs are enhanced and their RFs are enlarged, reflecting a greater number of more effective inputs. It appears that this central sensitization is produced by a cascade of events that starts with the nociceptive afferent barrage causing the release centrally of a number of chemical mediators, including glutamate and neuropeptides such as substance P. These substances prolong neuronal depolarization and increase the excitability of the neurons via actions at glutamate receptors and G-protein-coupled receptors. A loss of central inhibitory processes may also contribute to the increased neuronal excitability that is characteristic of central sensitization (Fig 5-4).[1,10,11,14]

The increased central excitatory state is dependent on peripheral nociceptive afferent input for its initiation. Central sensitization can last for days or even weeks and is thought to contribute to the persistent spontaneous pain and tenderness that characterize many clinical cases of injury or inflammation (see chapter 1). Central sensitization can explain the tenderness (ie, hyperalgesia) by virtue of the increase in the response of the central nociceptive neurons to nociceptive inputs. Similarly, enhanced responses to low-threshold mechanosensitive inputs (which are not normally associated with pain) in the nociceptive neurons could contribute to the allodynia that often is associated with pain conditions (see chapter 1). Recent evidence indicates that non-neuronal (glial) cells are also involved in central sensitization of Vc nociceptive neurons.[15,17] Peripheral inflammation or nerve injury produces activation of glia (eg, astrocytes and microglia) that release several

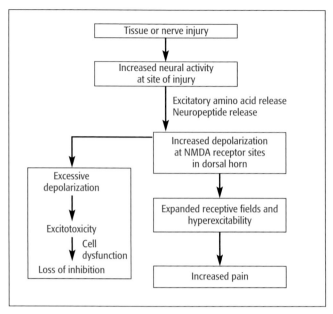

Fig 5-4 Outline of the cascade of events that may occur following peripheral tissue injury and inflammation or peripheral nerve injury. Note that the increased nociceptive afferent activity results in the central release of excitatory amino acids (eg, glutamate) and neuropeptides (eg, substance P, CGRP) that can lead to an increase in nociceptive neuronal excitability; a loss of central inhibitory influences may also contribute to the hyperexcitability. Modified with permission from Dubner.[16]

substances such as cytokines (eg, interleukin 1 β [IL-1β], interleukin 6 [IL-6], and tumor necrosis factor [TNF]) that activate specific receptors on neurons and lead to additional central sensitization (see Fig 5-3). Peripheral sensitization can also contribute to hyperalgesia and allodynia by increasing the excitability and decreasing the activation threshold of primary afferents (see chapters 1 and 6). Thus, many pain conditions may involve a mixture of peripheral and central sensitization phenomena.

Projections from the VBSNC

The nociceptive neurons and the LTM neurons throughout the VBSNC project to higher CNS centers such as the thalamus, cerebellum, and superior colliculus; and to the periaqueductal gray, spinal cord, reticular formation, and pontine parabrachial nucleus.[1–3,18] There are other nociceptive pathways, but their role in pain is still unclear.[1,18]

A portion of the V-thalamic projection is direct, but there are also multisynaptic paths that utilize connections in the reticular formation and adjacent brain stem areas (see Fig 5-1). Some of these connections are involved in endocrine responses, while others subserve brain stem autonomic reflex responses to noxious craniofacial stimuli, such as changes in salivation, respiration, heart rate, and blood pressure. Some neurons in the VBSNC serve as interneurons in craniofacial and cervical muscle reflexes, mastication and swallowing (see chapters 14 and 15).

Thalamocortical Nociceptive Transmission

The regions of the thalamus that receive and relay somatosensory information from the craniofacial region are the ventrobasal complex (or ventroposterior nucleus), the posterior group of nuclei, and the medial thalamus.[3,18] Most of the ventrobasal neurons are LTM neurons that are somatotopically organized. Those receiving and relaying tactile information from the face and mouth are concentrated in the medial portion (the nucleus ventralis posteromedialis), while neurons in the lateral portion of the ventrobasal thalamus relay somatosensory information from the trunk, neck, and limbs.

These thalamic regions also contain NS and WDR neurons. The properties of these neurons have been detailed in humans and experimental animals; they are similar to those described for comparable neurons in Vc, including convergence of cutaneous and deep afferent inputs. Most have RF and response properties, and connections with the overlying somatosensory cerebral cortex, which are indicative of a role in the sensory-discriminative dimension of pain. In contrast, nociceptive neurons in the more medial nuclei of the thalamus (eg, nucleus submedius, intralaminar nuclei, parafascicular nucleus) may be involved more in the affective or motivational dimensions of pain. They are connected with other higher brain areas that also participate in these functions (eg, hypothalamus, anterior cingulate cortex).

Some thalamic NS and WDR neurons project directly to the cerebral cortex, and NS and WDR neurons in the primary somatosensory cortical region (SI) respond to noxious stimuli in a manner that suggests that they play a role in the localization and discrimination of pain. They include SI neurons that may code the intensity of noxious thermal facial or tooth pulp stimuli.[18,19] Nociceptive neurons have also been described in other cortical regions such as the insular cortex, which appears to be involved in pain discrimination, and the anterior cingulate cortex, which has been implicated in the affective dimension of pain. Neural imaging in humans has greatly increased our knowledge of the distributed effects of noxious stimuli at multiple thalamic and cortical sites (see chapters 10 and 11).

Summary

This chapter has outlined some of the brain stem neural mechanisms that underlie orofacial pain. The RF and response properties of nociceptive neurons and associated neurochemical processes of the VBSNC were described. These neurons predominate in Vc but are also found in other components of the VBSNC, including the Vi/Vc transition zone, which appears to have a unique role in the responses to persistent deep tissue inputs. The patterns of afferent inputs to the brain stem nociceptive neurons and the associated brain stem circuitry are not hard-wired, but are plastic. Nociceptive afferent barrages can induce neuroplastic changes in neuronal properties, a process that has been termed *central sensitization*. Many of the clinical features of orofacial pain conditions seem to depend on a combination of central and peripheral sensitization. The properties of analogous nociceptive neurons at thalamic and cortical levels were also outlined, and their roles in different aspects of pain were noted.

References

1. Sessle BJ. Acute and chronic craniofacial pain: Brainstem mechanisms of nociceptive transmission and neuroplasticity, and their clinical correlates. Crit Rev Oral Biol Med 2000;11:57–91.
2. Darian-Smith I. Neural mechanisms of facial sensation. Int Rev Neurobiol 1966;9:301–395.
3. Dubner R, Sessle BJ, Storey AT (eds). The Neural Basis of Oral and Facial Function. New York: Plenum Press, 1978.

4. Gobel S, Hockfield S, Ruda MA. Anatomical similarities between medullary and spinal dorsal horns. In: Kawamura Y, Dubner R (eds). Oral-Facial Sensory and Motor Functions. Tokyo: Quintessence, 1981:211–223.

5. Gobel S, Bennett GJ, Allen B, et al. Synaptic connectivity of substantia gelatinosa neurons with references to potential termination sites of descending axons. In: Sjolund B, Bjorkland A (eds). Brain Stem Control of Spinal Mechanisms. New York: Elsevier/North Holland, 1982:135–158.

6. Johnson LR, Westrum LE, Henry MA. Anatomic organization of the trigeminal system and the effects of deafferentation. In: Fromm GH, Sessle BJ (eds). Trigeminal Neuralgia: Current Concepts Regarding Pathogenesis and Treatment. Stoneham: Butterworth-Heinemann, 1991:27–69.

7. Chiang CY, Park SJ, Kwan CL, Hu JW, Sessle BJ. NMDA receptor mechanisms contribute to neuroplasticity induced in caudalis nociceptive neurons by tooth pulp stimulation. J Neurophysiol 1998;80:2621–2631.

8. Dubner R. Recent advances in our understanding of pain. In: Klineberg I, Sessle BJ (eds). Oro-facial Pain and Neuromuscular Dysfunction: Mechanisms and Clinical Correlates. Oxford: Pergamon Press, 1985:3–19.

9. Sessle BJ. The neural basis of temporomandibular joint and masticatory muscle pain. J Orofac Pain 1999;13:238–245.

10. Dubner R, Basbaum AI. Spinal dorsal horn plasticity following tissue or nerve injury. In: Wall PD, Melzack R (eds). Textbook of Pain, ed 3. London: Churchill Livingstone, 1994:225–241.

11. Salter MW. Central neuroplasticit mechanisms mediating pain persistence. J Orofac Pain 2004;18:318–324.

12. Hargreaves KM, Goodis HE (eds). Seltzer and Bender's Dental Pulp. Chicago: Quintessence, 2002:184.

13. Bereiter DA, Bereiter DF, Hathaway CB. The NMDA receptor antagonist MK-801 reduces Fos-like immunoreactivity in central trigeminal neurons and blocks select endocrine and autonomic responses to corneal stimulation in the rat. Pain 1996;64:179–189.

14. Ren K, Dubner R. Central nervous system plasticity and persistent pain. J Orofac Pain 1999;13(3):155–163.

15. Guo W, Wang H, Watanabe M, et al. Glial-cytokine-neuronal interactions underlying the mechanisms of persistent pain. J Neurosci 2007;27:6006–6018.

16. Dubner R. Spinal cord neuronal plasticity: Mechanisms of persistent pain following tissue damage and nerve injury. In: Vecchiet L, Albe-Fessard D, Lindblom U (eds). New Trends in Referred Pain and Hyperalgesia. Pain Research and Clinical Management, vol 7. Amsterdam: Elsevier, 1993:109–117.

17. Chiang C-Y, Wang J, Xie Y-F, et al. Astroglial glutamate-glutamine shuttle is involved in central sensitization of nociceptive neurons in rat medullary dorsal horn. J Neurosci, 2007;27:9068–9076.

18. Dostrovsky JO, Craig AD. Ascending projection systems. In: MacMahon S, Koltzenburg M (eds). Wall & Melzack's Textbook of Pain. London: Churchill Livingstone, 2006:187–203.

19. Iwata K, Tsuboi Y, Tashiro A, Sakamoto M, Sumino R. Integration of tooth-pulp pain at the level of cerebral cortex. In: Nakamura Y, Sessle BJ (eds). Neurobiology of Mastication—From Molecular to Systems Approach. Amsterdam: Elsevier, 1999:471–481.

Neurochemical Factors in Injury and Inflammation of Orofacial Tissues

Asma A. Khan
Ke Ren
Kenneth M. Hargreaves

As reviewed in prior chapters, orofacial pain is one of the most common types of acute or chronic pain, with odontalgia alone occurring in about 12% of the adult population.[1] Many forms of orofacial pain have an inflammatory component. This chapter will discuss peripheral effects of injury, focusing on inflammatory pain and the role of peripheral neurons in inflammation and healing.

Peripheral Mechanisms of Pain, Hyperalgesia, and Allodynia

Two major theories for the detection of noxious stimuli by peripheral sensory neurons are the *specificity theory* and the *pattern theory* (see chapter 1). The former proposes that the perception of pain is due to activation of specialized sensory neurons (eg, nociceptors). The latter proposes that pain perception is due to intense stimuli that activate multiple classes of sensory neurons, producing a particular pattern of sensory input that results in pain. There is evidence for pain sensation occurring both by activation of specific nociceptors (ie, the specificity theory) as well as by combinations of nociceptors and non-nociceptors (ie, the pattern theory). Therefore, it is important to un-

derstand the contributions of both nociceptors and non-nociceptors to the perception of pain.

The response to tissue injury, infection, or inflammation is complex. Orofacial nociceptors can respond to tissue injury through several different ion channels and receptor processes (see chapter 4), but they may also respond to tissue infection. It has been demonstrated recently that a subclass of human trigeminal nociceptors, including those which innervate the pulp, express the toll-like receptor 4 (TLR-4) and cluster of differentiation 14 receptor (CD14) (Fig 6-1).[2] This finding supports the hypothesis that pulpal nociceptors can directly detect bacterial endotoxin, and it suggests a direct mechanism of pain resulting from bacterial infection. Ion channels and receptors are also involved in nociceptor responses to inflammation. The tissue response to inflammation involves the coordinated release of multiple classes of inflammatory chemical mediators that display distinct profiles of substance concentration over time.[3] In the inflamed peripheral tissue, the terminals of nociceptive primary afferents detect the presence of the mediators by receptors, that are expressed in the afferents' cell bodies and then are transported to the periphery. If the mediator reaches a sufficient concentration in the inflamed tissue to activate the

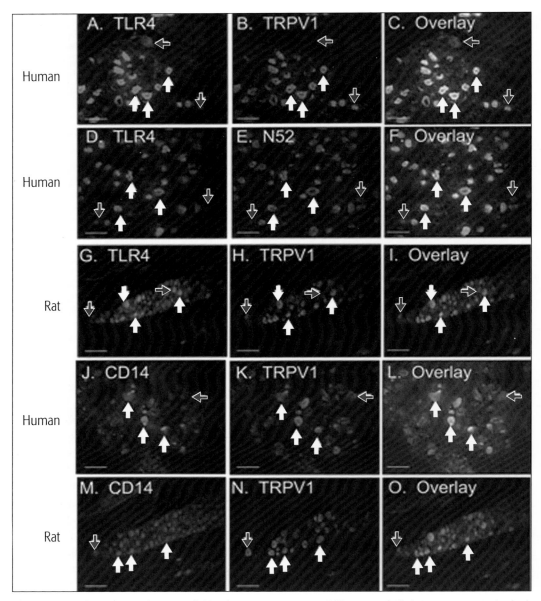

Fig 6-1 Expression patterns of TLR-4 and CD14 in V sensory neurons. *White arrows* indicate neurons expressing both markers, and *blue arrows* indicate neurons that express one but not both markers. Human V neurons were evaluated for co-localization of TLR-4 (panels A and D) and CD14 (panel J) with a marker for the capsaicin-sensitive subclass of nociceptors (TRPV1, panels B and C for TLR-4 and panels K and L for CD14), or a marker for myelinated sensory neurons (N52, panels E and F). Rat trigeminal neurons were evaluated for co-localization of TLR-4 with TRPV1 (panels G to I) and CD14 with TRPV1 (panels M to O). Reprinted with permission from Wadachi and Hargreaves.[2]

Table 6-1 Effect of inflammatory mediators on nociceptors and pain*

Mediator	Effect on nociceptors	Effect on human volunteers
Potassium	Activate	++
Protons	Activate	++
Serotonin	Activate	++
Bradykinin	Activate	+++
Histamine	Activate	+
Tumor necrosis factor α (TNF α)	Sensitize	+
Prostaglandins	Sensitize	±
Leukotrienes	Sensitize	±
Nerve growth factor (NGF)	Sensitize	++
Substance P	Sensitize	±
Interleukin 1 (IL-1)	Sensitize (?)	−
Endotoxin	Sensitize (?)	−
Prolactin	Sensitize	−
Proteases	Activate	−

*Modified with permission from Fields.[4]

receptors, then the nociceptors could become activated (ie, membrane depolarization with conduction of the signal into the central nervous system [CNS]) or sensitized. Some nociceptive afferents may indeed be "silent" and not sensitive to peripheral noxious stimuli unless they are sensitized by mediators (see also chapter 4). A sensitized nociceptor displays spontaneous depolarization, reduced threshold for depolarization, and increased after-discharges to suprathreshold stimuli. Table 6-1 illustrates the effects of various inflammatory mediators on these indices of nociceptor activity and on pain perception. Some of these mediators may produce persistent effects. For example, expression of nerve growth factor (NGF) and its receptor tropomyosin-related kinase A (trkA) is increased in inflamed dental pulp, and a single injection of NGF to humans can evoke pain and so-called allodynia that lasts up to 1 month. Furthermore, nociceptors may have receptors (eg, opioid or γ-aminobutyric acid) that can modulate their

excitability and the substances they release (see chapter 8).

There are important clinical implications in this process of peripheral (nociceptor) sensitization, since it contributes to the altered pain states of hyperalgesia and allodynia. *Hyperalgesia* is an increase in pain response to a suprathreshold stimulus and often occurs with *allodynia*, which is the sensation of pain that is produced by innocuous stimuli (see also Box 1-1). For example, a thermal burn or sunburn are common examples of allodynia; under these conditions even minor stimuli such as clothes rubbing on skin can produce pain. Hyperalgesia and allodynia are thought to be a result of both peripheral and central mechanisms.[5,6] The astute clinician tests for allodynia and hyperalgesia when performing a dental examination.[3] For example, percussing a normal tooth with a mirror handle is not painful, but it produces a pain sensation when nociceptors innervating the apical periodontal ligament are sensitized. This allodynic

---

Box 6-1 Peripheral mechanisms of hyperalgesia and allodynia

Changes in nociceptors
- Activation
- Sensitization
- Sprouting
- Protein expression
- Receptor or ion channel trafficking

Changes in peripheral tissue
- Concentration and composition of inflammatory mediators
- Tissue temperature
- Tissue pressure

Changes in non-nociceptors
- Perineuronal activation of satellite glial cells
- Sympathetic afferent sprouting/interactions with nociceptors
- A-β fiber sprouting and phenotype changes

---

response may lead to a diagnosis of acute apical periodontitis. Similarly, pulpal nociceptors can be sensitized and may exhibit a prolonged discharge after pulp vitality testing; a prolonged pain reaction to vitality testing leads to a diagnosis of irreversible pulpitis. Additional properties of sensitized pulpal nociceptors include a reduced mechanical threshold (eg, throbbing pain may be due to the pulsatile systolic increase in blood pressure) and reduced thermal threshold (eg, sensitized pulpal nociceptors activated at about 37°C [body temperature] may mediate spontaneous pulpal pain and be inhibited by patients cooling their inflamed teeth with ice water).[3] Thus, there is a firm biologic rationale for endodontic examinations.

Phenotypic changes can also occur in certain neurons hours to days after tissue inflammation or infection. For example, inflamed dental pulp and periradicular tissue exhibit sprouting of the terminal arborizations of afferent neurons and increased peripheral neuropeptide content within a few days of pulp exposure.[5] This increase in the density of peripheral innervation may predispose chronically inflamed tissue to lowered thresholds for sensation.

Other examples of such dynamic plasticity of peripheral neurons relate to ion channels such as the tetrodotoxin-resistant sodium channel Na_V 1.8 (also called SNS1/PN3) and the transient receptor potential V1 (TRPV1). Na_V 1.8 is upregulated in inflamed tissues, including dental pulp, and its activity is increased by inflammatory mediators such as prostaglandin E_2 (PGE_2) and NGF.[7,8] Since the sensitivity of Na_V 1.8 to lidocaine is about 25% of that of other sodium channels, it is thought to account, at least in part, for the increased failure of local anesthetics in inflamed tissues. TRPV1 transduces thermal and chemical stimuli and is thought to play an important role in the development of allodynia and hyperalgesia after inflammation. It has been hypothesized that peripheral sensitization reduces the activation threshold of TRPV1 from noxious temperatures (> 42°C) to close to body temperature. This may account for the clinical presentation of irreversible pulpitis where spontaneous pain is alleviated by application of cold. Recent studies suggest that in addition to TRPV1, other TRP channels may also play an important role in peripheral sensitization.[9]

Nociceptors are not the only type of peripheral neurons to exhibit phenotype switching after tissue injury. For example, a subpopulation of the large-diameter A-β fibers that normally encode for light tactile stimuli may express the neuropeptide substance P after inflammatory injury and can sprout their central terminals into lamina I of the spinal dorsal horn. The combined effect of expressing a new neuropeptide and terminating in a new central pathway has led to the hypothesis that A-β fibers may contribute to allodynia under conditions of tissue inflammation or infection. A second example of non-nociceptor changes after inflammation or nerve injury is the increase in perineuronal glial satellite cells.[10] Activated glia are known to release cytokines and trophic factors that, in turn, contribute to the development of hyperalgesia. Another example is the sprouting of sympathetic afferents after tissue injury or inflammation and activation of nociceptive afferents; but it is unclear to what extent, if any, these occur in orofacial tissues and contribute to orofacial pain. These proposed mechanisms are summarized in Box 6-1. Chapters 5 and 7 also outline these processes as well as additional mechanisms that are primarily based within the CNS.

Neurogenic Modulation in Inflammation and Wound Healing

Certain nociceptors not only signal the occurrence of tissue injury or inflammation but also regulate the subsequent inflammatory and healing responses of the injured tissue.[3] Thus, these neurons have both an afferent function (eg, signaling the CNS) and an efferent function (eg, peripheral release of neuropeptides and other neurochemicals such as excitatory amino acids). Injection of the excitatory amino acid glutamate into deep craniofacial tissues such as the masseter muscle activates nociceptors and induces pain in humans. These effects are mostly mediated by peripheral N-methyl-

D-aspartate (NMDA) receptors and are greater in women than in men.[11,12] Two neuropeptides that are released from peripheral terminals of certain nociceptors are substance P and calcitonin gene-related peptide (CGRP). In patients with pulpitis, the pulpal level of substance P is increased, and substance P receptors are expressed in human pulp tissue.[13,14] The release of substance P and CGRP into peripheral tissues may contribute to the neurogenic component of inflammation, since these neuropeptides have proinflammatory properties. For example, peripheral administration of these peptides produces vasodilatation and plasma extravasation in most tissues, and they can produce synergistic inflammatory effects when coadministered. In contrast, passive immunization with anti-substance P antisera or with anti-CGRP antisera can inhibit the development of inflammation.[15] Administration of substance P in vitro evokes the release of histamine from mast cells; PGE_2 and collagenase from synoviocytes; and cytokines such as interleukin 1 (IL-1), interleukin 6 (IL-6), and tumor necrosis factor α (TNF-α) from monocytes. Administration of substance P also activates p38 mitogen-activated protein kinase, which promotes IL-6 induction in dental pulp fibroblasts.[16] Moreover, local administration of substance P alters the functional and chemotactic activity of immune cells. Evidence indicates that electric stimulation of peripheral nerves produces plasma extravasation due, at least in part, to release of these neuropeptides. Extravasation permits the passage of blood-borne proteins (eg, albumin, kininogen) and fluid into the injured tissue, contributing to the further release of inflammatory mediators (eg, bradykinin) and to the development of edema. The release of neuropeptides can also be regulated by immune cells. Mast cell tryptase activates protease-activated receptors on neurons, leading to the release of substance P and CGRP and neurogenic inflammation. Considered together, these findings indicate a wide range of proinflammatory actions of neuropeptides (Table 6-2).

Table 6-2 Peripheral effects of substance P and CGRP on inflammation and wound healing processes

	Substance P	CGRP
Effects on inflammation		
Vasodilatation	+	+
Plasma extravasation	+	
Histamine release from mast cells	+	
PGE$_2$ and collagenase release from synoviocytes	+	
Cytokine release from monocytes (SP)	+	
Immune cell chemotaxis or activation (CGRP and SP)	+	+
Effects on wound healing processes		
Angiogenesis (SP)	+	
Dentinogenesis (CGRP)		+
Fibroblast proliferation (CGRP and SP)	+	+
Osteogenesis (SP)	+	

In addition to neurogenic inflammation, evidence exists to support the hypothesis that neuropeptides modulate the healing response to tissue injury. In whole animal studies, denervation or desensitization with capsaicin reduces the rate of healing of peripheral tissue (including surgical flaps) and increases the rate of pulp necrosis following tooth exposure.[5] In contrast, in both clinical trials and animal studies, electric stimulation of nerves increases the rate of healing.[17] These effects appear to be due, at least in part, to peripheral release of neuropeptides such as substance P and CGRP, since administration of neuropeptides to surgical wounds increases healing in most studies.[18] Thus, there is substantial evidence that peripheral neuropeptide release modulates healing in addition to inflammation.

The mechanisms for neuropeptide modulation of healing appear to include trophic effects on cells engaged in wound healing. For example, formation of new blood vessels (*angiogenesis*) is important in wound healing since the resulting neovascularization of the surgical site is an essential early event. This effect on healing is distinct from neuropeptide effects on inflammatory processes, since substance P induces angiogenesis at concentrations that do not elicit an immune response. Accordingly, attention has been directed to the mitogenic effect of neuropeptides on endothelial cells. Administration of substance P induces angiogenesis in vivo that is at least partially a result of a direct mechanism of action on endothelial cells since these cells express a substance P receptor.[19] Additional studies demonstrate that substance P evokes angiogenesis when administered at physiologic concentrations to endothelial cells in vitro. Collectively, these studies indicate that substance P has a direct effect on promoting wound healing via angiogenesis and endothelial migration.

Substance P and CGRP have additional roles in the regulation of wound healing. For example, depletion of neuropeptides to dental pulp causes a significant reduction in dentin formation, and CGRP facilitates the dentin bridge formation during the healing process after pulpotomy in rats.[18] These and other data suggest that neuropeptides regulate dentinogenesis, an important response to pulpal injury. In addition, both substance P and

CGRP induce the proliferation of pulpal fibroblasts in a concentration-dependent fashion. Finally, substance P has been shown to evoke osteogenesis in an in vitro assay. Accordingly, the efferent activity of certain sensory neurons plays an important role in regulating wound healing via the peripheral release of neuropeptides that act as trophic factors to selectively regulate the activation or proliferation of several cell types, including endothelium, odontoblasts, fibroblasts, and osteoblasts (see Table 6-2).

Summary

The classic view of peripheral nerves is that they function merely as telephone lines by simple transmission of signals generated from their peripheral terminals. However, this is an inaccurate oversimplification. This chapter has noted that peripheral nerves exhibit a dynamic plasticity after tissue injury, infection, or inflammation, with substantial alterations in functional properties and phenotype. The immediate alterations in functional properties are characterized as activation and sensitization. The delayed changes include phenotype switching, sprouting of peripheral and central terminals, and alterations in axonal transport of receptors or ion channels. Collectively, this dynamic plasticity contributes to the peripheral mechanisms of hyperalgesia and allodynia. This has clear clinical and scientific implications since the astute clinician uses this knowledge to interpret patients' symptoms and the results of diagnostic tests. Similarly, pain scientists are employing this knowledge to develop novel classes of analgesics or local anesthetics. In addition to their sensory properties, peripheral neurons regulate the development of neurogenic inflammation and wound healing by multiple mechanisms. The clinical implications of this knowledge are undoubtedly important and include potential interventions that may range in application from wound healing to pulp-capping procedures.

References

1. Lipton JA, Ship JA, Larach-Robinson D. Estimated prevalence and distribution of reported orofacial pain in the United States. J Am Dent Assoc 1993;124:115–121.
2. Wadachi R, Hargreaves KM. Trigeminal nociceptors express TLR-4 and CD14: A mechanism for pain due to infection. J Dent Res 2006;85:49–53.
3. Hargreaves KM. Endodontic pharmacology. In: Cohen S, Hargreaves KM (eds). Pathways of the Pulp, ed 9. St Louis: Mosby, 2006:668.
4. Fields HL. Pain. New York: McGraw-Hill, 1987, 32.
5. Byers MR, Närhi MV. Dental injury models: Experimental tools for understanding neuroinflammatory interactions and polymodal nociceptor functions. Crit Rev Oral Biol Med 1999:10:4–39.
6. Dubner R, Bennett GJ. Spinal and trigeminal mechanisms of nociception. Annu Rev Neurosci 1983;6:381–418.
7. Renton T, Yiangou Y, Plumpton C, Tate S, Bountra C, Anand P. Sodium channel Nav1.8 immunoreactivity in painful human dental pulp. BMC Oral Health 2005;5:5.
8. Gold MS, Reichling DB, Shuster MJ, Levine JD. Hyperalgesic agents increase a tetrodotoxin-resistant Na+ current in nociceptors. Proc Natl Acad Sci U S A 1996;93:1108–1112.
9. Numazaki M, Tominaga M. Nociception and TRP channels. Curr Drug Targets CNS Neurol Disord 2004;3:479–485.
10. Stephenson JL, Byers MR. GFAP immunoreactivity in trigeminal ganglion satellite cells after tooth injury in rats. Exp Neurol 1995;131:11–22.
11. Cairns BE, Hu JW, Arendt-Nielsen L, Sessle BJ, Svensson P. Sex-related differences in human pain and rat afferent discharge evoked by injection of glutamate into the masseter muscle. J Neurophysiol 2001;86:782–791.
12. Dong XD, Mann MK, Kumar U, et al. Sex-related differences in NMDA-evoked rat masseter muscle afferent discharge result from estrogen-mediated modulation of peripheral NMDA receptor activity. Neuroscience 2007;146:822–832.
13. Bowles WR, Withrow JC, Lepinski AM, Hargreaves KM. Tissue levels of immunoreactive substance P are increased in patients with irreversible pulpitis. J Endod 2003;29:265–267.
14. Caviedes-Bucheli J, Gutierrez-Guerra JE, Salazar F, Pichardo D, Moreno GC, Munoz HR. Substance P receptor expression in healthy and inflamed human pulp tissue. Int Endod J 2007;40:106–111.
15. Louis SM, Johnstone D, Russell NJ, Jamieson A, Dockray GJ. Antibodies to calcitonin-gene related peptide reduce inflammation induced by topical mustard oil but not that due to carrageenin in the rat. Neurosci Lett 1989;102:257–260.

16. Tokuda M, Miyamoto R, Sakuta T, Nagaoka S, Torii M. Substance P activates p38 mitogen-activated protein kinase to promote IL-6 induction in human dental pulp fibroblasts. Connect Tissue Res 2005;46:153–158.

17. Kjartansson J, Lundeberg T, Samuelson U, Dalsgaard C, Heden P. Calcitonin gene-related peptide (CGRP) and transcutaneous electrical nerve stimulation (TENS) increase cutaneous blood flow in a musculocutaneous flap in the rat. Acta Physiol Scand 1988;134:89–94.

18. Zhang M, Fukuyama H. CGRP immunohistochemistry in wound healing and dentin bridge formation following rat molar pulpotomy. Histochem Cell Biol 1999;112:325–333.

19. Ziche M, Morbidelli L, Pacini M, Geppetti P, Alessandri G,Maggi CA. Substance P stimulates neovascularization in vivo and proliferation of cultured endothelial cells. Microvasc Res 1990;40:264–278.

Mechanisms of Neuropathic Pain

Alain Woda
Michael W. Salter

The International Association for the Study of Pain defines *neuropathic pain* as "pain initiated or caused by a primary lesion or dysfunction in the nervous system."[1] Certain mechanisms such as peripheral sensitization of nociceptors or central sensitization (see chapters 5 and 6), which are known to occur in acute nociceptive pain, can participate in neuropathic pain in addition to the mechanisms appearing specifically after nerve injury. After a traumatic event involving peripheral neural tissues, spontaneous and evoked hyperalgesia can often be observed. This is frequently associated with allodynia, anesthesia, dysesthesia, or hypoesthesia (see chapter 1). A lesion of the inferior alveolar nerve following avulsion of the third molar is an example of such a traumatic event in the orofacial area. Models of chronic or persistent pain triggered by these nerve lesions exist in animals. A lesion of spinal or trigeminal (V) sensory nerves can lead to increased receptive field (RF) size and responses to noxious stimuli, decreased activation thresholds, abnormal spontaneous discharges of spinal or V central neurons, and pain behavior in animals.[2] Analogous neuronal changes can also be observed after even more discrete lesions such as a pulpotomy.[3,4] Such neuroplastic

changes may explain certain persistent pain conditions such as posttraumatic dysesthesia or atypical odontalgia, which can last for months or years after endodontic therapy of a tooth that had previously been symptom-free.[5]

These clinical and experimental effects of neural damage involve several mechanisms that are described in this chapter.

Ectopic Impulses from Damaged Primary Afferent Nerve Fibers

Several types of injury to primary afferents can lead to persistent pain and are common in the orofacial region.[2,6] Incisions, crush injury, or stretching or destruction by metabolic (eg, diabetes), chemical (eg, chemotherapy), or infective (eg, virus) diseases can lead to anterograde and retrograde degeneration as well as regeneration of the nerve fibers. Disorganization of the myelin sheath around myelinated fibers is another possible, sometimes concomitant, occurrence. As a result, abnormal activity or bursts of impulses that do not originate from nociceptor terminals may occur. These ectopic discharges may originate from large-diameter afferent fibers, small-diameter afferent fibers, the site of nerve damage, a focus of demyelinization, or even the cell body in the sensory ganglion. In addition, axon sprouting may occur following severance of peripheral nerve fibers. A great number of unmyelinated or thinly myelinated nerve fibers grow from the cut nerve trunk toward the original peripheral site. These sprouts can generate spontaneous discharges within days in the case of the myelinated fibers and within weeks for the unmyelinated fibers. These abnormal discharges persist until the target tissue is reached. If this does not occur because of the loss of the target or because of the presence of an obstacle, a neuroma can result. In this situation, many axons die; but those that remain may form a tangled mass of nervous tissue in conjunction with proliferated Schwann cells, which ensheath unmyelinated as well as myelinated axons of primary afferents.

In the neuroma, both myelinated and unmyelinated nerve fibers develop abnormal spontaneous and provoked activity, particularly following light tactile stimulation. A neuroma may also exhibit *ephaptic transmission*, which appears when two or more adjacent demyelinated or unmyelinated fibers of the damaged nerve form abnormal connections between or among them. Nerve fibers of all sizes may be involved. This ephaptic transmission process allows a very effective, though abnormal, transfer of impulses from one fiber type to another. Reverberating impulses may also be generated from focally demyelinated fibers. It has been shown that prolonged high-frequency discharges of "reflected" impulses can be generated by repeated stimulation, and impulses can be propagated both orthodromically (ie, toward the central nervous system [CNS]) and antidromically (ie, toward the peripheral tissues innervated by the fiber) from the demyelinated site. The nervi nervorum, which provides the innervation of the connective tissue sheath around the nerve, is thought by some authors to directly induce "nerve trunk pain" following damage to the nerve sheath, which may in turn induce discharge of impulses. Local inflammatory reactions and local sprouting may also occur around or from the nervi nervorum.

Involvement of the Sympathetic Nervous System

The relation between pain and the sympathetic nervous system has been known for a long time, and the clinical concept of sympathetically maintained pain reflects the belief that some pain conditions can be maintained by the sympathetic system.[7,8] The role of the sympathetic system is revealed by increased pain following the administration of agents that affect this system, decreased pain after administration of sympathetic antagonists (eg, that block α-adrenoreceptors) or guanethidine (a substance that acts by first releasing and then depleting norepinephrine from the sympathetic efferent terminals), or increased pain after the triggering of a sympathetic reflex. Moreover, one of the most common procedures in the treatment of these conditions is a local anesthetic block of the sympathetic ganglion, including the stellate ganglion in the case of some orofacial pains.

The underlying pathophysiologic mechanism seems to depend on a functional relationship between efferents of the sympathetic nervous system and somatic afferents, at least in the spinal somatosensory system. It has been shown that following peripheral spinal nerve injury, somatic primary afferent fibers, either myelinated or unmyelinated, express or upregulate α-adrenoreceptors. At the same time, sympathetic efferents become coupled with the afferents. Synaptic contacts can be established with the fiber at the lesion site or with the soma. For example, after a partial lesion of a spinal nerve, electric stimulation of a sympathetic trunk may activate or sensitize some nociceptors, and the somatic afferents may become sensitive to systemic catecholamines. Alternatively, following nerve injury, sympathetic efferent terminals sprout and form arborizations around some cell bodies in the spinal dorsal root ganglion; sympathetic efferent terminals are not normally present in this location. Some allodynia observed after peripheral axotomy is thought to be due to such coupling between sympathetic efferents and dorsal root ganglion neurons related to A-β fibers.[8] Whether this coupling occurs in the V ganglion is unclear.

Central Sprouting

Peripheral injury may also be associated with morphologic modification at the central endings of the primary afferent fibers. Sectioning a peripheral nerve results in reorganization of the central branches of axonal endings of A-β primary afferents. After sprouting, the terminals that were previously distributed in layers III and IV of the spinal dorsal horn may make synaptic contacts in more superficial layers of the dorsal horn. This could explain some types of allodynia, if the terminals of A-β afferents that transmit tactile messages were to make contact with nociceptive neurons present in these superficial layers.[2] It is likely that analogous brain stem changes occur in the V subnucleus caudalis.

Phenotypic Changes in Primary Afferents and Dorsal Horn Neurons

One of the most important advances in the knowledge of mechanisms of the pain that follows nerve injuries is the recognition of long-term alterations in gene expression. The best-documented phenotypic modifications are a decrease or increase in metabolic synthesis within neurons of ionic channel proteins, neurotransmitters, neuromodulators, neurotrophins, and their receptors. In response to axon injury, primary afferent neurons often show electrophysiologic changes: they develop or increase their baseline level of spontaneous activity, or they develop high-frequency bursts of action potentials. These changes in cellular functioning may be related to the spontaneous and/or paroxysmal pain episodes observed in some chronic pain patients after nerve lesions. Abnormal expression of sodium channel genes is one of the best-documented explanations of these signs of neuropathic pain. Many sodium channels with different properties exist; nerve injury can modify, increase, or decrease the expression of some of these channels. As a result, some sodium channels accumulate near the injured membrane of nociceptive primary afferents. This probably leads to an increased sodium conductance, which in turn participates in the neuronal hyperexcitability.[9] A sodium conductance increase also strongly contributes to the mechanisms of ectopic impulses previously described.

The changes that result from nerve injury are different from those that are seen after inflammation of long duration. In neuropathic conditions, expression of excitatory neurochemicals such as substance P and calcitonin gene-related peptide (CGRP) is typically decreased in small myelinated and unmyelinated fibers, although their expression can be increased following inflammation. Levels of other neurochemicals are also altered in spinal dorsal horn and caudalis neurons and/or dorsal root and trigeminal ganglion cells.[10] This occurs in addition to important phenotypic changes. For instance, peripheral as well as central excitatory amino acid receptor mechanisms play a role in central neuroplasticity through glutamate activation of α-amino-3-hydroxy-5-methyl-4-isoxazole-propionic acid (AMPA) and N-methyl-D-aspartate (NMDA) receptor subtypes (see chapter 5).[2,4] Neurotrophins such as nerve growth factor (NGF) and brain-derived neurotrophic factor (BDNF), which play a key role in somatosensory development, are also involved in the response of primary afferents to injury and are upregulated in the primary afferent neurons after peripheral axotomy.[11]

Microglial and Other Glial Cell Reactions

In addition to changes in neurons, it is becoming increasingly recognized that peripheral nerve injury produces responses in glial cells both at the site of injury and within the CNS. At the site of injury the extracellular microenvironment is rich in mediators, including cytokines, growth factors, and proteases. This microenvironment is highly regulated by Schwann cells, which also provide paracrine trophic support to the fibers. After injury, Schwann cells undergo dramatic phenotypic modulation, regaining capacity to proliferate, migrate, and secrete numerous factors that control repair and nerve regeneration.[12] Within the CNS, around the central endings of injured primary afferents, microglia and astrocytes respond with stereotyped patterns of change in morphology and gene expression.[13] A rapidly growing body of evidence indicates that microglia are actively involved in inducing and maintaining pain hypersensitivity through purinergic receptors, p38 mitogen-activated protein (MAP) kinase, and BDNF (see below). Astrocytes upregulate expression of glial fibrillary acidic protein (GFAP), and recent studies show that these cells are also involved in pain hypersensitivity after peripheral nerve injury or inflammation (see chapter 5).

Changes in Segmental Inhibitory Control

In the V brain stem nuclear complex (VBSNC) and spinal dorsal horn, input from A-β afferent fibers can control the transmission of input from A-β, A-δ and C-fibers to central pain pathways (Fig 7-1). Pain can occur when the inhibitory influence of large-fiber afferent input is reduced or when small-fiber afferent input is increased in such a way that an imbalance is created. It has been proposed that, following a traumatic lesion of peripheral nerve fibers and the consequent deafferentation, some neuropathic pain states may result from a lack of this so-called segmental inhibitory influence exerted by large-diameter fibers. Many therapeutic approaches are still based on this assumption. For example, transcutaneous electric nerve stimulation (TENS) uses high-frequency, low-intensity electric stimulation applied at or close to the affected dermatome. By recruiting large fibers, TENS is believed to induce analgesia by increasing the segmental inhibitory control of nociceptive neurons.

Segmental inhibitory control acts through inhibitory interneurons. It has been proposed that large amounts of excitatory amino acids are released after sensory nerve injury. These induce, through intense NMDA receptor activation, an excitotoxic effect on the postsynaptic inhibitory central interneurons that consequently could be altered or destroyed. The alteration or destruction of these inhibitory interneurons could lead to the development of hyperexcitability of the postsynaptic VBSNC or spinal neurons (see Fig 7-1).[2,15] Similarly, it is thought that the sectioning of the pulpal nerves associated with endodontic therapy causes degeneration-like alterations in the central endings of V primary afferents and in second-order VBSNC neurons. Prolonged impairment of the properties of VBSNC neurons has been noted after such endodontic approaches.[3,4]

In addition, the loss of segmental inhibitory control may result in the recruitment of normally ineffective synapses. The edge of the RF of individual VBSNC or spinal dorsal horn neurons is regulated by inhibitory or relatively ineffective synapses forming a subliminal fringe. The inhibitory influence could result from the same inhibitory interneurons noted previously. Nerve injury is believed to unmask these relatively inefficient synapses so that they become effective in exciting the neuron and contribute to the development of central sensitization.[4,16]

In addition to loss of inhibitory interneurons, a prominent mechanism for producing disinhibition is the loss of the effect of the inhibitory transmitters

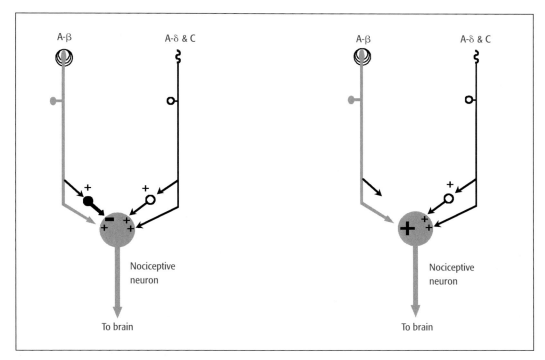

Fig 7-1 Schematic of the balance between excitatory and inhibitory influences from the periphery on the V or spinal nociceptive neurons in the CNS. *Left:* Equilibrium leading to normal transmission of nociception in the ascending pathways originating from the wide dynamic range neurons. Inhibitory interneurons *(black)* are triggered by activity in the large-diameter (A-β) afferent fibers and limit the influence of the excitatory input from small-diameter (A-δ and C) afferent fibers. *Right:* Persistent pain that results from loss of inhibitory interneurons. Reprinted with permission from Price et al.[14]

γ-aminobutynic acid (GABA) and glycine, by raising the concentration of Cl- in neurons in pain pathways. Normally, the intracellular concentration of Cl- is kept low by the action of the K+/Cl- co-transporter (KCC2).[17] Because of this, activation of GABA-A or glycine receptors causes hyperpolarization, as well as membrane shunting. However, after peripheral nerve injury, the expression of KCC2 is dramatically decreased in dorsal horn neurons in lamina I, which leads to a rise in intracellular Cl- concentration.[17] There is a resultant depolarizing shift in the equilibrium potential for Cl-. As a result, Cl- mediated postsynaptic responses to GABA and glycine become much less hyperpolarizing, causing disinhibition and, in about one-third of lamina

I neurons, net excitation. The rise in intracellular Cl- concentration is caused in part by BDNF, which is released, not from neurons, but rather from microglia activated following peripheral nerve injury.

The Concept of Peripherally Maintained Central Sensitization

Neuroplastic changes reflecting central sensitization (see chapter 5) can also be induced by peripheral nerve trauma. However, the central neuroplastic changes are progressively reversed over a period of several days or weeks, just as they are following the vast majority of clinical interventions (eg, following pulpectomy or lesion of a small nerve). However, several studies have suggested that the periphery can be involved in the maintenance of a central "pain state." Clinical cases have been described in which an old, nonpainful surgical scar in a limb contributes to a state of chronic pain in a region far from the scar. A local anesthetic injected into the scar site totally suppresses the pain, which, however, returns when the local anesthetic wears off. This suggests that the persistence of a weak sensory input into the CNS from the site of peripheral trauma may be sufficient to maintain the central hyperexcitability induced at the time of the traumatic event.[15]

Modulation of Central Sensitization Through Descending Controls

As pointed out in chapter 8, the excitability of VBSNC or spinal dorsal horn nociceptive neurons can also be modulated from the brain through descending inhibitory and excitatory controls. The activity of these neurons can be altered after nerve injury in addition to inflammatory processes. For this reason, it has been hypothesized that the increased pain responsiveness of certain patients (eg, those suffering from masticatory muscle and temporomandibular disorders, fibromyalgia, or low back pain) derives at least in part from an injury-induced central sensitization maintained by descending influences that have net excitatory effects.[15]

Mechanisms Implicated in Neuropathic Pain of the Orofacial Area

Examples of neuropathic orofacial pain entities include trigeminal neuralgia, postinjury neuralgia, atypical facial pain and other persistent idiopathic orofacial pain, complex regional pain syndrome, postherpetic neuralgia, neuropathic pain due to systemic disease, and central neuropathic pain. Many of the mechanisms described above have been implicated, but in most instances, the mechanisms involved are not known for certain. Several differing mechanisms may be at work depending on factors such as the evolutionary stage of the disease and genetic and environmental considerations (see chapter 9). In addition, it must be emphasized that different mechanisms may create the same disease and even the same symptom. For example, allodynia can result from central sensitization, phenotypic changes in the primary afferent fibers, central sprouting and reorganization of A-β fibers, lack of inhibitory controls, or more than one of the above mechanisms.

Summary

This chapter has noted that nervous tissue injury may be associated with several different mechanisms that can lead to the development of persistent neuropathic pain in the orofacial region. These mechanisms may include processes triggered by nociceptive or inflammatory stimuli applied to the periphery that result in peripheral (nociceptor) sensitization or in central sensitization. Nerve injury may also trigger different mechanisms that may directly activate the ascending pain pathways or maintain the central sensitization. These include the initiation of ectopic impulses, axon sprouting, neuroma formation, ephaptic transmission, reverberating impulses, or the action of the nervi nervorum. Other important possible changes involve functional contacts between sympathetic efferents and somatic afferents, reorganization of central terminals of primary afferents due to central sprouting, phenotypic changes in the primary afferents and spinal dorsal horn and V subnucleus caudalis neurons, changes in segmental and descending controls, and glia-neuron signaling.

References

1. Merskey H, Bogduk N (eds). Classification of Chronic Pain: Descriptions of Chronic Pain Syndromes and Definitions of Pain Terms, ed 2. Seattle: IASP Press, 1994:59–76.
2. Bennett GJ. Neuropathic pain. In: Wall PD, Melzack R, Bonica JJ (eds). Textbook of Pain, ed 3. New York: Churchill Livingstone, 1994:201–224.
3. Sessle BJ. Mechanisms of trigeminal and occipital pain. Pain Rev 1996;3:91–116.
4. Sessle BJ. Acute and chronic craniofacial pain: Brainstem mechanisms of nociceptive transmission and neuroplasticity, and their clinical correlates. Crit Rev Oral Biol Med 2000;11:57–91.
5. Woda A, Pionchon P. A unified concept of idiopathic orofacial pain: Clinical features. J Orofac Pain 1999;13:172–184.
6. Delcanho RE. Neuropathic implications of prosthodontic treatment. J Prosthet Dent 1995;73:146–152.
7. Stanton-Hicks M, Jänig W, Hassenbusch S, Haddox JD, Boas R, Wilson P. Reflex sympathetic dystrophy: Changing concepts and taxonomy. Pain 1995;63:127–133.
8. Baron R. The influence of sympathetic nerve activity and catecholamines on primary afferent neurons. IASP Newsletter 1998;May/June:3–8.
9. Waxman SG. The molecular pathophysiology of pain: Abnormal expression of sodium channel genes and its contributions to hyperexcitability of primary sensory neurons. Pain 1999;Aug(suppl 6):S133–S140.
10. Hökfelt T, Zhang X, Xu ZQ, et al. Cellular and synaptic mechanisms in transition of pain from acute to chronic. In: Jensen TS, Turner JA, Wiesenfeld-Hallin Z (eds). Proceedings of the 8th World Congress on Pain. Seattle: IASP Press, 1997;133–153.
11. Alvares D, Fitzgerald M. Building blocks of pain: The regulation of key molecules in spinal sensory neurons during development and following peripheral axotomy. Pain 1999;Aug(suppl 6):S71–S85.
12. Campana WM. Schwann cells: Activated peripheral glia and their role in neuropathic pain. Brain Behav Immun 2007;21:522–527.
13. Tsuda M, Inoue K, Salter MW. Neuropathic pain and spinal microglia: A big problem from molecules in "small" glia. Trends Neurosci 2005;28:101–107.
14. Price DD, Mao J, Mayer DJ. Central neural mechanisms of normal and abnormal pain states. In: Fields HL, Liebeskind JC (eds). Pharmacological Approaches to the Treatment of Chronic Pain: New Concepts and Critical Issues: The Bristol-Myers Squibb Symposium on Pain Research. Seattle: IASP Press, 1994:59–74.
15. Ren K, Dubner R. Central nervous system plasticity and persistent pain. J Orofac Pain 1999;13:155–163.
16. Wall PD. Recruitment of ineffective synapses after injury. In: Waxman SG (ed). Functional Recovery in Neurological Disease. Advances in Neurology, vol 47. New York: Raven Press, 1988;387–400.
17. Coull JA, Boudreau D, Bachand K, et al. Trans-synaptic shift in anion gradient in spinal lamina I neurons as a mechanism of neuropathic pain. Nature 2003;424:938–942.

Pain Modulatory Systems

William Maixner

Considering that pain has a neural basis, it is not surprising that much research in the area of pain modulation has focused on ways to alter pain perception by modifying or modulating the activity of several of the neural pathways described in chapters 5 and 11. Within recent years, it has become apparent that both pharmacologic agents (eg, opioids) and psychologic procedures (eg, the placebo effect, hypnosis, and distraction) can impair the perception of pain by modulating the neural systems that contribute to it. In this chapter, a brief overview of pain regulatory systems will be presented.

Sites and Processes that Modulate Pain Perception

Figure 8-1 displays a simplified model of several elements of the nervous system that have been implicated in pain transmission and pain modulation. The activity within and between these integrative elements gives rise to the sensory, affective, and emotional responses to noxious stimuli. Each site within this model represents important areas or pathways that influence the way in which nociceptive information is perceived and interpreted.

Modulation of nociceptor input

The peripheral terminals of A-δ and C-fiber afferents represent important areas where pain responses to tissue injury and inflammation are modulated (see Fig 8-1, site 1; see also chapters 4 and 6 for further review).[2–4] The administration of local anesthetics (eg, sodium channel blockers) to the peripheral nerve terminals or to the nerve trunk blocks nociceptive transmission and peripheral inflammatory responses. Similarly, nonsteroidal anti-inflammatory drugs such as aspirin and ibuprofen are capable of altering nociceptive afferent excitability and can alter the hyperalgesia associated with acute orofacial pain conditions. The peripheral terminals of nociceptive afferents also contain membrane-bound receptors (eg, opioid, γ-aminobutyric acid [GABA]). When, for example, the opioid receptors are stimulated by an opioid such as morphine, a reduction in the amount of substance P, calcitonin gene-related peptide (CGRP), and glutamate released from peripheral terminals by a noxious stimulus occurs. This process attenuates neurogenic inflammation and can suppress dental pain.[2–4] Endogenously released opioid peptides from the pituitary, adrenal medulla, and

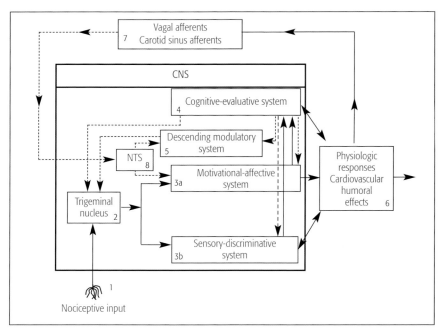

Fig 8-1 Diagram of peripheral and central nervous system (CNS) pathways involved in the transmission and modulation of pain. The model consists of four interactive units: nociceptive afferents, CNS integrative pathways, physiologic responses, and visceral afferents that respond to the physiologic responses evoked by noxious stimuli. Solid lines represent CNS pathways that contribute to the sensory, emotional, and physiologic responses to noxious stimulation. Dashed lines represent modulatory pathways capable of inhibiting or facilitating nociceptive transmission to the nucleus tractus solitarius (NTS). Reprinted with permission from Fillingim and Maixner.[1]

immune cells can also impair inflammatory responses by acting on opioid receptors located on the peripheral terminals.[4] The presence of opioid receptors on nociceptive afferent terminals has important implications especially apparent in the dentition, since teeth with an underlying pulpitis are frequently asymptomatic or nonpainful.

Modulation within the trigeminal brain stem complex

The synapses between primary afferents and neurons in the trigeminal brain stem nuclear complex (VBSNC) represent another important location for pain modulation (see Fig 8-1, site 2; see also chapter 5). The central terminals of nociceptive C-fibers also possess opioid receptors that, when stimulated, suppress the release of pain-producing neuromodulators.[3] These receptors are stimulated by exogenously administered opioids given in a clinical setting. It is also known that endogenous opioid peptides (eg, enkephalins) and the inhibitory amino acid GABA are stored and released by intrinsic neurons in such regions as the substantia gelatinosa of the VBSNC and the dorsal horn of the spinal cord.[2,5–7] The release of opioid peptides from these intrinsic or local inhibitory neurons acts to decrease the release of pain-producing substances from nociceptive afferents. In addition, endogenously released opioids, exogenously administrated opioids (eg, morphine), and GABA act directly on VBSNC and spinal nociceptive neurons that convey information to higher regions of the central nervous system (CNS). In this situation, more pain-producing substances from primary afferents are required to evoke neural transmission.

Motivational-affective, sensory-discriminative, and cognitive-evaluative systems

Several areas such as the thalamus, reticular system, limbic system, and various cortical regions play important roles in sculpting an individual's perceptual, autonomic, neuroendocrine, and emotional responses to tissue injury (see Fig 8-1, sites 3a, 3b, and 4).[8] The overall "mosaic" or composite of activity in these regions determines the perceptual experience, the emotional responses, and the meaning that we assign to painful stimuli. Given this knowledge, it is no wonder that pain is a highly personal experience that is susceptible to a variety of biologic, pharmacologic, and environmental influences (see chapter 11).

Descending modulatory system

Over the course of the last 50 years, a considerable amount of research has been conducted on control mechanisms that regulate the transmission of nociceptive information from the VBSNC and spinal dorsal horn to higher regions of the CNS. Perhaps the best studied of these systems are those commonly referred to as the *descending modulatory system*.[2,6,7,9,10]

The descending modulatory system is composed of a group of structures in the brain stem, midbrain, subcortex, and cortex that form a network of descending projections to the VBSNC and spinal dorsal horn. Many of the neurotransmitters released from the terminals of fibers of these descending projections inhibit sensory transmission by impairing the ability of nociceptive neurons in the VBSNC

and spinal cord to respond to noxious stimuli. Norepinephrine (NE) and serotonin (5-HT) are two such neurotransmitters whose cell bodies are located in brain stem sites. In addition to inhibitory neurotransmitters, descending control systems can also release neuroactive substances that augment the relay of sensory information through the VBSNC and spinal dorsal horn. One intrinsic substance that promotes the facilitation of nociceptive transmission is the endogenous opioid peptide *dynorphin*. This substance is synthesized and released in the VBSNC and spinal dorsal horn following the activation of descending facilitatory pathways.[10] The release of brain-derived neurotrophic factor, a neurotrophin, also results in the activation of descending facilitatory pathways.

The complex anatomic organization of the descending modulatory system (Fig 8-2; see Fig 8-1, site 5) permits a wide array of physiologic, emotional, and perceptual responses to tissue injury. This system provides the neural basis for the analgesic responses associated with the placebo effect. It is now known that increasing a patient's expectations that a drug will produce a powerful analgesic effect results in a substantial increase in the analgesic response. Increasing or modifying a patient's expectations is a cognitive process associated with alterations in the activity of neurons in cortical and subcortical structures that modulate the activity of components of the descending control system originating in the midbrain and brain stem (see chapter 5).

The perception of pain is greatly influenced by the context or environment in which the stimulus is experienced. The meaning ascribed to an environmental stimulus engages this powerful descending regulatory system to either upregulate or downregulate nociceptive transmission. Acute life-threatening events such as a battle or acute injury are frequently associated with pain perception that is greatly diminished until the threat no longer exists. In contrast, an anxious dental-phobic patient will experience more pain in the clinical setting than

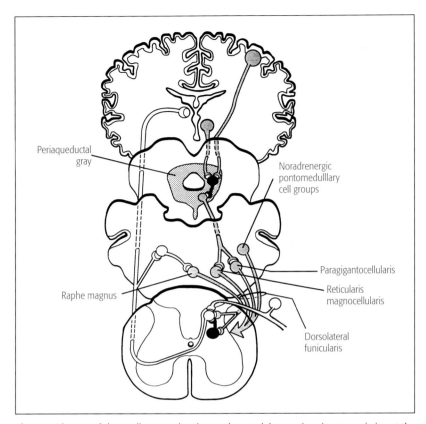

Fig 8-2 Diagram of descending neural pathways that modulate nociceptive transmission at the level of the VBSNC and spinal cord. Clear neurons represent cells that transmit nociceptive signals to the VBSNC, dorsal horn of the spinal cord, and supraspinal sites. The shaded lines represent neurons that descend to the VBSNC and spinal dorsal horn from supraspinal sites. The small dark interneurons release enkephalins when stimulated by neurotransmitters (eg, NE and 5-HT) released from the nerve terminals of fibers that contribute to the descending systems. The midbrain periaqueductal gray contains cell bodies that receive input from higher centers, and these cells send projections to the rostral ventrolateral medulla (noradrenergic pontomedullary cell groups, paragigantocellularis, and reticularis magnocellularis) and raphe magnus, which contains the cell bodies of 5-HT–producing neurons. These nuclear groups send projections or axons to the VBSNC and the spinal cord through the dorsolateral funiculus. Reprinted with permission from Bradley.[11]

a relaxed patient who has experienced painless dental procedures. One's psychologic state, previous life experiences, and personality influence the activity of descending pathways to produce net facilitation or inhibition, which in turn influences nociceptive transmission.

The responses of nociceptive neurons in the VBSNC and spinal dorsal horn can also be strongly inhibited by noxious stimuli applied to remote or distal sites. In the clinical dental setting, it has been shown that the application of a counterirritant to the arm or hand inhibits pain and diminishes the

Table 8-1 Endogenous opioid peptides and associated opioid receptors

Peptides	Receptors stimulated by peptide
Enkephalins	δ receptors > μ receptors
Endorphins	Both δ and μ receptors
Endomorphin	μ receptors
Dynorphins	κ receptors
Nociceptin/Orphanin FQ	Orphan receptor (ORL-1)

area of referral pain in patients experiencing a symptomatic pulpitis.[8] One mechanism by which counterirritants produce analgesia is by stimulating several of the descending pain inhibitory pathways shown in Fig 8-2. The stimulation of ascending nociceptive pathways activates powerful descending inhibitory systems located in the brain stem; these inhibit the transmission of nociceptive information in the VBSNC and spinal dorsal horn. Non-nociceptive afferent input may also induce inhibition of nociceptive transmission.

The analgesic effect of several centrally acting drugs such as morphine is also partially mediated by descending modulatory pathways.[6,9,10] Opioid receptors are localized on the cell bodies of neurons at almost all CNS levels contributing to these descending pathways. The systemic administration of an opioid such as morphine activates these receptors and will activate powerful inhibitory pathways to the VBSNC and spinal dorsal horn, thus blocking nociceptive transmission in these sensory relay sites (see Fig 8-2). Endogenous opioids such as enkephalins and endomorphin (see below) are also colocalized in nuclear regions that possess cell bodies with opioid receptors.[6,10] The analgesic effects mediated by the placebo effect, hypnosis, and acupuncture are in part mediated by this endogenous opioid system, since the administration of the opioid receptor antagonist naloxone can partially reverse the analgesic effects of these procedures.

Endogenous opioid and nonopioid pain regulatory systems

Modern understanding of the intrinsic or endogenous mechanisms that support analgesia began in the mid-1970s with the isolation and characterization of peptides from the guinea pig's ileum referred to as *enkephalins*; these exhibited biologic properties similar to morphine. Around the same time, peptides with morphine-like properties and associated receptor systems were identified and characterized in peripheral tissues and in the gray matter of spinal and supraspinal structures.[2,6,10] Several families of opioid peptides have been identified and characterized (Table 8-1). Enkephalins, endorphins, endomorphin, and dynorphins are synthesized as propeptides and are derived from separate genes.

At present, three families of opioid receptors (μ, δ, and κ) have been identified (see Table 8-1).[12–14] These receptors, like the opioid peptides, are derived from separate genes. Opioid receptors are distributed in regions of the nervous system that contain opioid peptides. Endorphins, enkephalins, and dynorphins show low to moderate receptor specificity. Endomorphin, unlike the other opioid peptides, shows high selectivity and specificity for the μ opioid receptor.[15]

Opioid peptides released from cells of the immune system and those released into the circulation from the adrenal medulla or other peripheral tissues (eg, gut, cardiac tissue) can inhibit the activation of nociceptive afferents by stimulating peripheral μ and δ receptors.[4] In addition, the activation of various descending modulatory systems (see Fig 8-1, site 5) regulates the activity of VBSNC and spinal enkephalin-containing neurons. This anatomic organization allows supraspinal processes to modulate pain transmission at the level of the VBSNC and spinal cord. In addition to spinal and VBSNC sites, small enkephalin-containing interneurons are located in brain stem, subcortical, and cerebral cortical regions; these interneurons inhibit neural transmission through other regions of the CNS that relay or transmit sensory information.

There is also considerable evidence for endogenous nonopioid systems.[6,16] The analgesic effects associated with the placebo effect, acupuncture, hypnosis, and certain physiologic and psychologic stressors are only partially blocked or reversed by pharmacologic agents that block opioid receptors. The remaining analgesia is thought to be mediated by nonopioid-dependent mechanisms. At present, researchers have a rather sparse understanding of the mediators, organization, and function of nonopioid processes. The inhibitory amino acid GABA is stored in small interneurons throughout the CNS; as noted previously, the release of GABA from small interneurons inhibits the release of neurotransmitters from primary afferent nociceptors and impairs the excitability of neurons that respond to tissue injury. The activation of various descending modulatory pathways (see Fig 8-1, site 5) adjusts the activity of VBSNC and spinal GABA-containing neurons, which allows supraspinal processes to modulate nociceptive transmission at the level of the VBSNC and spinal dorsal horn.

Although opioids are commonly viewed as agents that act to inhibit nociceptive transmission, it is becoming clearer that not all endogenous opioid peptides and associated receptor activation inhibit pain transmission under all physiologic and pathophysiologic conditions.[17–19] For example, the endogenous opioid peptide dynorphin increases the release of substance P from primary afferent C-fibers[2] by stimulating both κ opioid and N-methyl-D-aspartate (NMDA) receptors.[4,10,17] Under certain pathophysiologic conditions, especially those associated with inflammation, dynorphin appears to enhance nociceptive transmission.[10,17] The nonopioid peptide cholecystokinin, localized in both the VBSNC and spinal dorsal horn, inhibits the analgesic actions of opioids.[18] Finally, it has become increasingly recognized that the chronic use of opioids can produce paradoxic excitatory and hyperalgesic effects by stimulating a unique form of the μ opioid receptor and in response to β2-adrenergic stimulation.[18,19]

Pain modulatory systems activated by physiologic responses

Tissue injury not only affects sensory responses and negative feelings but also produces a variety of autonomic and neuroendocrine responses (see Fig 8-1, sites 6 to 8). These peripheral physiologic events occur in response to the stimulation of nociceptors, which results in the activation of CNS regions that regulate autonomic function and the secretion of various hormones from the pituitary gland. These events also influence sensory and emotional responses to tissue injury by activating visceral afferents.[8] The stimulation of these visceral afferents alters the excitability of the cerebral cortex and actually diminishes the arousal and emotional responses to sensory stimulation. These afferents are activated by a variety of substances such as the endogenous opioids (eg, morphine, nicotine, and cocaine). It is quite likely that a portion of the analgesic properties of these agents is mediated by the activation of specific receptors on the visceral afferents.[8]

In contrast to suppressing the sensory and emotional responses to pain, the activation of certain populations of visceral afferents may evoke exceptional negative feelings and sensations associated with tissue injury. For example, a noxious stimulus that evokes changes in gastric motility will produce gastric distress and the sensation of nausea. While not associated with sensations arising from the specific site of injury, these unpleasant sensations contribute to the overall emotional experience and affect the way pain is perceived and experienced.

The *nucleus tractus solitarius* (NTS) is an important brain stem region that relays visceral afferent input to other regions of the CNS that contribute to the ascending and descending modulation of pain transmission (see Fig 8-1, sites 3a, 3b, 5, and 8). This system represents an important pathway that allows visceral events to facilitate the way in which CNS pathways respond to noxious sensory input. It also contributes to the overall conscious experience of pain.

Genetic and Environmental Factors that Influence Pain Modulation

The circuitry presented in Fig 8-1 is an oversimplification of a very complex modulatory system. It is important that we do not view this system as a "hard-wired" immutable system that merely conveys information from one location to the next. The way the nervous system encodes and modulates sensory stimuli that are perceived as painful is affected by a number of individually determined genetic and environmental factors.[20,21] In recent years, it has become apparent that human pain sensitivity and its modulation is influenced by several subtle variances in genes that affect sensory processing of pain signals, inflammation, and psychologic states.[21]

In addition to predetermined genetic factors such as sex (see also chapters 9 and 13), envi-

ronmental factors and previous life and cultural experiences can also shape the way the nervous system modulates pain perception.[1] Intraoral pain may have a very different meaning and perceptual consequence to a patient who has recently been diagnosed with an oral cancer compared with a patient who experiences pain from an elective restorative procedure. Previous memories and cultural attributes or rites can also greatly influence cortical and subcortical structures that play a role in the way the peripheral nervous system and CNS formulate responses to tissue injury. Genetic and environmental factors work in concert to modulate the overall matrix of neural, autonomic, and endocrine responses to tissue injury and determine individuals' interpretation and appreciation of painful sensations (see chapter 9).[8,21]

Summary

This chapter has outlined several processes within the CNS involved in the modulation of pain. A number of mechanisms at several levels contribute to the transmission, integration, and regulation of nociceptive signals. These include descending modulatory pathways in the CNS are involved in a number of physiologic responses and therapeutic approaches associated with pain modulation, endogenous opioids, and nonopioid chemical processes (eg, GABA) that are connected with analgesia and hyperalgesia. Finally, neural mechanisms associated with genetic and environmental factors that influence pain and its control were considered, and the importance of individual genetic factors, as well as previous life and cultural experiences, to the perception and modulation of pain were emphasized.

Acknowledgments

This work was supported by NIDCR grants DE07509, DE11661, DE16558, DE017018, and NS045685.

References

1. Fillingim RB, Maixner W. Gender differences in the responses to noxious stimuli. Pain Forum 1995;4:209–221.
2. Scholz J, Woolf CJ. Can we conquer pain? Nat Neurosci 2002;(5 suppl):1062–1067.
3. Likar R, Sittl R, Gragger K, et al. Peripheral morphine analgesia in dental surgery. Pain 1998;76:145–150.
4. Stein C, Cabot PJ, Schafer M. Peripheral opioid analgesia: Mechanisms and clinical implications. In: Stein C (ed). Opioids in Pain Control: Basic and Clinical Aspects. Cambridge: Cambridge Univ Press, 1999:96–108.
5. Dubner R, Bennett GJ. Spinal and trigeminal mechanisms of nociception. Annu Rev Neurosci 1983;6:381–418.
6. Yaksh T. Central pharmacology of nociceptive transmission. In: Wall PD, Melzack R (eds). Textbook of Pain, ed 4. New York: Churchill Livingstone, 1999:253–308.
7. Sessle BJ. Acute and chronic craniofacial pain: Brainstem mechanisms of nociceptive transmission and neuroplasticity, and their clinical correlates. Crit Rev Oral Biol Med 2000;11:57–91.
8. Maixner W, Sigurdsson A, Fillingim R, Lundeen T, Booker D. Regulation of acute and chronic orofacial pain. In: Fricton JR, Dubner RB (eds). Orofacial Pain and Temporomandibular Disorders. New York: Raven Press, 1995:85–102.
9. Fields HL, Basbaum AI. Central nervous system mechanisms of pain modulation. In: Wall PD, Melzack R (eds). Textbook of Pain, ed 4. New York: Churchill Livingstone, 1999:309–329.
10. Millan MJ. Descending control of pain. Prog Neurobiol 2002;66:355–474.
11. Bradley RM. Essentials of Oral Physiology. St Louis: Mosby, 1995.
12. Wu SY, Dun SL, Wright MT, Chang JK, Dun NJ. Endoinhibition of substantia gelatinosa neurons in vitro. Neuroscience 1999;89:317–321.
13. Roques BP, Noble F, Fournie-Zaluski MC. Endogenous opioid peptides and analgesia. In: Stein C (ed). Opioids in Pain Control: Basic and Clinical Aspects. Cambridge: Cambridge Univ Press, 1999:21–45.
14. Gaveriaux-Ruff C, Kieffer B. Opioid receptors: Gene structure and function. In: Stein C (ed). Opioids in Pain Control: Basic and Clinical Aspects. Cambridge: Cambridge Univ Press, 1999:1–20.
15. Stone LS, Fairbanks CA, Laughlin TM, et al. Spinal analgesic actions of the new endogenous opioid peptides endomorphin-1 and -2. Neuroreport 1997;8:3131–3135.
16. Wiesenfeld-Hallin Z, Xu XJ. Opioid-nonopioid interactions. In: Stein C (ed). Opioids in Pain Control: Basic and Clinical Aspects. Cambridge: Cambridge Univ Press, 1999:131–142.
17. Arcaya JL, Cano G, Gomez G, Maixner W, Suarez-Roca H. Dynorphin A increases substance P release from trigeminal primary afferent C-fibers. Eur J Pharmacol 1999;366:27–34.
18. Suarez-Roca H, Maixner W. Morphine produces a multiphasic effect on the release of substance P from rat trigeminal nucleus caudalis slices by activating different opioid receptor subtypes. Brain Res 1992;579:195–203.
19. Liang DY, Liao G, Wang J, et al. A genetic analysis of opioid-induced hyperalgesia in mice. Anesthesiology 2006;104:1054–1062.
20. Mogil JS. The genetic mediation of individual differences in sensitivity to pain and its inhibition. Proc Natl Acad Sci U S A 1999;96:7744–7751.
21. Diatchenko L, Nackley AG, Slade GD, Fillingim RB, Maixner W. Idiopathic pain disorders—Pathways of vulnerability. Pain 2006;123:226–230.

Pain and Genetics

Ze'ev Seltzer

Jeffrey S. Mogil

As shown throughout this book, chronic pain syndromes affecting the craniofacial region constitute an unsolved clinical problem because they are common, cause incalculable suffering and incapacitation, and are difficult to treat by existing therapies. Available painkillers currently provide only partial pain relief that is compromised by side effects. A clinically driven subfield in pain genetics is the focus of this chapter since it seeks genetic factors that explain interindividual differences in the susceptibility to develop chronic orofacial pain in order to account for the variance and also to identify new drug targets. On this basis, this chapter introduces the reader to pain genetics, describes the rationale and some methodological considerations that underlie studies in pain genetics, and explains the background for the forecast that genetics may discover new treatment targets. For a broader perspective with greater detail, see Mogil.[1]

Why Is the Variance in Chronic Orofacial Pain Important?

Any number of outcomes may emerge when an anatomically complex region responds to injury, disease, or exposure to toxins. Therefore, it should come as no surprise that there are large interindividual differences in chronic orofacial pain. Each patient presents with a unique combination of spontaneous pain, stimulus-evoked pain, and pain aggravated by movement. Individuals with the same pathology may present highly variable pain intensity, the location where pain is felt, duration and frequency of pain episodes, and affective-emotional impact of chronic orofacial pain on quality of life and daily activities; even the description of what the pain feels like (eg, burning, crushing) may be different, as well as the analgesic efficacy derived from painkillers (for examples, see Aubrun et al[2]).

Figure 9-1 provides an example of the variability in chronic pain intensity presented by 228 traumatic leg amputees. After controlling for confounding variables such as height of the amputation, years since amputation, and ethnicity, enormous differences in phantom leg pain levels are apparent. While about 25% of the amputees never suffered from pain in the missing leg, approximately 75% reported having pain episodes occurring at relatively regular times, with the same episode duration and typical intensity within individuals. A few amputees only had very faint pain, a few others

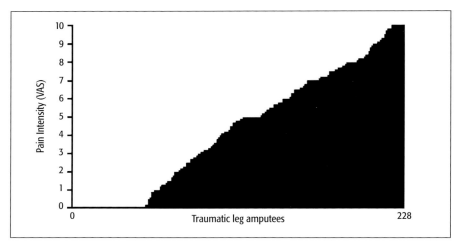

Fig 9-1 The typical intensity of phantom leg pain as reported by 228 leg amputees using a visual analog scale (VAS), where 0 represents "No pain" and 10 represents "The most intense pain imaginable." (Seltzer, unpublished data).

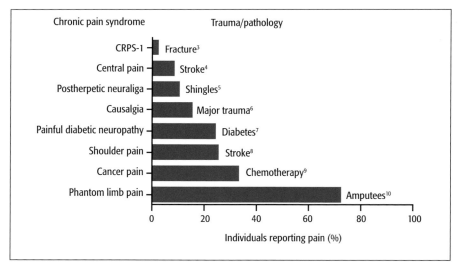

Fig 9-2 Percentage of individuals experiencing the traumas or pathologies listed on the right who developed the chronic pain syndromes on the left. CRPS-I = complex regional pain syndrome, type I.

suffered from maximal pain, and the rest presented with pain ranging between these extremes. Note that in this example, the majority of amputees reported phantom pain. This is an exception; in most cases the percentage of individuals developing chronic pain after some insult is lower, as Fig 9-2 suggests.

Is Chronic Orofacial Pain a Heritable Trait?

The enormous variance in attributes describing chronic pain and the excess of females presenting with chronic orofacial pain (see chapters 1 and 13) suggest that the susceptibility to develop such pain may be heritable, that is, passed on from one generation to the next via genetic mechanisms. The following equation shows that, like any biologic trait, the phenotypic variance of chronic orofacial pain (VAR_P) is produced by genetic (VAR_G) and environmental or nongenetic sources (VAR_E), and their interaction (VAR_I):

$$VAR_P = VAR_G + VAR_E + VAR_I$$

A *phenotype* is any measurable or categorizable trait that describes some feature of an organism (eg, height), whereas a *genotype* refers to the genetic constitution of an individual within its species.

Studies on the incidence of trigeminal neuralgia and familial migraine in twin pairs and pedigrees demonstrate the involvement of genetic factors.[11] A few reports have already identified chromosomal regions, and even a small number of specific genes and single mutations affecting migraines, headaches, and chronic orofacial pain,[12,13] as well as chronic pain in body parts other than the head.[14–16] Studies in animal models of painful neuropathies have established that levels of chronic pain are considerably heritable.[17–20] Furthermore, manipulations of individual genes by overexpression, deletion (in transgenic "knock-out" experiments), or inhibition of expression using small interfering ribonucleic acid (siRNA) or antisense oligodeoxynucleotide injections have identified more than 240 rodent genes that have some demonstrated role in pain.[21–23]

What Is the Size of the Heritable Component in Chronic Orofacial Pain?

Estimating heritability in chronic orofacial pain is not simple because the only measurable variance is that of the pain (VAR_P). However, the use of sophisticated statistics to analyze data from the incidence of chronic pain in closely related individuals has enabled researchers to measure the genetic and environmental variance in several chronic pain syndromes, thereby estimating the *broad-sense heritability (H^2)*, a value that reflects all genetic contributions to a population's phenotypic variance. This is depicted in the following equation:

$$H^2 = VAR_G / VAR_P$$

The importance of estimating heritability in chronic orofacial pain is in the ability to forecast the extent to which pain could be treated if pharmacologically addressing the genetic component. Figure 9-3 shows data from studies that estimated the size of H^2 in various chronic pain syndromes. On average, genetic factors account for approximately 40% of the variance in chronic pain levels, similar to the average value in animal models of painful neuropathies.[24] This calculation carries an optimistic message for pain patients, because it suggests that drugs developed on the basis of genetic knowledge could provide meaningful pain relief.

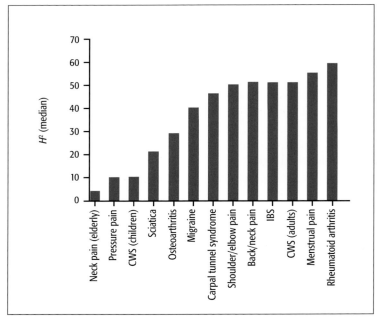

Fig 9-3 Broad-sense heritability estimates *(H²)* of a number of painful disorders (see MacGregor[11]). Where multiple estimates have been reported for the same syndrome, the median value is plotted. Note that it is unclear in many cases whether the *H²* value represents the heritability of developing the painful pathology or the heritability of pain within the pathology. CWS = chronic widespread pain; IBS = irritable bowel syndrome.

How Can We Find Orofacial Pain Genes?

Phenomics of chronic orofacial pain

The overall goal in discovering pain genes is to provide evidence of a statistically significant "association" between a pain trait and some genetic marker (usually single nucleotide polymorphisms [SNPs]) in or near these genes. Thus, "genes for pain" are nothing more than genes associated with variability in the phenotypes collected from participants in a given cohort. Each pain syndrome is a unique and complex experience characterized by multiple sensory-discriminative, affective-emotional and cognitive-evaluative variables; therefore, to faithfully represent the pain, a clinician should characterize it in as much detail as is practical. It is not enough to determine whether a patient does or does not have pain and limit the description to pain intensity. *Pain phenomics* is the research field that constructs questionnaires for quantifying phenotypic pain data for genetic studies. Phenomic questionnaires for chronic orofacial pain are currently unavailable.

Collecting DNA samples

Since there are no available national or international repositories of deoxyribonucleic acid (DNA) samples that would enable interested researchers to get samples for a genetic study, they must collect their own cohorts, a process that generally takes years. For several reasons related to statistical power, a researcher needs to recruit several hundreds of genetically unrelated pain patients with the same syndrome and hundreds of controls matched for age, ethnicity, sex, etc, who have had the same surgery, disease, or trauma but did not develop chronic pain. Such cohorts are sufficient to discover genes that have major effects on pain levels. Identifying smaller-effect "modifier" genes necessitates a larger study group measured in thousands rather than hundreds of participants.

Following approval by Institutional Ethics Review Boards to conduct genetic experiments in humans, potential participants are recruited. Every recruited participant signs an informed consent form and undergoes an interview to fill out a structured and validated pain phenotyping questionnaire. DNA for genetic studies is usually extracted from white blood cells. DNA from a venipunctured blood sample of 10 to 20 mL is enough for many hundreds of genotypings. But even this quantity of genotypings is limited. Because collecting a cohort of pain patients and their matched controls is so laborious and expensive, some investigators invest in *whole genome amplification*, a process that provides as many copies of the whole genome as is affordable or needed. Other investigators "immortalize" the DNA by introducing it into a cell line of lymphoblasts that continuously produce donor DNA. The lymphoblasts may also be used for messenger ribonucleic acid (mRNA) expression analyses as a substitute for the patient's tissues. It is also advisable to keep the plasma of the blood sample and store it for future analyses of proteins, peptides, and cytokines whose levels are possibly affected by the genes studied and can therefore be used as indicators of changes occurring in the trigeminal system during chronic orofacial pain. When venipuncturing for a blood sample is not possible, a clinician could use commercially available kits to extract high quantities of good-quality DNA from saliva.[25]

Genotyping DNA in search of chronic orofacial pain genes

Two types of polymorphic genetic markers *(marker loci)* are currently used for genotyping individuals in a cohort: short tandem repeats (STRs)—also called *microsatellites*—and SNPs. Each individual carries two identical (ie, homozygous) or different (ie, heterozygous) alleles at each marker locus (eg, aa, ab, and bb genotypes). The level of significance of the statistical association between the frequency of carriers of these three genotypes and levels of the trait that characterize chronic orofacial pain is interpreted as a preliminary indication that a causative gene or its part (in the case of microsatellite markers), or causative SNP (when using SNP markers), is nearby. An additional step of positional refinement is then needed to identify the point mutation(s) responsible for the pain trait. This is done by comparing sequences of the relevant DNA interval, seeking mismatches that segregate with pain levels.

SNPs that control chronic orofacial pain may be identified in one ethnic group but not in others. Therefore, meeting treatment needs of peoples of various ethnic origins necessitates studying many ethnic groups. Failure to control for ethnicity can also confound genetic association studies via "population stratification."[26]

It should be noted that much genomic variation is not produced by SNPs at all but by copy number variants and other more complex polymorphisms.[27] If no sequence mismatches in a gene under study are found to segregate with chronic pain levels, it is possible that the gene is still implicated in the variance of the pain trait by other genetic mechanisms, (eg, by controlling gene expression levels). In one such scenario, another gene could affect splice variation and editing of the mRNA transcript of the pain gene, which determines how many copies of the mRNA of this gene are to be produced and what type of protein is to be produced. Identification of such mechanisms necessitates quantification of mRNA expression levels in situ (ie, in neural structures where the gene is expressed). Since human material is usually unavailable for research, animal models may serve as surrogates, complemented if needed by comparing mRNA expression levels of lymphoblasts with immortalized DNA of patients with chronic orofacial pain and controls.

Two genotyping approaches can be used to identify chronic orofacial pain genes: (1) studying candidate genes implicated in chronic pain by prior information, and (2) an unbiased scan of all genes in the genome, screened at once in a single run (called genome-wide association study [GWAS]), followed by studying identified candidates.

Candidate gene approach

This approach tests the hypothesis that SNPs on one or more genes of known identity segregate in the tested cohort with traits related to chronic orofacial pain. The candidacy of such genes is inferred from the literature as having a known or potential role in pain mechanisms[28] (for example, see Diatchenko et al[16]).

Genome-wide association study

Screening candidate genes by looking "under the streetlight" at known pain-relevant genes carries the risk of missing many other genes for which no knowledge exists to date. This disadvantage is avoided when using the unbiased GWAS approach, which genotypes polymorphisms on approximately 500,000 to 1,000,000 SNPs preselected as capable of detecting nearby mutation(s) affecting a trait under investigation in all genes on the genome. The markers are arranged as microarrays on "chips" that can identify all the chronic orofacial pain genes an individual carries. The chips are commercially available from several producers but are still not economically feasible.

How Can Pain Medicine Advance in the Postgenomic Era?

When all major genetic variations that affect chronic orofacial pain are discovered, novel diagnostic kits will be developed to identify the risk an individual carries for developing chronic orofacial pain; this type of knowledge will be useful in planning treatment choices if, for example, that individual will undergo maxillofacial surgery. The same knowledge is expected to result in the development of prognostic kits that could identify which treatment is genetically most beneficial for an individual. Similar kits could select better subjects for clinical trials, thereby minimizing costs and shortening drug development times. Novel preventive treatments could provide effective "preemptive analgesia" and better postoperative care. New chronic orofacial pain mechanisms could be discovered by studying neurons or glial cells expressing the identified pain genes, and better animal models could be developed based on their relevance to human orofacial pain genes. Finally, applying gene therapy could "patch" the genome of individuals born with "bad" gene variants that carry the risk for chronic orofacial pain. The rapid advancements made in the Human Genome Project raise the hope that this futuristic scenario may become a reality in our lifetime.

Summary

This chapter has emphasized the importance of clinically observable interindividual variability in chronic orofacial pain conditions as a clue suggesting that these syndromes are complex heritable traits. This means that these conditions are controlled by genetic determinants that interact with the environment. The chapter also provided estimations that the size of the heritable component in chronic pain is approximately 40%, indicating that drugs based on genomic knowledge could be effective painkillers. Next, the primary molecular approaches currently used to discover genes for chronic pain were introduced. Finally, several practical outcomes that are likely to result from the Human Genome Project were described, thereby highlighting the clinical relevance of pain genetics to orofacial pain conditions.

References

1. Mogil JS (ed). Progress in Pain Research and Management, Vol 28: The Genetics of Pain. Seattle: IASP Press, 2004:349.
2. Aubrun F, Langeron O, Quesnel C, Coriat P, Riou B. Relationships between measurement of pain using visual analog score and morphine requirements during postoperative intravenous morphine titration. Anesthesiology 2003;98:1415–1421.
3. Veldman PH, Reynen HM, Arntz IE, Goris RJ. Signs and symptoms of reflex sympathetic dystrophy: Prospective study of 829 patients. Lancet 1993;342:1012–1016.
4. Andersen G, Vestergaard K, Ingeman-Nielsen M, Jensen TS. Incidence of central post-stroke pain. Pain 1995;61: 187–193.
5. Cluff RS, Rowbotham MC. Pain caused by herpes zoster infection. Neurol Clin 1998;16:813–832.
6. Richards RL. Causalgia. A centennial review. Arch Neuro. 1967;16:339–350.
7. Schmader KE. Epidemiology and impact on quality of life of postherpetic neuralgia and painful diabetic neuropathy. Clin J Pain 2002;18:350–354.
8. Gamble GE, Barberan E, Bowsher D, Tyrrell PJ, Jones AK. Post stroke shoulder pain: More common than previously realized. Eur J Pain 2000;4:313–315.
9. Foley KM. Controlling cancer pain. Hosp Pract (Menneap) 2000;35:101–108, 111–112.
10. Dijkstra PU, Geertzen JH, Stewart R, van der Schans CP. Phantom pain and risk factors: A multivariate analysis. J Pain Symptom Manage 2002;24:578–585.
11. MacGregor AJ. The heritability of pain in humans. In: Mogil JS (ed). Progress in Pain Research and Management, Vol 28: The Genetics of Pain. Seattle: IASP Press, 2004:151–170.
12. van den Maagdenberg AM, Haan J, Terwindt GM, Ferrari MD. Migraine: Gene mutations and functional consequences. Curr Opin Neurol 2007;20:299–305.
13. Diatchenko L, Slade GD, Nackley AG, et al. Genetic basis for individual variations in pain perception and the development of a chronic pain condition. Hum Mol Genet 2005;14:135–143.
14. Mailis A, Wade J. Profile of Caucasian women with possible genetic predisposition to reflex sympathetic dystrophy: A pilot study. Clin J Pain 1994;10:210–217.
15. Waxman SG, Dib-Hajj S. Erythermalgia: Molecular basis for an inherited pain syndrome. Trends Mol Med 2005; 11:555–562.
16. Diatchenko L, Anderson AD, Slade GD, et al. Three major haplotypes of the b2 adrenergic receptor define psychological profile, blood pressure, and the risk for development of a common musculoskeletal pain disorder. Am J Med Genet B Neuropsychiatr Genet 2006;141:449–462.
17. Devor M, Raber P. Heritability of symptoms in an experimental model of neuropathic pain. Pain 1990;42:51–67.
18. Mogil JS, Wilson SG, Bon K, et al. Heritability of nociception I: Responses of 11 inbred mouse strains on 12 measures of nociception. Pain 1999;80:67–82.
19. Seltzer Z, Wu T, Max MB, Diehl SR. Mapping a gene for neuropathic pain-related behavior following peripheral neurectomy in the mouse. Pain 2001;93:101–106.
20. Shir Y, Zeltser R, Vatine JJ, et al. Correlation of intact sensibility and neuropathic pain-related behaviors in eight inbred and outbred rat strains and selection lines. Pain 2001;90:75–82.
21. Mogil JS, Yu L, Basbaum AI. Pain genes?: Natural variation and transgenic mutants. Annu Rev Neurosci 2000;23: 777–811.
22. Hatcher JP, Chessell IP. Transgenic models of pain: A brief review. Curr Opin Investig Drugs 2006;7:647–652.
23. LaCroix-Fralish ML, Ledoux JB, Mogil JS. The Pain Genes Database: An interactive web browser of pain-related transgenic knockout studies. Pain 2007;131:3.e1–4.
24. Mogil JS, Seltzer Z, Devor M. Social and environmental influences on pain: Implications for pain genetics. In: Mogil JS (ed). Progress in Pain Research and Management, Vol 28: The Genetics of Pain. Seattle: IASP Press, 2004:257–282.
25. Rogers NL, Cole SA, Lan HC, Crossa A, Demerath EW. New saliva DNA collection method compared to buccal cell collection techniques for epidemiological studies. Am J Hum Biol 2007;19:319–326.
26. Freedman ML, Reich D, Penney KL, et al. Assessing the impact of population stratification on genetic association studies. Nat Genet 2004;36:388–393.
27. Beckmann JS, Estivill X, Antonarakis SE. Copy number variants and genetic traits: Closer to the resolution of phenotypic to genotypic variability. Nat Rev Genet 2007; 8:639–646.
28. Belfer I, Wu T, Kingman A, Krishnaraju RK, Goldman D, Max MB. Candidate gene studies of human pain mechanisms: Methods for optimizing choice of polymorphisms and sample size. Anesthesiology 2004;100:1562–1572.

Section III

Pain and Behavior

Measurement of Pain

Pierre Rainville

Pain in the oral region is a major reason people consult their dentist, and the clinician should acknowledge this simple fact by specifically asking about pain as a part of the basic dental examination. The assessment of pain symptoms may provide valuable clues to the differential diagnosis, to the evolution of an underlying pathology, to the treatment efficacy, and most importantly, to the patient's wellbeing. Pain may also have a variety of effects on other biologic and psychosocial functions. The assessment of pain should therefore be considered indispensable to provide optimal care and service.

The definition proposed by the International Association for the Study of Pain (IASP) emphasizes both sensory and affective-emotional aspects of pain and implies that clinicians evaluate both of these dimensions in their patients. A variety of measurement techniques are described in the following pages that rely on subjective report to evaluate these basic aspects of pain perception. Complementary behavioral and physiologic measures that offer additional indices of pain states are also briefly described. Recent advances in medical imaging that provide measurements of pain-related brain responses are discussed to further demonstrate that self-reports of pain reflect pain-related activity within the central nervous system (CNS).

Basic Characteristics of Measures

The gold standard for measurement of clinical or experimentally induced pain must fulfill a series of criteria.[1] A valid pain measure should be sensitive to changes in pain produced by variations in nociceptive input or by effective analgesic procedures (*criterion-related validity*). It should also enable a clinician to discriminate different pain conditions (eg, inflammatory vs neuropathic pain) in patients (*discriminant validity*). Pain measures should also be reliable—ie, stable in time and not affected by the experimenter testing a human volunteer in a pain experiment or the clinician taking the measurement from a pain patient. In addition to being highly valid and reliable,[2] a good pain measure should *(1)* allow for a comparison of the magnitude of changes in pain across treatments and pain conditions, *(2)* be relatively free of bias, *(3)* be useful for assessing both experimental and clinical pain, *(4)* allow for comparisons with neurobiologic measures in humans and animals to study underlying mechanisms, and *(5)* be relatively easy to use. In the broader context of clinical pain assessment, valid sets of measures should further sample the various dimensions of the pain experience and its effect on the patient's ability to function (*content validity*).

Box 10-1 Pain measurements

Self-report

- Pain threshold: the least experience of pain that a subject can recognize; the lowest stimulus intensity at which a subject perceives pain

- Pain tolerance: the greatest level of pain a subject is prepared to tolerate

- Pain scales (see Fig 10-1)

    Nominal and ordinal scales: translation of the pain experience according to discrete categories

    Magnitude estimation scales: translation of the pain experience on a continuum

    Pain questionnaires: evaluation of multiple dimensions of the pain experience via a combination of scales

Spontaneous motor/behavioral responses

- Facial: pain and emotional expression

- Vocal: nonverbal oral expression (eg, crying in neonates)

- Motor/behavioral: reduced motility, postural adjustments, changes in gait, protective behaviors, pain complaints, analgesic consumption

Physiologic responses

- Motor: nociceptive withdrawal reflex

- Autonomic: sympathetic and parasympathetic responses

- Endocrine: neurohormonal responses

- Neurophysiologic: activity within primary afferent nerve fibers, motor and sympathetic efferents, and the CNS

Subjective Reporting

The first category of measures relies on the collaboration with the subject to produce a response that reflects the pain experience as precisely as possible (Box 10-1).

Pain threshold and tolerance

Threshold measurement is the simple detection of pain in response to a stimulus. Pain thresholds can be measured by asking subjects to report when they feel pain during a gradual and controlled increase in stimulus intensity (method of limits), or in response to the repeated administration of discrete stimuli of different intensities (method of constant stimulus). The threshold is defined as the average point at which subjects start to feel pain, or as the stimulus intensity at which pain is felt in 50% of the trials. Reliable thresholds have been obtained with a variety of stimuli applied to skin, muscle, gingiva, and tooth pulp.[2,3] The clinical application of such reliable, quantifiable approaches has revealed, for example, that temporomandibular disorder (TMD) patients display abnormally low pressure pain thresholds both within and outside the region reported to be painful, which indicates the presence of allodynia and suggests that central mechanisms underlie the allodynia.[3] This approach is a good example of the value of using similar pre-

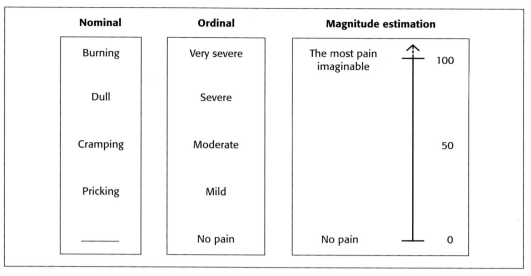

Nominal	Ordinal	Magnitude estimation
Burning	Very severe	The most pain imaginable — 100
Dull	Severe	
Cramping	Moderate	50
Pricking	Mild	
——	No pain	No pain — 0

Fig 10-1 Three types of pain scales relying on self-report. *Nominal scales* can be used to assess the quality of the sensation. *Ordinal scales* are designed to capture the level of pain experienced based on rank-ordered categories organized along a given dimension (eg, pain, pain sensation, pain unpleasantness). *Magnitude estimation* relies on the report of pain along a continuum typically represented by a line, numbers, or both. Verbal labels are generally assigned to both ends of the scale to indicate the extremes of the continuum. Exceeding the upper limit on numeric magnitude-estimation scales may be allowed to minimize potential regression biases (dotted arrow = unbounded estimation).

cise quantitative measurements in the laboratory and the clinic because it allows inferences to be drawn about underlying pathologic processes.

Pain tolerance measurements have been developed to quantify the other end of the continuum of pain experience[2] (see Box 10-1). Tolerance is most often measured experimentally by immersion of a subject's hand in near-freezing water (the *cold pressor test*) or by the temporary interruption of blood circulation in the arm *(ischemic pain)*. In these tests, tolerance is the maximum duration or the maximum intensity that a subject can willingly endure.

Threshold and tolerance measures are easy to use in experimental settings and can be easily adapted to test pain perception in patients. Their main limitation is the minimal information that each provides on a very restricted range of pain experience. They may also be less sensitive than magnitude estimation, and they are not adapted to the adequate description of spontaneous clinical pain.

Nominal and ordinal scales

Nominal and ordinal (category) scales are commonly used to evaluate clinical pain as well as treatment efficacy (Fig 10-1). In nominal scales, patients are asked to choose words from a list that most closely describe their pain. Nominal scales are best at describing the quality of pain and can be used to distinguish between various clinical conditions (eg, neuropathic vs inflammatory pain).

In ordinal scales, numbers, verbal labels, or images (eg, graded facial expressions) can represent different pain levels. Each scale is ideally associated with a single pain dimension (eg, quality, intensity, unpleasantness, pain-related anxiety).

The simplicity of nominal and ordinal scales explains their widespread use in clinical research and practice, but these methods have important limitations. First, the nominal scales may not include descriptors that cover all the possible pain experiences, thereby forcing patients to choose words that may not correspond precisely to their experience. Moreover, different people may interpret the same words differently, while the same people may use words differently depending on their condition.[4,5] When ordinal scales are used, the failure to control for the repartition of the different categories, paired with the tendency of subjects to distribute responses evenly between categories, may also lead to an important scaling bias.[2] Furthermore, the magnitude of the interval between categories is usually unknown, so that differences between groups and treatments or changes over time cannot be quantified and analyzed using the most powerful parametric statistical methods. To circumvent some of the problems associated with verbal-category nominal and ordinal scales, alternative methods of subjective reports have been developed that rely on magnitude estimation.

Magnitude estimation

Magnitude estimation requires subjects to indicate the level of pain experienced along a continuum represented in another modality such as loudness of a sound or handgrip strength[2] (cross-modality matching). Subjects may be asked to mark their pain level on a visual analog scale (VAS) or a numeric scale that represents pain sensory intensity or pain unpleasantness[6] (see Fig 10-1). Psychophysical functions can be estimated over a large range of stimulus and pain magnitudes by the use of these methods (Fig 10-2), and data obtained

allow for the estimation of absolute magnitude of changes (ratio properties). This is essential to establish a parallel between pain perception and physiologic activity and between clinical and experimental pain[7] (see Fig 10-2).

Magnitude-estimation scales are subject to various forms of bias. For example, in experimental settings, subjects tend to spread their responses across the entire range of the scale. Ratings of intense painful experiences may also be compressed at the upper end of scales that have an upper limit (bounded scales) so that a given increase in sensation is not represented uniformly along the full range of the scale (regression bias). Simple variations of these scales have been developed to reduce bias effects further by combining visual, numeric, verbal-descriptors category, and/or unbounded-scale properties to provide enhanced reliability and validity.

Multidimensional evaluation

Quantitative sensory testing (QST) uses several measurement methods (eg, threshold, tolerance, and magnitude-estimation) across several modalities (eg, touch, pressure, thermal pain) to provide a more comprehensive assessment of normal and abnormal pain perception. These tests are ideally designed and combined to examine specific pain-related neurophysiologic mechanisms (eg, temporal summation of pain to test central sensitization). QST thereby contributes to the characterization of the neuropathophysiologic changes associated with a variety of pain-related conditions (eg, neuropathic pain).

More complete pain assessment tools are typically in the form of a questionnaire or a series of magnitude-estimation scales.[8] The McGill Pain Questionnaire (MPQ) is the best-known assessment instrument and relies on multiple verbal-category scales.[9,10] After drawing the location of their pain on an outline of the body, subjects select words that best represent their experience of pain from a

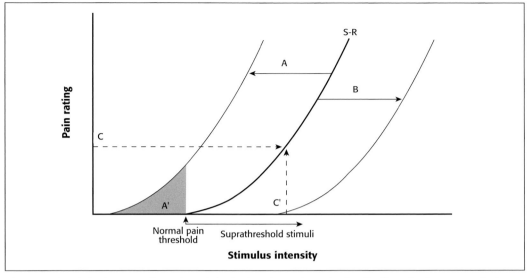

Fig 10-2a The relation between pain (y-axis) and stimulus intensity (x-axis) can be described by a stimulus-response (S-R) curve starting at pain threshold and typically increasing following a power function. Leftward shift of the curve indicates hyperalgesia (A); rightward shift of the curve indicates analgesia (B). Allodynia corresponds to the experience of pain in response to a stimulus that does not normally provoke pain (shaded area A'). Tests can also be used to match a patient's pain with a level of experimental pain. According to this method, a setup describing clinical pain (C) can be projected onto the S-R curve to infer the corresponding level of experimental pain (C'), as described in Fig 10-2b.

Fig 10-2b Stimulus-response (S-R) function used to establish a parallel between clinical and experimental pain. In the triangulation procedure, the S-R function is first calculated by asking patients to rate experimental pain over a broad intensity range (eg, electric stimulation of the tooth pulp). Using the same pain-rating scale, patients also rate their clinical pain or the pain evoked by a clinically relevant stimulus (eg, cold spray applied to the dentin) (C). Patients are further asked to find the level of experimental pain that best matches the clinical pain by adjusting the intensity of the experimental stimulus (eg, electric stimulation) (C'). Patients have been shown to produce highly consistent pain estimations attested by the convergence of clinical pain evaluation using pain rating and stimulus adjustment methods on the S-R function. Such observations provide concurrent validation to the scaling methods used.

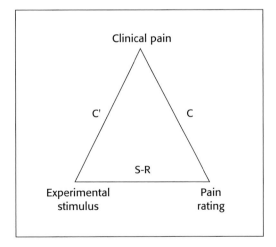

comprehensive list. Words are organized into several categories intended to reflect sensory (eg, pounding, cramping, burning), affective (eg, exhausting, terrifying, cruel), and evaluative (eg, intense, radiating) aspects of the experience. The temporal dynamic of pain is assessed separately using words describing the persistence, frequency, and duration of pain. Finally, patients rate the actual, least, and worst pain on an ordinal intensity scale ranging from 0 (mild) to 5 (excruciating). The MPQ has been adapted to a wide variety of clinical and experimental pain conditions and translated into several languages.

Several other pain assessment tools have been developed to thoroughly assess the multiple dimensions of pain.[11] Additional measures may be included in questionnaires to describe cognitive variables (eg, expectation of relief), pain-related behaviors (eg, moaning), and psychosocial factors (eg, how often do others express sympathy) known to interact with pain.[12] Finally, measures of functional activity, quality of life, treatment seeking, etc, can be included in assessments to describe the impact of pain on patient's lives and social interactions.

Behavioral and Physiologic Responses

Subjective reports have a limited application in many populations. They cannot be used in animals and preverbal infants, and their use is limited in children and in adults with language deficits or severe cognitive impairments. Alternative approaches have been developed that rely on the observation and quantification of spontaneous behavioral responses evoked during pain (see Box 10-1). These behavioral indices have shown various levels of sensitivity to interventions to diminish pain. One main challenge in the development of nonverbal indices of pain is to understand how they relate to other verbal and physiologic measures.

Physiologic measures also provide an important complementary approach to assess pain (see Box 10-1). For example, electromyographic (EMG) recordings of nociceptive reflexes and autonomic responses to noxious stimuli can be sensitive to various analgesic interventions and may be used to characterize abnormal pain responses. However, there are many problems in using those indices alone: (1) They are not specific to pain and may be observed in a variety of stressful situations; (2) some responses might be reversed in some conditions (eg, bradycardia in response to stimulation of the trigeminal region); (3) variability between individuals is usually large; (4) responses may habituate or sensitize with repetitive or sustained stimulation; and (5) they are only modestly correlated with subjective reports. Although physiologic indices are useful in group studies and are essential for comprehension of pain mechanisms, their weaknesses limit their use in a clinical context (see Mohl et al[13]).

Functional Brain Imaging

Medical imaging techniques have recently been developed to study the cerebral processes underlying pain.[14] Consistent with electrophysiologic recordings made in animals (see chapter 5), these studies have shown activation of primary and secondary somatosensory cortices, the insula, and anterior cingulate cortex during acute pain. The measured responses are proportional to the intensity of the nociceptive stimulus and to the intensity of the pain reported by the subjects.[15] Changes in pain induced by various interventions (eg, opiate drug, hypnosis, placebo) also reflect a modulation of the activity within those brain areas (see chapter 11). Brain-imaging investigations of sustained clinical pain states have provided more equivocal results, but several studies have shown abnormal activity within the same brain areas.[14]

Summary

This chapter has outlined the considerable advances that have been made in pain measurements in the past few decades. The usefulness of systematic pain assessment is now widely recognized. Quantitative psychophysical methods adapted to both experimental and clinical studies have been developed to describe multiple aspects of the pain experience. Elaborate questionnaires have also been validated to assess both the sensory-affective and the complex psychosocial aspects of pain. More recently, brain-imaging techniques have provided powerful means to assess neurophysiologic responses associated with pain. Although the self-report measures of pain are often thought to suffer from their subjective nature, brain-imaging studies have demonstrated that they reliably reflect brain activity.

No simple rule governs the choice of pain measurements, and different methods and pain scales are best adapted as necessary to different clinical and experimental conditions. Clinicians and researchers must therefore select the instruments and methods that best respond to their specific needs and questions.

References

1. Gracely RH. Studies of pain in human subjects. In: McMahon S, Kaltzenburg M (eds). Wall and Melzack's Textbook of Pain, ed 5. London: Elsevier, 2006:267–290.

2. Harris G, Rollman GB. The validity of experimental pain-measures. Pain 1983;17:369–376.

3. Reid KI, Gracely RH, Dubner R. The influence of time, facial side, and location on pain-pressure thresholds in chronic myogenous temporomandibular disorder. J Orofac Pain 1994;8:258–265.

4. Urban BJ, Keefe FJ, France RD. A study of psychophysical scaling in chronic pain patients. Pain 1984;20:157–168.

5. Fernandez E, Towery S. A parsimonious set of verbal descriptors of pain sensation derived from the McGill Pain Questionnaire. Pain 1996;66:31–37.

6. Price DD, McGrath PA, Rafii A, Buckingham B. The validation of visual analogue scales as ratio scale measures for chronic and experimental pain. Pain 1983;17:45–56.

7. Heft MW, Gracely RH, Dubner R, McGrath PA. A validation model for verbal descriptor scaling of human clinical pain. Pain 1980;9:363–373.

8. Wade JB, Dougherty LM, Archer CR, Price DD. Assessing the stages of pain processing: A multivariate analytical approach. Pain 1996;68:157–167.

9. Melzack R. The McGill Pain Questionnaire: Major properties and scoring methods. Pain 1975;1:277–299.

10. Melzack R. The short-form McGill Pain Questionnaire. Pain 1987;30:191–197.

11. Turk DC, Melzack R. Handbook of Pain Assessment, ed 2. New York: Guilford Press, 2001.

12. Thomas RJ, McEwen J, Asbury AJ. The Glasgow Pain Questionnaire: A new generic measure of pain; development and testing. Int J Epidemiol 1996;25:1060–1067.

13. Mohl ND, Lund JP, Widmer CG, McCall WD Jr. Devices for the diagnosis and treatment of temporomandibular disorders. Part II: Electromyography and sonography. J Prosthet Dent 1990;63(3):332–336 [erratum 1990;63(5):13].

14. Apkarian AV, Bushnell MC, Treede RD, Zubieta JK. Human brain mechanisms of pain perception and regulation in health and disease. Eur J Pain 2005;9:463–484.

15. Coghill RC, McHaffie JG, Yen YF. Neural correlates of interindividual differences in the subjective experience of pain. Proc Natl Acad Sci U S A 2003;100:8538–8542.

Psychologic State and Pain Perception

Petra Schweinhardt
Marco L. Loggia
Chantal Villemure
M. Catherine Bushnell

Why do some people experience terrible pain during a dental procedure, whereas others experience little or no pain during the same procedure? Are some patients just less tolerant than others, or does the pain experience actually differ from person to person? For many reasons, including individual genetic makeup and life experiences, not everyone experiences a painful stimulus in the same way. Evidence now shows that the varied perceptual experiences of pain are based on different levels of activity in pain-transmission and pain-modulation pathways in the brain. This chapter will address how the psychologic states of people can affect the processing of nociceptive information in the brain and, therefore, their perceptions of pain.

There have always been anecdotal accounts of people apparently experiencing little or no pain in situations that most of us would find intolerable, yet Western medicine has given little credence to a patient's ability to modify pain, focusing instead on the pharmacologic control of pain. For this reason, the majority of research on pain control has concentrated on peripheral and spinal cord mechanisms of opioid and anti-inflammatory analgesic therapy. Nevertheless, researchers are increasingly recognizing that a variety of pain-modulation mechanisms exist within the nervous system and that these can be accessed either pharmacologically or through contextual and/or psychologic manipulation.[1] Variables such as attentional state, emotional context, empathy, hypnotic suggestions, attitudes, and expectations, including the placebo response, now have been shown to alter both pain processing in the brain and pain perception. Techniques that modify these variables can preferentially alter sensory and/or affective aspects of pain perception. The associated modulation of pain-evoked neural activity occurs in limbic and/or sensory brain regions, suggesting multiple endogenous pain-modulation systems (see chapter 8).

Focusing on Pain Can Make It Worse

Attentional state is probably the most widely studied psychologic variable that modifies the pain experience. A number of clinical and experimental studies show that pain is perceived as less intense when a person is distracted from the pain (see Villemure and Bushnell[2] and Apkarian et al[3] for a review). Distraction was achieved in these studies by asking subjects to focus on something else. In a clinical setting, patients may be given music to listen to or videos to watch. However, a few studies indicate that focusing on pain may actually have the paradoxic effect of reducing its perceived intensity in certain individuals. For example, Hadjistavropoulos et al[4] observed that chronic pain patients who were particularly health anxious reported less anxiety and pain when they focused on the physical sensations. Thus, the effect of attention and/or distraction on pain may not be uniformly predictable but rather influenced by such variables as personality type.

In some studies, subjects were asked to rate separately how intense the pain sensation was and how much it bothered them (ie, pain intensity versus pain unpleasantness). These studies have shown that attending to another sensory modality during pain results in parallel reductions in both perceived intensity and unpleasantness of the pain, sometimes with a greater modulation of pain intensity.[5] Correspondingly, attention-related modulation of neural activity evoked by noxious stimuli has been observed in pain-related pathways throughout the brain. At the level of the cerebral cortex, imaging studies have shown attention-related modulation of pain-evoked responses in both sensory and limbic cortical areas, including the primary (SI) and secondary (SII) somatosensory cortices, the anterior cingulate cortex, and the insular cortex; these structures showed greater activation when the subject was attending to pain (see Apkarian et al[3] for a review). Figure 11-1 shows that the SI cortex is more activated by noxious stimuli when subjects are required to attend to the pain than when they attend to an auditory stimulus. Thus, simply distracting a patient from pain can have profound consequences in how the pain is processed in the brain.

Our Emotions Affect Our Perception of Pain

Mood and emotional state also affect pain perception; negative emotions lead to more pain than positive emotions. Clinical studies have shown that emotional states and attitudes of patients influence pain that is associated with chronic diseases.[7] In the experimental context, manipulations that positively affect mood or emotional state, such as pleasant music, odors, pictures, and humorous films, generally reduce pain perception; whereas those that negatively affect mood and induce negative emotions, such as anxiety, increase pain perception.[2]

What Are the Mechanisms by Which Attention and Emotions Alter Pain?

The neural mechanisms underlying attentional and emotional modulation of pain and the changes in activity of the cortical areas subserving pain perception are not fully known, but they most likely involve various levels of the central nervous system (CNS). An opiate-sensitive descending pathway from the frontal cortex to the amygdala, periaqueductal gray (PAG), rostral ventral medulla, and trigeminal brain stem sensory nuclear complex (VBSNC) and spinal cord dorsal horn has been implicated in psychologic modulation of pain (see chapter 8). Some researchers have suggested that this pathway is involved in attentional modulation of pain, but these studies have typically used tasks that simultaneously altered attention and emotions. For example, Valet and colleagues[8] found an activation of the frontal cortex–PAG pathway when subjects were distracted from their pain. However, they used the incongruent color-word Stroop task as the distractor, which is distracting but also stressful and increases arousal. Thus, both emotional and attentional states were probably altered. When odors were used to manipulate attention to pain and emotional state independently, it was found that the PAG is preferentially implicated in emotional modulation of pain, whereas the superior posterior parietal cortex is more important for attentional modulation.[9]

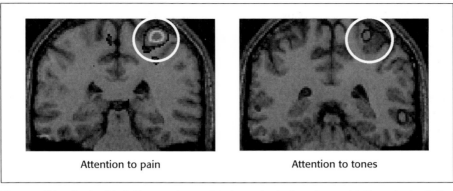

Attention to pain   Attention to tones

Fig 11-1 Pain-related activity in SI cortex when a subject's attention is directed to a painful heat stimulus *(left)* or to an auditory stimulus *(right)*. Activity was determined by subtracting positron emission tomography (PET) data recorded when a warm stimulus (32°C to 38°C) was presented from those recorded when a painfully hot stimulus (46.5°C to 48.5°C) was presented during each attentional state. Adapted from Bushnell et al.[6]

How Can the Clinician Use Attention and Emotions to Reduce a Patient's Pain?

Dental procedures are often a source of anxiety in patients. The prevalence of dental anxiety in the general population is in the range of 4% to 20%, independent of population, culture, and country; its incidence is not reduced by improving dental treatment.[10] Since it appears that both distraction and a positive emotional state alter pain, and they do so through separate modulatory systems, any activity that both diverts attention from a painful procedure and helps improve a patient's emotional state could be particularly useful in a dental setting. Because anxiety and stress increase pain perception, it seems particularly important to use interventions that reduce anxiety and improve mood, in addition to distracting the patient. A number of methods can be easily implemented in the dental clinic setting, eg, playing music, showing humorous films on a monitor installed above the dental chair, or filling the room with pleasant odors. Such methods have been shown to be effective in reducing dental pain.[11,12,13]

Social Influences on Pain

Although pain is commonly referred to as a private experience, research shows that social interaction influences how we perceive and/or communicate our pain. For instance, the mere presence of another individual in pain can modify pain behaviors by promoting a form of imitative learning termed *social modeling*. A number of years ago, Craig et al[14] showed that when subjects are tested in a room where an actor is purportedly receiving painful stimulation, they will increase or decrease their pain behavior to match that of the actor: if the actor exhibits tolerance to pain, subjects will tolerate more pain and will rate the pain as less intense, and vice versa if the actor exhibits low tolerance.

People around us can also influence our pain behavior with their attitudes toward our pain. Illness or pain behaviors can in fact be inadvertently reinforced if their occurrence is accompanied by special attention from others (eg, family) or offers the opportunity to avoid unpleasant situations. For instance, solicitous attention from parents predicted slower recovery from oral surgery in adolescent patients.[15]

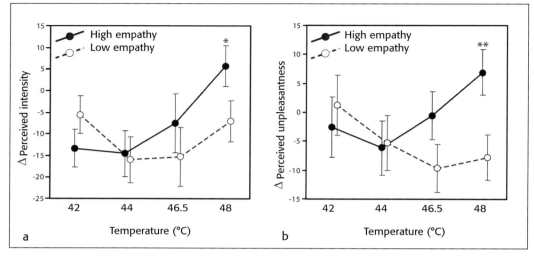

Fig 11-2 Effects of empathy on pain perception. Increased empathy resulted in increased perceived (a) intensity and (b) unpleasantness of painful stimuli but not for nonpainful stimuli. The high empathy group reported the 48°C stimulus as significantly more intense and unpleasant than the low empathy group. Graphs show the average rating for each temperature while the participants watched the testing video minus the baseline rating recorded while the participants watched the neutral cityscape video. Bars represent mean ± SEM. $P = .06$; $*P < .05$; $**P < .01$. Adapted with permission from Loggia et al.[17]

"I feel your pain": Empathy can increase pain

There is now evidence that witnessing the distress of others can alter pain perception, independent of imitative behavior. Langford and colleagues[16] showed that if a mouse is exposed to another mouse in pain, it displays increased pain sensitivity, but only if the two mice have had previous social contact with each other. The authors showed evidence that this social modulation of pain cannot be explained by imitation. They instead proposed that empathy, or a precursory form of it, can induce an increase in pain perception.

A similar phenomenon has now been shown in humans. In one study,[17] participants' sensitivity to nonpainful and painful heat stimuli applied to the hand was measured during exposure to a neutral cityscape video to establish their baseline response. Then subjects were divided into two groups. A state of high empathy was induced by having one group of subjects watch a video of an actor telling a sad personal story, whereas a state of low empathy was induced in the other group of subjects with a video of the same actor describing how he managed to dupe somebody out of money. Thermal sensitivity was measured again while participants watched the video of the actor receiving painful or innocuous heat stimuli. Subjects in the high empathy group rated painful heat stimuli as more intense and unpleasant than did subjects in the low empathy group, but ratings of nonpainful heat did not differ between groups (Fig 11-2). As in the mice, the increased pain could not be explained by imitative behavior.

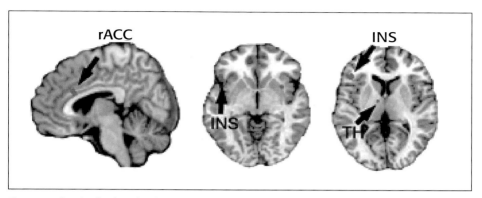

Fig 11-3 Pain-related regions showing correlations between placebo effects in reported pain and placebo effects in pain-related neural activity. *(left)* When painful shock was presented to the subjects, the rostral anterior cingulate cortex (rACC) was activated more during the control condition than during placebo. *(middle and right)* Similar effects were observed in the insular cortex (INS) and thalamus (TH). Adapted with permission from Wager et al.[19]

Why does empathizing with others affect our own pain perception?

A number of studies using functional magnetic resonance imaging (fMRI) of the brain have shown that watching somebody in pain leads to the activation of brain areas involved in first-person perception of pain, such as the anterior cingulate cortex and rostral insula.[18] It appears that empathy can sensitize pain pathways of the brain.

Placebo and Orofacial Pain

Placebo analgesia refers to the reduction of pain sensations after administration of an inert agent, ie, one that does not possess any specific activity for the condition being treated. As discussed above, psychosocial factors, such as faith in the therapeutic procedure or desire for pain relief, play a role in the effectiveness of *any* medical or dental treatment. The administration of a placebo reveals the effects of these factors that are normally entangled with the specific effects of the active treatment. Brain imaging has been extremely useful in estab-

lishing that placebo analgesia is indeed real by showing that placebo-induced pain relief is associated with a concomitant decrease of brain activity in pain-processing areas such as the thalamus and the insular cortex[19] (Fig 11-3). This means that reported pain reductions following placebos are real effects rather than being merely due to changes in pain reporting or compliance with experimental instructions.

How do placebos exert their analgesic effects?

About 30 years ago, Levine and colleagues[20] showed that pain relief induced by administration of a placebo after dental surgery could be blocked by the opioid-receptor antagonist naloxone. Since then, numerous reports have supported the idea that endogenous opioids are important for placebo analgesia. Endogenous opioids are essential for the descending inhibitory control of pain. The brain stem PAG and rostroventral medulla are two key areas for descending pain control,[1] and as noted above and in chapter 8, this circuitry is probably involved in the emotional modulation of pain.

These regions project to the VBSNC and spinal cord and inhibit incoming nociceptive signals. Human imaging studies show increased activation of brain stem structures during placebo analgesia; the anterior cingulate and prefrontal cortices, which are activated by placebo procedures, may play a role in placebo analgesia by tapping into the descending pain modulatory system via their projections to the PAG.[19]

Summary

This chapter has referred to the extensive evidence that psychologic factors influence pain perception. Neuroimaging studies show that activity in pain pathways is altered by attentional state, positive and negative emotions, stress, empathy, and the administration of a placebo. The same psychologic factors activate intrinsic modulatory systems in the brain, including those stimulated when opiates are given for pain relief. It is important for both the patient and the clinician to be aware of the effect of psychologic state on pain transmission so that patients can learn to participate in their own pain control and clinicians can create an environment that helps their patients reduce anxiety, improve mood, and focus attention away from the pain.

References

1. Fields HL. Pain modulation: Expectation, opioid analgesia and virtual pain. Prog Brain Res 2000;122:245–253.
2. Villemure C, Bushnell MC. Cognitive modulation of pain: How do attention and emotion influence pain processing? Pain 2002;95:195–199.
3. Apkarian AV, Bushnell MC, Treede RD, Zubieta JK. Human brain mechanisms of pain perception and regulation in health and disease. Eur J Pain 2005;9:463–484.
4. Hadjistavropoulos HD, Hadjistavropoulos T, Quine A. Health anxiety moderates the effects of distraction versus attention to pain. Behav Res Ther 2000;38:425–438.
5. Villemure C, Slotnick BM, Bushnell MC. Effects of odors on pain perception: Deciphering the roles of emotion and attention. Pain 2003;106:101–108.
6. Bushnell MC, Duncan GH, Hofbauer RK, Ha B, Chen JI, Carrier B. Pain perception: Is there a role for primary somatosensory cortex? Proc Natl Acad Sci U S A 1999; 96:7705–7709.
7. Haythornthwaite JA, Benrud-Larson LM. Psychological aspects of neuropathic pain. Clin J Pain 2000;16(2 suppl):S101–S105.
8. Valet M, Sprenger T, Boecker H, et al. Distraction modulates connectivity of the cingulo-frontal cortex and the midbrain during pain—An fMRI analysis. Pain 2004;109: 399–408.
9. Villemure C, Bushnell MC. Mood and attention influence supra-spinal pain processing differentially. J Neurosci 2008 (in press).
10. Skaret E, Soevdsnes EK. Behavioural science in dentistry. The role of the dental hygienist in prevention and treatment of the fearful dental patient. Int J Dent Hyg 2005; 3:2–6.
11. Satoh Y, Nagai E, Kitamura K, et al. Relaxation effect of an audiovisual system on dental patients. Part 2. Palus-amplitude. J Nihon Univ Sch Dent 1995;37:138–145.
12. Aitken JC, Wilson S, Coury D, Moursi AM. The effect of music distraction on pain, anxiety and behavior in pediatric dental patients. Pediatr Dent 2002;24:114–118.
13. Lehrner J, Marwinski G, Lehr S, Johren P, Deecke L. Ambient odors of orange and lavender reduce anxiety and improve mood in a dental office. Physiol Behav 2005; 86:92–95.
14. Craig KD, Weiss SM. Vicarious influences on pain-threshold determinations. J Pers Soc Psychol 1971;19: 53–59.
15. Gidron Y, McGrath PJ, Goodday R. The physical and psychosocial predictors of adolescents' recovery from oral surgery. J Behav Med 1995;18:385–399.
16. Langford DJ, Crager SE, Shehzad Z, et al. Social modulation of pain as evidence for empathy in mice. Science 2006;312:1967–1970.
17. Loggia ML, Mogil JS, Bushnell MC. Empathy hurts: Compassion for another increases both sensory and affective components of pain perception. Pain 2008 (in press).
18. Singer T. The neuronal basis and ontogeny of empathy and mind reading: Review of literature and implications for future research. Neurosci Biobehav Rev 2006;30: 855–863.
19. Wager TD, Rilling JK, Smith EE, et al. Placebo-induced changes in FMRI in the anticipation and experience of pain. Science 2004;303:1162–1167.
20. Levine JD, Gordon NC, Fields HL. The mechanism of placebo analgesia. Lancet 1978;2:654–657.

12

Psychosocial Factors

Samuel F. Dworkin

There is abundant evidence from epidemiologic and clinical research, and more recently from behavioral neuroscience (supported by brain imaging studies), that the psychosocial environment contains potent risk factors for pain, especially chronic pain.[1,2] The term *psychosocial* encompasses both factors within the individual (eg, anxiety, depression) and factors in the environment that influence how patients might express pain and/or seek treatment. These factors may be as diverse as the availability of dental treatment and pain medications or the way in which prior experience (learning and memory), culture, and society shape how people reveal their pain experience. Most importantly, an understanding of the psychosocial aspects of the pain experience expands possibilities for pain management by creating opportunities for biobehaviorally based treatments that can modify the emotional, cognitive (thinking), and behavioral status of a patient to achieve the following objectives:

1. Produce a more compliant and better informed patient
2. Eliminate or minimize negative physiologic and emotional states—especially depression, anxiety, fear, and the anticipation of pain

3. Potentiate the action of sedative, analgesic, and anesthetic pharmacologic agents used to control pain and anxiety
4. Introduce cognitive-behavioral methods to assist the patient in self-management and enhanced self-control for both acute and chronic pain, with and without analgesic or sedative medications

This chapter addresses the perceptions, appraisals, and behaviors shown by people reporting dental and orofacial pain. Some biobehaviorally based approaches to the management of acute pain are discussed in chapter 11, while those applicable to persistent or chronic pain are interwoven throughout the chapters in section IV, Management of Orofacial Pain: Principles and Practices. It is important to remember that the stomatognathic system is responsible for several life-sustaining physiologic processes, including eating, breathing, swallowing, and verbal as well as nonverbal communication. Psychologic factors play an important—some would say a central—role in the perceptions, appraisals, and behaviors of people when pain arises in such a biologically and personally important part of the body as the face and mouth.[3,4]

Types of Pain

Patients seek out dentists for relief of pain arising from toothache or periapical inflammation that can reach excruciating levels, and many are driven to dentists for relief of diffuse longer-lasting orofacial pain caused by neurologic or musculoskeletal factors.

Acute pain

The expectation that the dentist can relieve pain has been strongly positive for dentistry, and dentistry has in fact learned a great deal about pain and pain control, especially when the pain is acute. Alleviation of the pain of dental procedures has been developed to a high degree, and for most people requiring routine dental care, pain associated with treatment is largely preventable. Each clinician must learn how best to respond to the anxiety or other emotions that accompany a patient's experience; evidence shows that these psychologic processes have a direct influence on acute pain threshold and tolerance levels. This is true whether the pain is associated with treatments or is postoperative, and whether it accompanies dental, medical, surgical, or invasive diagnostic procedures.[4]

Chronic pain

Chronic neuropathic and musculoskeletal pains are not only perceived by patients as more diffuse and more persistent types of pain than more common acute dental pain but, as the name implies, remain more resistant to quick or simple resolution (see subsequent chapters on pain management). The amount and even the location of chronic pain, as well as the behaviors of the patient, are only poorly predicted by physical events. Atypical odontalgia, for example, is usually associated with poorly defined pathologic markers inconsistent with expressed pain perception and behavior. Similarly,

myalgia can be a source of minor inconvenience to some patients; for others, it can become a major decades-long disorganizing force associated with significant depression and disruption of everyday activities—yet, there may be no detectable physical change to distinguish the two conditions. So, the impact of persistent pain often cannot be understood in terms of pathology. It is the deleterious and life-changing quality of chronic orofacial pain that makes it such an important area for study and action by researchers and clinicians alike.

Biomedical Models of Pain

The subjectivity of pain means that many biomedically oriented health care providers do not believe that it is critical to attend to patients' descriptions of how pain affects their daily lives, since such descriptions are not biologically based. Often, interest in psychosocial factors is equated with the assumption that the pain experience is imaginary/not real or is being made up by the patient, especially when the clinician cannot find a biologically plausible explanation for the pain.

Thus, mechanistic and strictly biomedical views of pain, while appealing because of their deceptive simplicity, are scientifically unwarranted. For example, it is not considered likely that a single "pain gene" will be discovered which, in isolation, determines the varied ways in which people around the world express complex conditions such as chronic pain (see chapter 9).[5,6] The biomedical model has been succeeded by a biopsychosocial model (more thorough discussion follows) that clarifies how physical events in the body can give rise to pain and pain relief–seeking behaviors that are influenced by the patients' pain history, gender, and ethnicity as well as to factors in the environment (eg, having to go to the dentist) that are equated with pain or the potential for pain.

The Neurologic and Psychosocial Interface

Current neurophysiology and cognitive neuro-science provide a biologic basis for understanding how emotional, cognitive, and behavioral processes can become linked and stored, preserving memories and belief systems that influence the pain experience and guide actions we take to cope with pain. There is increased acceptance among patients and clinicians alike that the complex, hard-to-understand pain-related behaviors are real bodily processes that result from complex central processing of pain information. It is important to understand that pain, while it is in the brain, is not "all in the head" given the pejorative and highly judgmental sense the latter phrase unfortunately conveys.

Biopsychosocial Model of Pain

Figure 12-1 presents a schematic for integration of physiologic or pathophysiologic activity with associated psychologic states and socially and culturally determined behavior. The model, known as the *biopsychosocial model*, is currently accepted as the basis for understanding complex physiologic and psychosocial interactions evident in all disease and illness. The model has been applied to the understanding of chronic pain and has served as the basis for extensive research into chronic orofacial pain.[7] The stages of the pain experience offered by this model reflect normal mechanisms through which individuals come to experience pain, attempt to make sense of the pain, and adapt to deal with the pain appropriately. These same higher-order processes are subject to distortions and maladaptive responses as well. Following are some examples for each level at which it is possible to analyze complex expressions of pain within the framework of this biopsychosocial model.

Nociception

Nociception involves the physiologic events in the pain-transmission system that, among other things, provide pain information to higher centers dealing with attention, memory, emotions, decision-making, and motor preparedness. The topic of nociception is discussed in earlier chapters dealing with peripheral and central biologic mechanisms for pain (see chapters 4 to 8).

Perception

Perception is the initial stage of forming a pain response and identifying the physical qualities of the pain experience. It is dealt with at some length in chapter 11.

Appraisal

Appraisal involves higher-order integrative mental operations attaching cognitive and emotional meaning to the sensations being perceived. Appraisal is crucial for attaching attitudes, beliefs, expectations, and emotional arousal to those pain sensations—in short, this is the level at which meaning is attributed to the physical experience. Inappropriate attribution of meaning, influenced by attention and memory, may yield pain-related catastrophizing thoughts, anxiety or phobia, depression, or somatization, ie, the tendency for a person to label readily detected nonspecific physical sensations as symptoms of disease.

Behavior

Observable pain-related behaviors are either contributory to pain (eg, myoclonus) or the result of pain (eg, verbal and nonverbal expressions of pain, inactivity, or diet modification). Fordyce's[8] introduction of the notion of pain behaviors into the rehabilitation of chronic pain patients called attention to the possibility that chronic pain can become

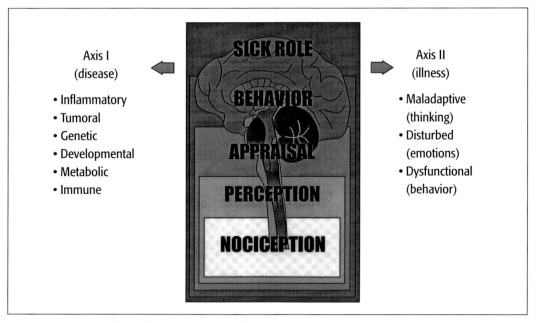

Axis I
(disease)

- Inflammatory
- Tumoral
- Genetic
- Developmental
- Metabolic
- Immune

SICK ROLE

BEHAVIOR

APPRAISAL

PERCEPTION

NOCICEPTION

Axis II
(illness)

- Maladaptive
  (thinking)
- Disturbed
  (emotions)
- Dysfunctional
  (behavior)

Fig 12-1 Biopsychosocial model for pain. The model's five-stage process integrates physiologic or pathophysiologic activity with associated psychologic states and socially and culturally determined behavior.

associated with maladaptive patterns of work or social avoidance and that treatment should not focus exclusively on uncovering difficult-to-observe pathophysiology but should employ behaviorally based methods for returning the pain patient to a more productive lifestyle. Regarding acute pain, inappropriate behavior may include avoidance of dental care except under crisis conditions. The persistence of oral behaviors such as thumb sucking or bruxism may become associated with chronic pain and/or dental deformations.

Sick role

Social expectations and rules shape how we express our pain. Sanctioning of different sick roles for men and women in response to pain is an important example of the influence that social factors

can play in determining manifestations of pain (eg, that it is "unmanly" to acknowledge being in pain). Patients with the most treatment-resistant forms of temporomandibular disorders (TMDs) are at risk for abusing health care services, including excessive treatment-seeking behavior and the repeated demand for narcotic pain medications, both often examples of dysfunctional chronic pain behaviors.

The biopsychosocial model, as its name implies, reflects our growing understanding that illnesses and cures are indeed complex; to understand how and when we experience pain and how we will respond to treatment, a host of factors in addition to biology must be considered. This model does not seek to compete with, let alone to replace, scientifically derived biologic models or current clinical practices.

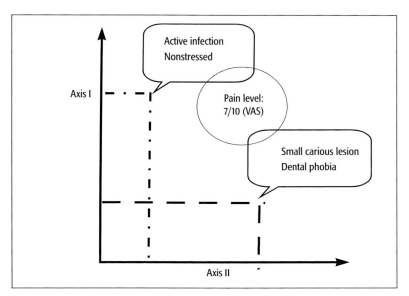

Fig 12-2 Dual-axis schematic for pain assessment. Axis I represents the status of a patient's biomedical, physical, and clinical factors that may yield a biologically based diagnosis; Axis II represents a patient's psychologic, emotional, and behavioral status. VAS = visual analog scale.

A Dual-Axis Approach to Assessment of Dental and Orofacial Pain

The pragmatic application of a biopsychosocial model of pain for dentistry is to avoid thinking of pain as either solely physical or mental, simply biologic or psychologic, either in the body, hence "real," or in the mind, hence "imagined." Instead of trying to force a particular patient with pain onto one end or the other of a single psychologic versus somatic continuum, at least two axes are conceptualized for characterizing patients in pain. Each patient should be located on one axis that reflects the status of physical/clinical factors that may yield a biologically based diagnosis, and on a second axis that reflects psychologic, emotional, or behavioral status.[9] Figure 12-2 presents a schematic for such a dual-axis approach to assessing, diagnosing, and treating orofacial pain.

Assessing Pain-Relevant Psychologic and Psychosocial Factors

Because chronic pain is such an enigmatic challenge and because TMDs are the overwhelmingly most common form of chronic orofacial pain,[3,10] the remainder of this chapter will draw examples primarily from TMDs to provide guides to the integrated and comprehensive biobehavioral assessment and diagnosis.

When assessing the contribution of Axis II psychologic and psychosocial factors (see Fig 12-2), four domains are recommended: (1) pain history and response to prior treatment; (2) parafunctional oral behaviors (eg, assessment of bruxism, pernicious oral habits); (3) psychologic screening; and (4) dysfunctional behaviors that interfere with daily activities and/or compromise quality of life. The assessment of these biobehavioral domains is possible largely through routine history and examination methods described in chapter 17. Because psychologic upset and pain-related disability are such common features of chronic orofacial pain, a brief discussion is provided of readily available methods that dentists can use to assess psychologic and psychosocial disability.

Psychologic status

Recommended screening assessments for psychologic status include those for depression, anxiety, and the presence of multiple nonspecific physical symptoms referred to in psychiatry as *somatization*.[11,12] Formal assessment requires specialized measurement instruments and/or diagnostic interview schedules beyond the training and clinical expertise of most dentists. However, the routine inclusion of relatively straightforward measures[9,11,13] in a clinical database minimizes patients' resistance to the perception that attention is being unduly given to psychologic factors when they present with a physical pain problem. Such measures are appropriate only as screening aids and allow impressions to be formed concerning the need for more specialized psychologic assessment by a psychiatrist or clinical psychologist. Depression commonly co-occurs with chronic pain conditions and has been extensively documented in TMD clinic populations. Similarly, the reporting of widespread, nonspecific physical symptoms is present in a significant minority of TMD patients, and such long-standing nonspecific physical symptoms represent an important obstacle to successful treatment.[14]

Regarding acute dental and orofacial pain, anxiety and panic are emotional disturbances seen in phobic dental patients and patients who find any form of invasive dental procedure so intensely aversive that they may avoid all but the most urgent dental care. The paradox here is that such dental neglect virtually assures chronic dental and orofacial infection or inflammation, which will cause

more acute pain than the relevant dental treatment so assiduously being avoided by these dentally anxious or phobic individuals.[4,15]

Psychosocial functioning and quality of life

The Graded Chronic Pain Scale (GCPS) has been validated for assessing the current level of psychosocial functioning.[16] It has been used primarily in conjunction with Axis II assessment of chronic orofacial pain patients by relating pain intensity levels to extent of pain-related interference with activities of daily living and extent of health care utilization. Prognosis is more guarded when self-reported activity limitations are high and when pain interferes appreciably with the ability to discharge responsibilities at home, school, or work, and/or when it limits social activities. The assessment of both psychologic status and level of psychosocial function is viewed as essential to allowing rational management of any chronic pain condition, including TMDs.[17]

A guide to the content, administration, scoring, and interpretation of the depression, somatization, and GCPS is available from the International Consortium for RDC/TMD-Based Research (http://www.rdc-tmdinternational.org/). In addition, the National Institutes for Health provide an interactive text (http://symptomresearch.nih.gov/chapter_22/index.htm) on research and management of clinically important symptoms, such as fatigue, somatization, cardiac pain, and TMDs.

Oral Health–Related Quality of Life

Oral health–related quality of life measures, including the oral health impact profile, assess how oral health status relates to the ability to actively control, participate in, and enjoy one's personal and social life. Such broader approaches to assessment of the personal functioning of patients with orofacial pain are relatively new but have already yielded promising insights into how pain deters lifestyle.[18]

Summary

This chapter has introduced the biologically plausible biopsychosocial model for pain. Its corollary, the dual-axis approach to evaluating dental or orofacial pain, provides a scientific underpinning from both the biologic and behavioral sciences for *(1)* maintaining a multidisciplinary perspective when evaluating pain and *(2)* incorporating psychologic and psychosocial measures into patients' comprehensive history and clinical examination. The focus of the chapter has been directed at elucidating underlying global concepts and methods for assessing whether or not psychosocial aspects of pain are impacting lives of dental patients. Much evidence has accumulated that attests to the effectiveness of behaviorally based treatments for chronic pain, either in conjunction with medical/surgical interventions or as "stand-alone" therapies. Excellent sources of additional information for concerned clinicians are available, including evidence-based biobehavioral interventions that are suitable for incorporation into dental practice.[4,11,17–20]

References

1. Blyth FM, Macfarlane G, Nicholas MK. The contribution of psychosocial factors to the development of chronic pain: The key to better outcomes for patients? Pain 2007; 129:8–11.
2. Wright AR, Gatchel RJ, Wildenstein L, Riggs R, Buschang P, Ellis E. Biopsychosocial differences in high-risk and low-risk patients with acute TMD-related pain. J Am Diet Assoc 2004;135:474–483.
3. Dworkin SF. Chronic orofacial pain: Biobehavioral perspectives. In: Mostofsky DI, Forgione AG, Giddon DB (eds). Behavioral Dentistry. Ames, IA: Blackwell Munksgaard, 2006:99–114.
4. Eli I. Oral Psychophysiology: Stress, Pain, and Behavior in Dental Care. Boca Raton, FL: CRC Press, 1992.
5. Zubieta JK, Heitzeg MM, Smith YR, et al. COMT val158met genotype affects mu-opioid neurotransmitter responses to a pain stressor. Science 2003;299: 1240–1243.
6. Davey Smith G, Ebrahim S, Lewis S, Hansell AL, Palmer LJ, Burton PR. Genetic epidemiology and public health: Hope, hype, and future prospects. Lancet. 2005;366 (9495):1484–1498.
7. Dworkin SF, Von Korff M, LeResche L. Epidemiologic studies of chronic pain: A dynamic-ecologic perspective. Ann Behav Med 1992;14:3–11.
8. Fordyce WE. Behavioral Methods for Chronic Pain and Illness. St Louis: Mosby, 1976.
9. Dworkin SF, LeResche L. Research diagnostic criteria for temporomandibular disorders: Review, criteria, examinations and specifications, critique. J Craniomandib Disord 1992;6:301–355.
10. Greene CS. Concepts of TMD etiology: Effects on diagnosis and treatment. In: Laskin DM, Greene CS, Hylander WL (eds). Temporomandibular Disorders: An Evidence-Based Approach to Diagnosis and Treatment. Chicago: Quintessence, 2006:219–228.
11. Turner JA, Dworkin SF. Screening for psychosocial risk factors in patients with chronic orofacial pain: Recent advances. J Am Diet Assoc 2004;135:1119–1125.
12. American Psychiatric Association; Task Force on DSM-IV. Diagnostic and Statistical Manual of Mental Disorders: DSM-IV, ed 4. Washington, DC: American Psychiatric Association, 1994.
13. Derogatis LR. SCL-90-R: Administration, Scoring and Procedures Manual, ed 2. Towson, MD: Clinical Psychometric Research, 1983.
14. Yap AU, Chua EK, Tan KB, Chan YH. Relationships between depression/somatization and self-reports of pain and disability. J Orofac Pain 2004;18:220–225.
15. Heaton LJ, Carlson CR, Smith TA, Baer RA, de Leeuw R. Predicting anxiety during dental treatment using patients' self-reports: Less is more. J Am Dent Assoc 2007; 138(2):188–195.
16. Von Korff M, Ormel J, Keefe FJ, Dworkin SF. Grading the severity of chronic pain. Pain 1992;50:133–149.
17. Garofalo JP, Wesley AL. Research diagnostic criteria for temporomandibular disorders: Reflection of the physical-psychological interface. APS Bulletin 1997;7(3):4–16.
18. John MT, Reissmann DR, Schierz O, Wassell RW. Oral health-related quality of life in patients with temporomandibular disorders. J Orofac Pain 2007;21:46–54.
19. Dworkin SF, Huggins KH, Wilson L, et al. A randomized clinical trial using research diagnostic criteria for temporomandibular disorders-Axis II to target clinic cases for a tailored self-care TMD treatment program. J Orofac Pain 2002;16:48–63.
20. Sherman JJ, Turk DC. Nonpharmacologic approaches to the management of myofascial temporomandibular disorders. Curr Pain Headache Rep 2001;5:421–431.

Pain and Gender

Thuan T. T. Dao

Given the anatomic and genetic differences between men and women, most people would intuitively believe in the differential predisposition and responses of the two genders to various sensory afflictions, including pain experiences. However, there is little consensus on whether these apparent differences are mainly due to sociocultural, psychologic, or biologic factors, or to dynamic interactions between these[1] (Fig 13-1). This chapter will review these controversies and discuss some of the proposed hypotheses on gender differences in pain mechanisms. In the following, *gender* is defined as the genetic sex with which one identifies.

Clinical Pain

Prevalence of clinical pain in women

A review of the literature indicates that women report more severe pain, more frequent pain, and pain of longer duration than do men.[2,3] Several conditions in which chronic pain is a prominent component appear to be associated with a higher female prevalence, and the list of painful disorders that affect women is more than twice as long as that for men.[4] Interestingly, many of the pain conditions that affect mostly women are still of unknown

etiology (Table 13-1). Some involve the cardiovascular system (eg, migraine headaches without aura, Raynaud disease) or gastrointestinal system (eg, irritable bowel syndrome, chronic constipation), while a large number are expressed at the level of the head and neck. These include the various conditions that make up temporomandibular disorders (TMDs), various types of headaches (with the exception of cluster and posttraumatic headaches that have a male predilection), and many other pain disorders of unknown origin (see Table 13-1). From Table 13-1, it is interesting to see that only one disease at the head and neck level (periapical periodontitis and abscess) is caused by an identifiable local pathology. Most of the others would be classified as neurogenic or neuropathic pain. With the exception of back pain, which may be more strongly related to occupation than gender, women also report more musculoskeletal pain than do men. However, it is important to note that pain disorders do not always have a female predilection. The disorders with no gender predilection and those with higher male prevalence added together outnumber those associated with female predominance.[4] Furthermore, the gender prevalence of some disorders appears to be dependent on age. For instance, osteoarthritis is more prevalent in women after age 60 but is predominant in men before they reach 60.

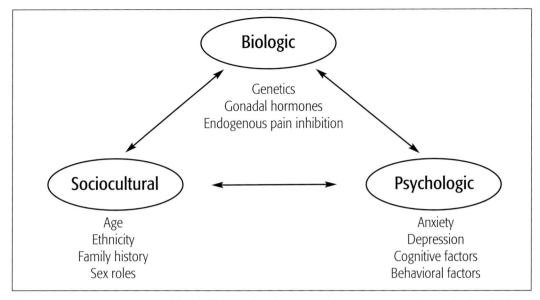

Fig 13-1 Numerous factors may explain the differences in pain perception between women and men. Reprinted with permission from Fillingim.[1]

Diseases with gender-specific signs and symptoms

There is also evidence that certain signs and symptoms of several diseases are gender specific.[4] For instance, the aura associated with migraine headache is twice as prevalent in men as in women. Similarly, men are significantly more likely than women to complain about neck, back, and jaw pains and the nausea associated with acute myocardial infarction. With regard to pain induced by dental treatments, the perception of general pain intensity, analgesic consumption, pain when eating, and the influence of discomfort on daily life were reported to be all significantly greater in girls than in boys receiving orthodontic treatment.[2] Risk factors and predictors of diseases also display gender differences. For instance, risk of low back pain increases with height among men but not among women. Similarly, chest pain is a much poorer predictor of coronary artery disease in women with abnormal angiography than in men.

Methodological issues

While these data show the uneven gender distribution of pain disorders and symptoms, they do not allow us to explain the nature of the differences and the causes of this discrepancy. Instead, the literature is mostly descriptive, and the findings are often noted by chance in studies not originally designed to address the gender issue. Typically, gender is included as a sociodemographic variable and may not even be included in the data analysis. Even when gender differences are well described, the studies are rarely designed to provide explanations for the findings. The interpretation of the extensive literature on clinical pain prevalence is further

Table 13-1 Gender prevalence in some pain disorders*

Pain disorders	Female predominance	Male predominance
Head and neck pain	Atypical odontalgia[u]	Cluster headache[u]
	Burning tongue[u]	Posttraumatic headache[t]
	Cervicogenic headache[de]	Raeder paratrigeminal syndrome[u]
	Chronic tension-type headache[d]	Short-lasting, unilateral, neuralgiform
	Chronic paroxysmal hemicrania[u]	headache with conjunctival injection
	Hemicrania continua[u]	and tearing (SUNCT) syndrome[u]
	Occipital neuralgia[u]	
	Periapical periodontitis and abscess[inf]	
	Postdural puncture headache	
	Temporal arteritis[infl]	
	Tic douloureux[u]	
	Temporomandibular disorders[u]	
Relatively generalized	Carpal tunnel syndrome[de,m]	Ankylosing spondylitis[u]
syndromes	Fibromyalgia[u]	
	Rheumatoid arthritis[infl]	
Limb pain	Chronic venous insufficiency[m,n]	Brachial plexus avulsion[t]
	Raynaud disease[d]	Lateral femoral cutaneous neuropathy[t]
Visceral pain	Gallbladder disease[m]	Abdominal migraine[d]
	Irritable bowel syndrome[d]	Duodenal ulcer[infl]
	Oesophagitis[infl]	
	Reflux oesophagitis with peptic ulcer[infl]	

*Data from Merskey and Bogduk[5]; this information needs further validation.
Suggested etiology: d = dysfunctional; de = degenerative; inf = infective; infl = inflammatory; m = mechanical; n = neoplasm; nep = neuropathic; t = traumatic; u = unknown.

complicated by other methodological considerations, including the accuracy of pain reports, the validity and reliability of pain-measuring methods, and the restrictiveness of the study sample.

Experimental Pain

Gender differences in pain perception have also been extensively studied in the laboratory, where standardized protocols allow some variables that confound the interpretation of clinical studies to be controlled. A large number of psychophysical studies concluded that women exhibit greater sensitivity to laboratory pain than do men,[6] but the findings are not always consistent across studies.[4]

The lack of consistency in animal as well as human studies is not surprising given the differences in the experimental protocols and the diversity of noxious stimuli that have been employed, including electric and thermal stimuli, mechanical pressure pain, cold pressor pain, and ischemic pain. The results may also differ depending on the dimension of pain being assessed and the environment in which the experiment takes place. For instance, it is well known that threshold and tolerance measures are susceptible to social environmental factors that include the gender of the experimenter, the presence of other people, their status and pain attitudes, instructional set, and the clinical relevance of the laboratory settings.[7] In addition, responses to threshold and tolerance tests may be modulated by the subject's state of anxiety and expectation of pain tolerance, which have been shown to differ between men and women.[8] There are other reasons why experimental data should be interpreted with caution. For instance, experimental pains are usually acute and do not reflect the persistent or recurrent nature of chronic pain conditions. Thus, they do not constitute a threat to the subject's health or cause a state of distress or disability that may affect the subject's perception and description of the pain signals. Furthermore, the majority of ex-perimental studies have used stimuli delivered to the skin, while chronic endogenous pains are mostly felt in deep structures, such as muscles, joints, or visceral organs. Given the numerous interacting variables that may shape responses to pain, it is difficult to impute the differences to gender alone.

Sociocultural and Psychosocial Factors Proposed for Gender Differences in Pain

The mass of evidence does suggest that women and men are not affected in the same way by pain disorders. One explanation that has been offered for the overrepresentation of women with chronic orofacial pain in clinical samples is that female patients more readily seek treatment.[2] The proponents of this hypothesis suggest that women have a greater awareness or interest in symptoms than do men and an increased readiness to perceive physical sensations of pain as indicative of illness or serious pathology. They may attend to pain sooner in an effort to minimize its intrusiveness because they have multiple primary role obligations.[2] In contrast, some societies regard male pain endurance and insensitivity to pain as measures of virility. Anxiety, hypervigilance, and past pain experiences have also been proposed as factors that may explain gender differences in pain.[8] Given the number of pain conditions with a male predominance, the sometimes conflicting female/male prevalence, the changes in female/male prevalence with age, and evidence mentioned above that some signs, risk factors, and predictors of diseases may be gender-specific, these assumptions are certainly not tenable in all cases.

While the previous hypotheses emerge from the concept that gender responses to pain may be shaped differentially by psychologic and sociologic factors, other explanations reflect the prejudicial attitudes of some health care providers toward

---

Box 13-1 Biologic factors underlying the gender differences in pain

Differences in the pelvic reproductive organs

Chronobiology of sex hormones

    Effects of puberty and the menstrual cycle

    Effects of exogenous hormones

    Interactions between sex hormones and various neuroactive agents

Differences in peripheral and central neural mechanisms

    Differences in opioid and nonopioid analgesic mechanisms

    Differences in structural organization and function of the sympathetic nervous system

---

women. For instance, some physicians believe that women have more psychosomatic illnesses, more emotional liability, and more complaints due to emotional factors than do men.[9] The claim that pain in women is a "leap of the head" may be motivated by clinical observations that pain complaints in women often cannot be substantiated with any "objective" signs or measures, mainly because many recurrent pain disorders with a higher female prevalence are still of unknown origin, and gender-specific pains due to anatomic and hormonal differences (eg, pains associated with menstruation, ovulation, pregnancy, and childbirth) are more often nonpathologic in women than in men. There is also mounting evidence that gender differences in pain may have biologic causes, as discussed in the rest of this chapter.

Potential Biologic Factors Underlying Gender Differences in Pain

While debate continues about the various biologic factors (Box 13-1) that may contribute to gender differences in pain, it is difficult to disagree with Berkley[4] that "females and males do differ virtually absolutely and unarguably in three aspects of their productive biology. Their pelvic reproductive organs differ and their hormonal conditions differ chronobiologically and compositionally."

Differences in the pelvic reproductive organs

The vagina and cervix could contribute to gender differences in pain because they represent an additional bodily entrance for viral and other pathologic agents.[4] Based on data derived from animal studies, it is hypothesized that these infective agents may in turn trigger a sequence of local events that lead to the spread and referral of pain and hyperalgesia outside the original site of injury. These events include the diffusion of viral agents along C fibers from the site of entry to remote segments of the spinal cord and the brain, central sensitization that outlasts the initial pathology, projection of neurons from the entire spinal cord to those in the higher central nervous system (CNS) levels involved in orofacial pain, and sensitization of nociceptors induced by the interactions between afferent fibers and efferent sympathetic fibers. This hypothesis may explain why pathologic conditions that affect the vaginal canal may degenerate into fibromyalgia, various headaches, and facial/trigeminal pain. Although each neurologic phenomenon has been well documented, it is important to note that the cascade of events linking chronic pain conditions to remote sources of injury remains hypothetical.

Differences related to chronobiology of sex hormones

Effects of puberty and the menstrual cycle on experimental pain

The importance of reproductive hormones to pain states is illustrated by recent evidence that pubertal development has significant but different effects in boys and girls on back pain, headache, and TMDs.[10] The periodic fluctuation of some pain conditions across the menstrual cycle was one of the first clues that reproductive hormones are implicated in pain mechanisms. These include non-pathologic pains associated with the female reproductive cycle, ie, menstruation and ovulation, and various medical conditions exacerbated at specific phases of the menstrual cycle (eg, menstrual headaches, rheumatoid arthritis, diabetes, and irritable bowel syndrome). For instance, headache worsens around the premenstrual period in approximately 60% of female migraine sufferers, and 14% of women with migraine experience headache only with menses.[9] Similarly, TMD pain has been reported to worsen during the menstrual and premenstrual periods.[11] Pain sensitivity to noxious stimuli has also been shown to vary across the menstrual cycle. However, there is no consensus regarding the phase of the hormonal cycle associated with greatest pain sensitivity (ie, lowest pain threshold).[12]

Effects of exogenous hormones on pain

A role for gonadal hormones in pain mechanisms is also supported by data showing the effects of exogenous hormones on both clinical and experimental pains. In postmenopausal women, estrogen replacement therapy can exacerbate migraine[13] and has been shown to increase the prevalence of TMDs by 30%.[14] Similarly, women receiving hormone replacement therapy have a significantly higher prevalence of lower back pain than nonusers.[15]

Comparable effects have been observed with the use of oral contraceptives (OC). Users of OC are at higher risk of TMDs,[14] and OC can change the character and frequency of migraine by either inducing, changing, or alleviating the headache crises.[13] Interestingly, the cyclic fluctuations of both clinical and experimentally delivered pains during the unregulated menstrual cycle are not observed in subjects whose hormonal fluctuations have been stabilized with OC.[11,16]

Interactions between neuroactive agents and gonadal hormones

Gonadal hormones interact with various neuroactive agents that are involved in inflammation and nociception. Variations in estrogen plasma levels are accompanied by changes in neurotransmitters such as serotonin, acetylcholine, dopamine, and β-endorphin.[17] At the trigeminal level, the fluctuation of headaches has been reported to be associated with variations in serotonin and epinephrin levels across the menstrual cycle.[18] Interactions between estrogen and nerve growth factor,[19] γ-aminobutyric acid,[17] and peripheral effects of glutamate and opioids[20] have also been suggested as important in the modulation of pain, including TMDs.

Differences in peripheral and central neural mechanisms

While there is emerging evidence that glutamate and opioids may be involved in peripheral mechanisms underlying gender differences in pain,[20] imaging studies of the brain have shown differences between men and women in the spatial pattern and intensity of CNS responses to acute pain.[21] Intrinsic descending pain inhibitory systems, such as those responsible for opioid and nonopioid stress-induced analgesia, also appear to be influenced by both gender and the cyclic fluctuations of hormones. Furthermore, there is growing evidence that opioid analgesia may show a gender preference for women, since the administration of drugs that act on κ-opioid receptors produced better analgesia in women than in men.[22]

Differences in the structural organization and function of the sympathetic nervous system may also partially explain gender differences in pain. Many functions of the sympathetic nervous system are influenced by gender, including lower levels of resting sympathetic activity to skeletal muscles in women, higher sympathetic output to the skin in women, and differences in cardiovascular responses to various stressors. Other autonomic activities that are strongly influenced by the menstrual cycle and may be related to cutaneous and muscle pains include sweating, skin blood flow, and reflex postural vasoconstriction. In addition, plastic changes in the autonomic nervous system may occur differently in women than in men. Since neuroplastic changes are sometimes associated with the development of chronic pain (see chapter 7), extrapolation of such data may explain the large female predominance in the occurrence of chronic pain disorders associated with the sympathetic nervous system, such as sympathetically maintained pain, causalgia, or reflex sympathetic dystrophy.[4]

Summary

This chapter has noted that women report higher levels of endogenous pain in more bodily regions than do men. Furthermore, when the gender question was brought to the laboratory, it was substantiated by experimental data showing gender disparity in the responses to noxious stimuli. Distinct anatomic, neural, and hormonal differences in women and men provide compelling clues that their pains might be modulated in a differential manner by a number of biologic factors. These ob-

servations should help to counteract prejudicial attitudes toward female patients that can lead to inadequate care. Debates about the importance of biologic and psychosocial factors to gender differences in pain continue, but the answer is unlikely to fall into any one category since the two factors are certainly interrelated. In any case, the evaluation and treatment of pain patients should be performed on an individual basis. After all, the main issue is not whether gender differences in pain exist. Our ultimate objective is to use the available information about these differences in a judicious manner to improve treatment strategies and the quality of life for those who experience pain.

References

1. Fillingim RB. Sex, gender and pain: A biopsychosocial framework. In: Fillingim RB (ed). Sex, Gender, and Pain. Seattle: IASP Press; 2000:1–4.
2. Dao TT, LeResche L. Gender differences in pain. J Orofac Pain 2000;14:169–184; discussion 184–195.
3. Fillingim RB (ed). Sex, Gender, and Pain. Seattle: IASP Press; 2000.
4. Berkley KJ. Sex differences in pain. Behav Brain Sci 1997;20:371–380.
5. Merskey H, Bogduk N. Classification of Chronic Pain. Descriptions of Chronic Pain Syndromes and Definitions of Pain Terms, ed 2. Seattle: IASP Press; 1994.
6. Fillingim RB, Maixner W. Gender differences in the responses to noxious stimuli. Pain Forum 1995;4:209–221.
7. LeResche L. Gender differences in pain. Epidemiologic perspectives. Pain Forum 1995;4:228–230.
8. Rollman GB, Abdel-Shaheed J, Gillespie JM, Jones KS. Does past pain influence current pain: Biological and psychosocial models of sex differences. Eur J Pain 2004; 8:427–433.
9. Colameco S, Becker LA, Simpson M. Sex bias in the assessment of patient complaints. J Fam Pract 1983;16: 1117–1121.
10. LeResche L, Mancl LA, Drangsholt MT, Saunders K, Korff MV. Relationship of pain and symptoms to pubertal development in adolescents. Pain 2005;118:201–209.
11. LeResche L, Mancl L, Sherman JJ, Gandara B, Dworkin SF. Changes in temporomandibular pain and other symptoms across the menstrual cycle. Pain 2003;106:253–261.
12. Sherman JJ, LeResche L, Mancl LA, Huggins K, Sage JC, Dworkin SF. Cyclic effects on experimental pain response in women with temporomandibular disorders. J Orofac Pain 2005;19:133–143.

13. Loder E, Rizzoli P, Golub J. Hormonal management of migraine associated with menses and the menopause: A clinical review. Headache 2007;47:329–340.

14. LeResche L, Saunders K, Von Korff MR, Barlow W, Dworkin SF. Use of exogenous hormones and risk of temporomandibular disorder pain. Pain 1997;69:153–160.

15. Brynhildsen JO, Bjors E, Skarsgard C, Hammar ML. Is hormone replacement therapy a risk factor for low back pain among postmenopausal women? Spine 1998;23:809–813.

16. Dao TT, Knight K, Ton-That V. Modulation of myofascial pain by the reproductive hormones: A preliminary report. J Prosthet Dent 1998;79:663–670.

17. Aloisi AM, Bonifazi M. Sex hormones, central nervous system and pain. Horm Behav 2006;50:1–7.

18. Marcus DA. Interrelationships of neurochemicals, estrogen, and recurring headache. Pain 1995;62:129–139.

19. Stohler CS. Masticatory myalgias. Emphasis on the nerve growth factor-estrogen link. Pain Forum 1997;6(3):176–180.

20. Cairns BE, Sessle BJ. Peripheral mechanisms contribute to innate biological sex differences in pain. IASP: Sex, gender and pain SIG newsletter 2005;October:2–3.

21. Wiesenfeld-Hallin Z. Sex differences in pain perception. Gend Med 2005;2:137–145.

22. Fillingim RB, Gear RW. Sex differences in opioid analgesia: Clinical and experimental findings. Eur J Pain 2004;8:413–425.

Pain and Motor Reflexes

James P. Lund
Greg Murray
Peter Svensson

Other chapters in this book describe the many recent advances in the search to manage pain. Much of the thinking about the etiology and treatment of chronic pain conditions over the last century has focused on the interrelationship between pain and the motor disability that is a common accompaniment. Movements vary from the most complex, voluntary movements (eg, speech, piano playing) to repetitive rhythmic movements (eg, chewing, swallowing) to the simplest spinal cord and brain stem reflexes. Brain stem reflexes (eg, facial-blink reflexes, jaw-opening reflexes) are used to test the functional integrity of cranial nerve afferent and efferent pathways and to help identify and localize lesions (eg, tumors, infarcts) of the reflex loops or central systems that control them.[1,2] This chapter will focus on motor reflex responses to acute orofacial pain and the effects of clinical and experimental pain on the jaw muscle reflexes in particular. Acute orofacial pain can also evoke autonomic reflexes with important physiologic effects (eg, salivary, cardiorespiratory), but these reflexes will not be discussed.

It should also be noted that the jaw-closing muscles are equivalent to the extensors of the legs and arms because they resist the pull of gravity and determine mandibular postural position. The suprahyoid muscles (mylohyoid and digastric) are the jaw flexors (ie, jaw openers). Mastication, like other rhythmic movements (eg, respiration, locomotion), is controlled by a central pattern generator (CPG), which is a primitive neural network that generates a rhythmic motor pattern when driven by tonic inputs from sensory receptors and/or higher centers. In mammals, CPGs are in the brain stem (for mastication, respiration, swallowing) or spinal cord (for locomotion). The CPG for mastication consists of neurons in the brain stem reticular formation, the trigeminal (V) main sensory nucleus, and the spinal subnucleus oralis. When discussing the effects of stimulating nociceptors during chewing, it is important to consider that these neurons produce the rhythm of mastication and generate the bursts of motor neuron activity in the cranial nerve motor nuclei controlling the orofacial muscles (for reviews, see Lund et al[3,4]).

Nociceptive Reflexes

The jaw-opening reflex

When nociceptors are suddenly stimulated, reflexes are evoked that tend to remove the affected body part from the source of pain. If you burn your fingers, nociceptor activation causes the flexion-withdrawal reflex that activates arm flexors and inhibits extensors. The jaw-opening reflex (JOR) is the oral equivalent of this response. It is triggered by the stimulation of nociceptors throughout the oral cavity, tooth pulp, jaw muscles, temporomandibular joint (TMJ), and perioral skin, and also by strong activation of orofacial mechanoreceptors, including periodontal mechanoreceptors. Figure 14-1 illustrates this basic pathway in the rabbit and shows that the JOR in animals consists of activation of jaw-opening muscles and inhibition of jaw-closing muscles. Injection of algesic chemicals into the TMJ, muscle, or other orofacial tissues of anesthetized rats can evoke simultaneous increases in the activity of jaw-closing as well as jaw-opening muscles.[6,7] However, in humans, the JOR is essentially inhibition of jaw-closing muscles with little evidence for excitation of jaw-opening muscles. The sudden cessation of the jaw-closing movement during biting and chewing happens before we know it. The JOR is usually self-activated by biting on something hard or sharp, on a cracked or abscessed tooth, or on the tongue (see Fig 14-1). Noxious stimulation of the tongue reflexly evokes tongue retraction at the same time as the JOR, to remove it from the source of damage.

During biting and chewing, the brain receives a barrage of information from many orofacial mechanoreceptors: mucosal, periodontal, muscle, and joint. With the jaw at rest, such non-noxious afferent activity can evoke the JOR, but if the JOR were activated during the closing phase of mastication, it would be impossible to close the jaws. This is one example of why reflex responses have to change drastically during movement. Animal experiments have revealed that the masticatory CPG can inhibit JOR interneurons that are supplied by non-noxious afferents[8] (Fig 14-2), which explains how we can chew through food without evoking an unwanted JOR. However, the CPG cannot simply shut down the JOR during mastication because the JOR is needed to protect against self-injury (see Fig 14-1). In fact, when orofacial nociceptors are activated during jaw closing, the jaw-closing muscles are strongly inhibited very quickly. This, together with a large digastric response, suddenly cuts short the closing phase and minimizes tissue damage. All this is driven by the masticatory CPG that facilitates the nociceptor interneurons in the JOR circuits during the jaw-closing phase. It is very unlikely that nociceptors will be stimulated during jaw opening; this is why the reflex response during opening is small (see Fig 14-2).

Other orofacial reflexes: Facial-blink reflex, tongue reflexes

Noxious stimuli applied to various orofacial sites can evoke numerous other orofacial reflexes in addition to jaw reflexes.[1,7] Examples include the well-known facial-blink or corneal reflex, which functions to protect the eyes by rapidly closing the eyelids following corneal receptor activation. Others include tongue reflexes that are evoked by stimulation of the tongue and other orofacial sites; for example, accidental biting of the tongue activates mucosal nociceptors that excite hypoglossal (cranial nerve XII) motor neurons as well as a JOR (see Fig 14-1). This reflex retracts the tongue from the noxious stimulus.

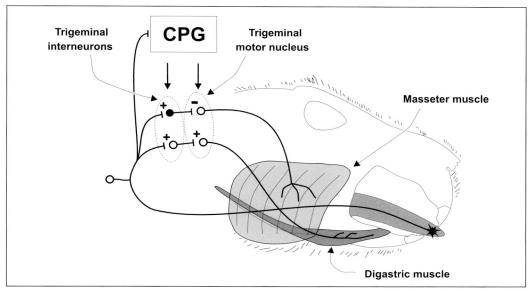

Fig 14-1 Effect of biting the tongue during mastication. A noxious stimulus to the tongue activates mucosal nociceptors; action potentials are conveyed to the V subnucleus caudalis (Vc), to higher centers for pain perception, and to interneurons. For the JOR, there are two types of interneurons: excitatory interneurons *(open circle)* that cause excitation of digastric motor neurons and inhibitory interneurons *(filled circle)* that cause inhibition of jaw-closing motor neurons (only masseter is shown). Tongue reflexes can also be evoked by the noxious stimulus. The CPG for mastication influences the excitability of the interneurons and α-motor neurons. + = excitatory synapse; − = inhibitory synapse. Reprinted with permission from Lund.[5]

Fig 14-2 Modulation of the JOR during mastication. The low threshold (T) test reflex response is the control JOR response in the digastric muscle evoked by activation of low-threshold (ie, nonpainful) orofacial afferents when there is no chewing. During the closing phase of the chewing cycle, the masticatory CPG depresses the response from nonpainful afferent activation—note the reduced size of the JOR during closing and occlusal phases. In contrast, the JOR evoked by the stimulation of nociceptive afferents (high T) is actually *enhanced* during the closing phase of chewing. There is also a corresponding marked inhibition of the jaw closers. Therefore, during jaw closing and chewing, the system has a heightened "awareness" of the possibility of damage to the system (eg, biting the tongue, further cracking of a partially cracked tooth, biting down on an ulcer under a denture). Reprinted with permission from Lund and Olsson.[8]

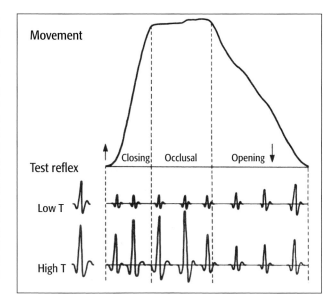

Effects of Nociception on Jaw Reflexes

Activation of nociceptors not only triggers reflexes but can also modify ongoing motor activity, which includes reflexes. Many clinical researchers have investigated these interactions by measuring reflex responses in chronic pain patients and control patients and comparing the results; others have studied reflexes during experimental pain induced in normal subjects by chemical means (eg, hypertonic saline, glutamate, capsaicin), pressure activation of jaw muscle, or cutaneous nociceptors. Studies have focused on the JOR and the jaw-closing reflex (JCR); there is little information on lateral (horizontal) jaw reflexes.

Jaw-opening reflex

As discussed earlier, the human JOR has usually been studied during tonic contraction of the jaw-closing muscles, during which brief stimulation of nociceptors and some mechanoreceptors (eg, periodontal) causes a relatively long-lasting reduction in firing of motor neurons and electromyographic (EMG) activity that is termed *exteroceptive suppression (ES)*. ES is sometimes also called the *silent period*, but this is a confusing term because *silent period* also refers to the fall in EMG activity following the JCR. The ES consists usually of three components: early and late periods of inhibition (ES1, ES2) separated by a period of increased activity, the *intersuppression period (ISP)*.[8] Numerous experiments have examined the influence of experimental pain on ES in human jaw-closing muscles. In the example shown (Fig 14-3), ES1 was unchanged during masseter pain, but the duration and area of ES2 were decreased. This seems to correspond to a reduction in inhibition. Although it is clear that ES1 reflects true motor neuron inhibition, changes in the subsequent peaks and troughs are difficult to interpret because all the motor neurons are synchronously inhibited at the start of ES1. Therefore, they all tend to fire again at about the same time during ISP and then fall silent during ES2, even if inhibition does not continue.

It is much easier to interpret the reflex responses of single motor units. Svensson et al[9] showed that tonic masseter pain reduced the duration of inhibition caused by mental nerve stimulation in human masseter motor units (Fig 14-4). This is good evidence that jaw muscle nociceptor activation suppresses nociceptive reflexes in the same muscle. Similar effects can be observed when arms or legs are painfully stimulated, which suggests the involvement of endogenous pain modulatory systems (see chapter 8).

Although several attempts have been made to use changes in one or more parameters of ES (eg, total ES duration, presence/absence of ES2) in the diagnosis of temporomandibular disorders (TMDs), this has not been successful.[11] Each parameter of the ES can vary considerably; most importantly, ES duration is inversely related to jaw-closing force. Therefore, reports of a prolonged ES duration in TMD patients most likely reflect the difficulty that these patients have in maintaining jaw-closing force.[11] Brain stem reflexes have been studied in patients with persistent orofacial pain because it was hoped that these reflexes might provide a simple diagnostic tool. However, most jaw reflex studies in patients with persistent orofacial pain have been hampered by the lack of stringent diagnostic criteria, insufficiently matched control groups, and poor control of experimental parameters; the results should therefore be interpreted cautiously. At the present time, ES has no value in the diagnosis of any orofacial pain condition.[12]

Jaw-closing reflex

The JCR is a stretch reflex classically evoked by a downward chin tap to the relaxed mandible. This stretches jaw-closing muscle spindles (hence the name *stretch reflex*) and causes a brief volley of

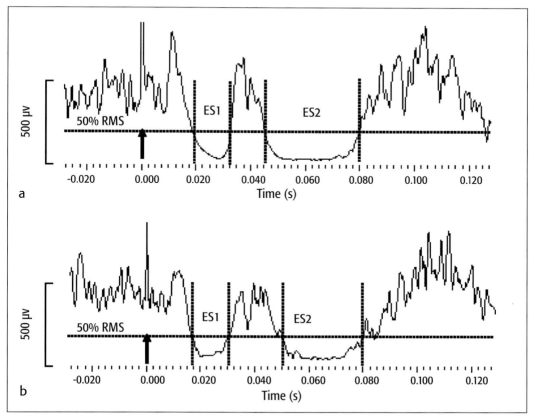

Fig 14-3 Exteroceptive suppression (ES) periods in the EMG activity of the left masseter muscle elicited by 1 ms electric shocks to the mental nerve *(arrow)*. *(a)* Control data show the average of 16 repeated sweeps taken before pain was induced by hypertonic saline injection into the same muscle. *(b)* In the presence of pain, ES2 was shorter. RMS = root mean square. (Reproduced with permission from Wang et al.[9])

action potentials in spindle primary afferents. These afferents influence the activity of α-motor neurons in the brain stem V motor nucleus. The tap results in a brief synchronous activation of jaw-closing muscle motor units at very short latency (~ 10 ms), which elevates the jaw. Slower stretches evoke additional long-latency responses. Muscle spindle afferents provide servocontrol of muscle length during biting and mastication, while the jaw-closing muscle maintains mandibular postural position in relation to the skull during vigorous movements of the body.[13]

The JCR is facilitated by experimental jaw muscle pain, but not by a remote similar pain (Fig 14-5).[14,15] A similar finding has been reported for limb muscle stretch reflexes. Since there is good evidence that the hypertonic saline used to induce the pain does not make motor neurons more excitable[14,15] (see chapter 15), it was suggested that experimental muscle pain causes an increase in the sensitivity of muscle spindle afferents to stretch through an increase in γ-motor neuron activity. However, animal experiments designed to test this hypothesis have been rather inconclusive, with both

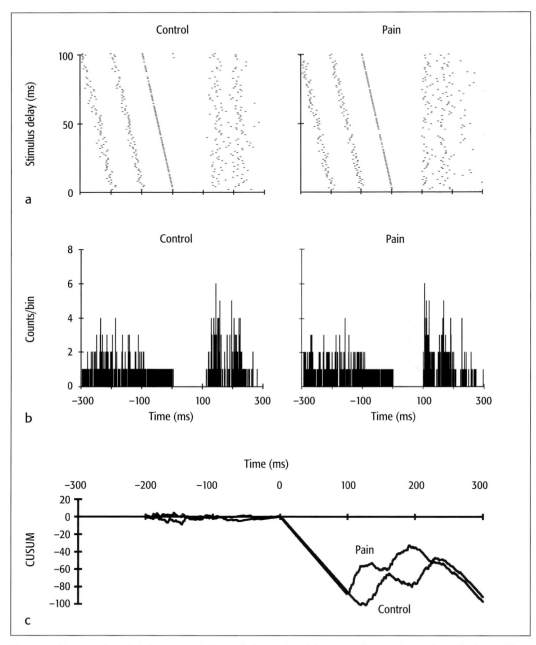

Fig 14-4 *(a)* Raster plots of single motor unit (SMU) discharges from left masseter in control (prepain) and pain conditions. The mental nerve was stimulated at time 0. Each dot in each horizontal row of dots is an SMU action potential, and rows were arranged in order of the delay between the last action potential and the shock. Note that firing resumes at a time that is independent of the delay. *(b)* Cumulative histograms show that firing is suppressed for a shorter period of time in the presence of pain compared with the control. *(c)* The control and pain data are presented in the cumulative sum (CUSUM) format. (Reproduced with permission from Svensson et al.[10])

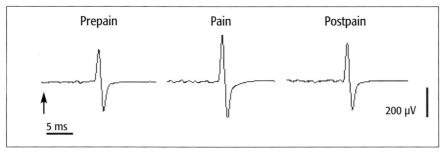

Fig 14-5 Effect of noxious stimulation on the JCR response in the masseter muscle. Typical examples of averaged JCR responses in the masseter muscle before, during, and after pain. The subject is biting on a device capable of stretching the jaw very fast (10 ms ramp time, 1 mm displacement) that elicits a short-latency reflex response (latency about 8 to 9 ms). During painful stimulation of the masseter, reflex amplitude increases when compared to the amplitude before or after painful stimulation. Reprinted with permission from Wang et al.[14]

increases and decreases in spindle sensitivity reported after algesic chemical injection into muscles.

Since tonic experimental pain increases the amplitude of the JCR, it is surprising that the JCR amplitude appears to be depressed in patients with TMDs[11] and patients with neuropathic pain,[16] while other studies do not find significant differences between patients and controls. However, the JCR amplitude varies greatly between individuals and between right and left sides, and it is highly dependent on the force and direction of the chin tap, the sex and age of the subject, and the level of background EMG activity. Therefore, it is likely that any JCR parameter will have very poor sensitivity, specificity, and positive predictive value for detecting chronic pain conditions.[11,17,18] Nonetheless, unilateral absence of or clear differences in JCR latency between right and left sides could indicate an underlying neurologic disease.

Summary

This chapter first outlined animal data pointing to the effects of noxious orofacial stimuli in eliciting reflex activity in the jaw-opening and jaw-closing muscles and other muscles. It then noted that some of the jaw reflexes that can be evoked by non-noxious stimuli need to be suppressed during mastication so that chewing can continue unhindered; noxious stimulation, however, will still evoke the JOR to stop the chewing cycle. Other nociceptive orofacial reflexes were briefly presented, and the chapter concluded with a discussion of the effects of pain on jaw reflexes. Clinical researchers have studied brain stem reflexes for many years because it was thought that changes in latency or amplitude of EMG signals could be used as a simple way of diagnosing patients with various types of pain, including TMDs. However, they have not provided convincing evidence that jaw reflexes are useful aids in the diagnosis and treatment of persistent orofacial pain. Nevertheless, experimental pain models have been used to advance our knowledge of jaw reflexes and their control, although it has not yet been possible to use this knowledge to build new rigorous pathophysiologic models of orofacial pain. Although the use of jaw motor reflexes in the detection of brain stem and cranial nerve lesions is well supported, it seems unlikely that they will be useful tools in the diagnosis and management of the common forms of persistent orofacial pain.

References

1. Aramideh M, Ongerboer de Visser BW. Brainstem reflexes: Electrodiagnostic techniques, physiology, normative data, and clinical applications. Muscle Nerve 2002;26:14–30.
2. Cruccu G, Iannetti GD, Marx JJ, et al. Brainstem reflex circuits revisited. Brain 2005;128(pt 2):386–394.
3. Lund JP, Kolta A, Westberg KG, Scott G. Brainstem mechanisms underlying feeding behaviors. Curr Opin Neurobiol 1998;8:718–724.
4. Lund JP, Kolta A, Sessle BJ. Trigeminal motor system. In: Squire LR (ed). New Encyclopedia of Neuroscience. Oxford: Elsevier (in press).
5. Lund JP. Pain and movement. In: Lund JP, Lavigne G, Dubner R, Sessle BJ (eds). Orofacial Pain: From Basic Science to Clinical Management. Chicago: Quintessence, 2001:151–163.
6. Yu XM, Sessle BJ, Vernon H, Hu JW. Effects of inflammatory irritant application to the rat temporomandibular joint on jaw and neck muscle activity. Pain 1995;60:143–149.
7. Sessle BJ. Acute and chronic craniofacial pain: Brainstem mechanisms of nociceptive transmission and neuroplasticity, and their clinical correlates. Crit Rev Oral Biol Med 2000;11:57–91.
8. Lund JP, Olsson KA. The importance of reflexes and their control during jaw movement. Trends Neurosci 1983;6:458–463.
9. Wang K, Svensson P, Arendt-Nielsen L. Modulation of exteroceptive suppression periods in human jaw-closing muscles by local and remote experimental muscle pain. Pain 1999;82:253–262.
10. Svensson P, McMillan AS, Graven-Nielsen T, Wang K, Arendt-Nielsen L. Modulation of an inhibitory reflex in single motor units in human masseter by tonic painful stimulation. Pain 1999;83:441–446.
11. De Laat A, Svensson P, Macaluso GM. Are jaw and facial reflexes modulated during clinical or experimental orofacial pain? J Orofac Pain 1998;12:260–271.
12. Svensson P. Masseter reflexes modulated by pain. Mov Disord 2002;17(suppl 2):S45–S48.
13. Miles TS, Nauntofte B, Svensson P. Clinical Oral Physiology. Chicago: Quintessence, 2004.
14. Wang K, Svensson P, Arendt-Nielsen L. Effect of tonic muscle pain on short-latency jaw-stretch reflexes in humans. Pain 2000;88:189–197.
15. Peddireddy A, Wang K, Svensson P, Arendt-Nielsen L. Effect of experimental posterior temporalis muscle pain on human brainstem reflexes. Clin Neurophysiol 2005;116:1611–1620.
16. Bodéré C, Tèa SH, Giroux-Metges MA, Woda A. Activity of masticatory muscles in subjects with different orofacial pain conditions. Pain 2005;116:33–41.
17. Cruccu G, Frisardi G, Pauletti G, Romaniello A, Manfredi M. Excitability of the central masticatory pathways in patients with painful temporomandibular disorders. Pain 1997;73:447–454.
18. Lund JP, Widmer CG. An evaluation of the use of surface electromyography in the diagnosis, documentation, and treatment of dental patients. J Craniomandib Disord 1989;3:125–137.

Persistent Pain and Motor Dysfunction

James P. Lund

This chapter builds upon the information provided in chapter 14 concerning the reflex effects of transient pain and outlines the effects that persistent pain may have on motor function. It especially focuses on the applicability of two major concepts postulated to account for these effects—the *vicious cycle theory* and the *pain-adaptation model*—and considers them in the particular context of the jaw musculature.

The Vicious Cycle Theory

At the turn of the 20th century, it was thought that common forms of muscle pain were caused by abnormal movement patterns that led to hyperactivity, spasm, fatigue, and pain. Later, Travel[1] suggested that chronic muscle pain could be explained if pain itself caused or maintained hyperactivity. Despite the lack of evidence, this suggestion became the *pain-spasm-pain* or *vicious cycle theory* of chronic pain and dysfunction (Fig 15-1a). Although really an untested hypothesis, the vicious cycle theory was quickly co-opted to explain the etiology of chronic lower back pain (CLBP), fibromyalgia, myofascial pain, tension-type headaches, and postexercise muscle soreness (for review, see Lund et al[2] and Stohler[3]). Many authors adapted the hypothe-

sis to support their belief that almost anything that caused pain in muscles or joints and altered movements or increased muscle activity could initiate temporomandibular disorders (TMDs). They reinforced the idea that conditions such as TMDs have a multifactorial etiology and provided a hypothetic framework for treatments aimed at reducing muscle activity either directly (eg, with biofeedback) or indirectly by correcting "abnormal" anatomy (eg, with occlusal splints, occlusal adjustments, orthodontics, and joint and orthognathic surgery).

The way in which the vicious cycle hypothesis has been incorporated into two philosophic approaches to TMDs is illustrated in Fig 15-1b. Those who emphasize the importance of the dental occlusion consider TMDs are caused by occlusal interferences,[4] while advocates of neuromuscular dentistry and craniomandibular orthopedics believe that TMDs arise because the mandible and maxilla are misaligned.[5] Both indicate that abnormal dentoskeletal anatomy leads to abnormal patterns of movement and muscular hyperactivity, leading to pain. Once pain occurs, the vicious cycle kicks in. Note that both groups believe that myalgic forms of TMDs can lead to progressive intracapsular pathology via hyperactivity especially of the lateral pterygoid muscle.

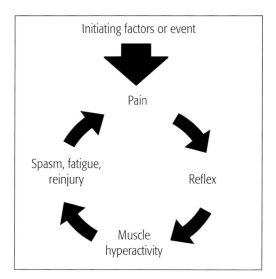

Fig 15-1a The vicious cycle. This diagram shows the pain-spasm-pain cycle first described by Travel.[1] It is based on the concept that activation of muscle nociceptors can lead to chronic pain because activation of nociceptors causes a tonic reflex contraction of all muscles.

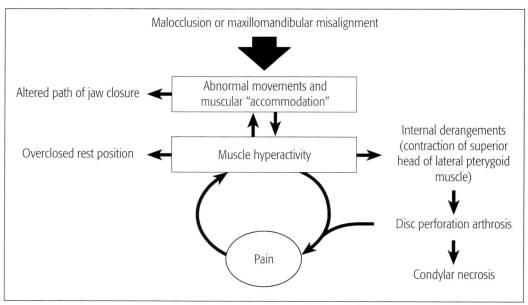

Fig 15-1b The vicious cycle hypothesis adapted to gnathology, neuromuscular dentistry, and craniomandibular orthopedics.

Assessment of pain models based on the vicious cycle

All such models for TMDs and similar human conditions are based on two premises: *(1)* that mus-cle hyperactivity can lead to pain, and *(2)* that pain leads to tonic muscle hyperactivity. The first is true, as everyone has experienced sore muscles after heavy exercise. However, the evidence from clinical and experimental studies shows that persistent pain in humans does not usually cause hyperactivity and that tonic muscle hyperactivity is unlikely to be the cause of most chronic musculoskeletal pain.

Fatigue, postexercise muscle soreness, bruxism, and myoclonus

When muscles are voluntarily contracted at high tension for long periods, the fibers begin to fatigue, which causes progressive changes in muscle fiber function. Tension drops, and the electromyographic (EMG) signal shifts to low frequencies of higher mean amplitude. Pain finally sets in, probably because the muscle fibers release algesic metabolites. However, the jaw-closing muscles are inherently resistant to fatigue because even the most rapidly contracting fibers have a high oxidative capacity. Only long-lasting clenching causes pain in the jaw and cranial muscles, and true mechanical fatigue is very difficult to induce.[6] The pain goes away quickly once the contraction stops. However, pain can return if exercise was particularly heavy or if muscles were untrained. This postexercise pain is called *delayed-onset or postexercise muscle soreness (PEMS)*. It develops gradually over several hours and then slowly diminishes. The pain is probably caused by inflammation that follows the mechanical breakdown of myofibrils and perhaps connective tissues as well (for review, see Lund et al[2] and Stohler[3]).

Nocturnal bruxers or those with various forms of orofacial myoclonus who awaken with pain in their jaw muscles (see chapter 16) probably suffer from PEMS. On the other hand, many bruxers with badly worn teeth and hypertrophied muscles have no pain. One possible explanation for this is that their jaw muscles have adapted to heavy work.

Although high levels of muscle activity may cause persistent pain, this does not lead to an increase in tonic contraction in the affected muscle as the vicious cycle theory postulates. For instance, when heavy exercise was used to induce PEMS in the biceps, there was no difference in levels of EMG activity recorded before and during pain (for review, see Lund et al[2] and Stohler[3]). The authors of these studies were surprised because the sore arms showed signs usually interpreted as evidence of muscle tension: they were slightly flexed at rest and tense to palpation. The authors speculated that these signs were caused by local edema. This may explain why areas of pain, tightness, taut bands, and trigger points, which are usually assumed to be caused by contraction of muscle fibers, are not regions of high electric activity (for examples, see Jensen et al[7] and Peterson et al[8]).

In addition, pain does not seem to increase muscle activity in bruxism. There is no difference between the levels of resting masseter EMG activity in bruxers with or without pain, although the masseters of bruxers are more active than those of age-matched and sex-matched controls.[9] These data suggest strongly that the higher resting activity in bruxers is due to the hypertrophy of the muscles, not to pain.

TMDs and related conditions

Many studies have been carried out to see if the muscles of patient groups suffering from TMDs, CLBP, tension-type headache, or fibromyalgia are more active than normal. Although it would be better to discuss the myalgic and arthralgic forms of TMDs separately, this is not possible because they were not differentiated in most publications. To make a proper comparison, EMG activity recorded over painful muscles in patients should be compared to recordings from similar sites in appropriate control subjects. When such comparisons were carried out for fibromyalgia, headache, neck/shoulder pain, and back pain, the results were very clear: there was no significant difference between the groups in almost all of the published reports (for review, see Lund et al[2] and Stohler[3]). A recent study[10] of females compared surface EMG levels from the trapezius, neck, temporalis, and frontalis of fibromyalgia patients, chronic shoulder-neck pain patients, and age-matched female control subjects at rest and during stressful tasks. There were no differences between groups, and EMG levels were not related to intensity of pain.

Early studies of TMDs did show that resting EMG activity of masseter and anterior temporalis muscles was slightly higher in a group of patients with TMDs.[2,3] However, the control groups contained mainly young men, while the patient groups were made up of women of up to middle age. Two later studies using age- and sex-matched controls also found slightly higher resting EMG levels in the pain group; but two others in which groups were matched for age, sex, and bruxism did not. In one of these studies, the pain patients did not have higher resting activity than their respective control groups[9] (bruxers with pain vs bruxers with no pain; other TMDs with pain vs non-TMD controls). Another factor that must be taken into account is that EMG electrodes on the skin over jaw muscles may also record from facial muscles, and the activity of many of these clearly goes up during pain.

The lateral pterygoid muscle and intracapsular disorders

The superior head of the lateral pterygoid muscle occupies a special place in many clinicians' concept of TMDs. They believe that hyperactivity in this muscle can lead to a progression from an initial myalgia/muscle dysfunction to internal derangements of the temporomandibular joint (TMJ), to arthritis, and even to necrosis of the condyle (see Fig 15-1b). Anterior displacement of the disc was assumed to occur because of either tonic contraction of the superior head or lack of coordination of the superior and inferior heads of the muscle. Many textbooks include cartoons of the muscle in which the superior head inserts exclusively into the articular disc, while the inferior head inserts below the head of the condyle. More careful descriptions of the two heads of the muscle and the structures of the TMJ show that no muscle fibers enter the

disc at all in some human specimens, and even when small bundles do enter the disc, pulling on them does not displace the disc relative to the condyle.[11] Furthermore, recent studies using intramuscular EMG recordings have shown that the two heads function as one,[12] and there is no evidence that the lateral pterygoid behaves abnormally in TMD patients. It is therefore unlikely that abnormal activity in this muscle could have any role in intracapsular disorders. Its frequent tenderness in pain patients cannot be used as a marker of TMD pain because the same symptom is found in about 50% of the general population.[7]

The Effect of Persistent Pain on Biting and Mastication

Many TMD patients complain that biting and chewing not only hurt but are more difficult to do when they are in pain. Some also report that they cannot open their mouth wide and that their bite has changed.[13] Several researchers have looked at the relationship between maximum voluntary contraction (MVC) and pain. Molin found that maximum biting force of female TMD patients was 40% lower than in age-matched controls.[14] Pain elsewhere in the body has similar effects. For instance, patients with fibromyalgia have significantly less strength in the hands and legs than control subjects, and subjects with CLBP cannot contract the paraspinal muscles as forcefully as controls. Although detraining of muscles undoubtedly occurs in patients with chronic pain, tonic nociceptor input also seems to contribute to a reduced MVC. Maximum biting force decreases while experiencing pain following third molar extraction; and when postsurgical pain in the knee is blocked, MVC goes up by more than 400% (for review, see Lund et al[2] and Stohler[3]).

Pain in the legs and back changes the way that we walk. Patients with CLBP walk more slowly than control subjects. Their steps are shorter, their gait

Fig 15-2 Comparison of the EMG activity recorded over the left paraspinal muscles at L4 in a 35-year-old male control subject *(top and bottom)* with a male CLBP patient *(middle)*. Note that the participant's muscle was very active when both feet were in contact with the ground but almost inactive during the swing phase in the control state *(top)*. In the CLBP patient, the muscle did not become inactive during the swing phases *(middle)*, and this same pattern was seen in the control participant after 5% saline had been injected into the back muscles on the right side to cause pain *(bottom)*. LTO = left toe off; LHS = left heel strike; RTO = right toe off. Adapted with permission from Arendt-Nielsen et al.[15]

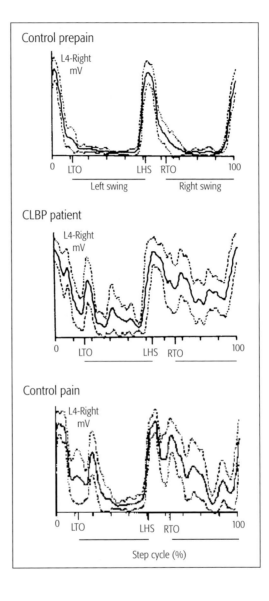

tends to be asymmetric (eg, limping), and the normal pattern of alternating periods of activity (stance phase) and inactivity (swing phase) in lumbar paraspinal muscles is disturbed: the muscles are significantly more active during swing in the pain group than in controls[15] (Fig 15-2). Stohler et al[16] showed that a similar phenomenon occurs during mastication. The masticatory movements of a patient group were significantly more irregular than controls. They also compared painful and nonpainful chewing strokes in the patients and found that jaw-closing muscles were significantly more active in the painful strokes but only during the jaw-opening phase when they were acting as antagonists to jaw opening.

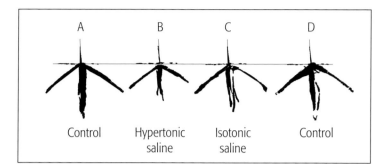

Fig 15-3 Examples of Gothic arch traces taken (A) before pain, (B) during moderate pain caused by hypertonic saline, (C) during an injection of isotonic saline that caused a little pain, and (D) after pain. Adapted with permission from Obrez and Stohler.[17]

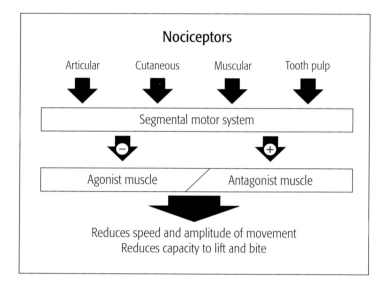

Fig 15-4 Pain-adaptation model of chronic pain and dysfunction. This model in built on the premise that the effect of tonic stimulation of nociceptors on segmental motor systems is not dependent on the tissue of origin. All lead to a reduction in the output of agonist motor neurons and an increase in antagonist activity. Adapted with permission from Lund et al.[2]

We now know that the major motor signs and symptoms that accompany several chronic pain states can be induced experimentally by painful infusions of hypertonic saline or other algesic chemicals into normal muscles. For instance, normal subjects adopt the gait and EMG pattern of patients with CLBP when 5% saline is injected into the paraspinal muscles[15] (see Fig 15-2). Experimental muscle pain also brings on signs of TMDs, since pain in the masseter muscle reduces the amplitude and velocity of experimental mastication,[18] and similar pain reduces the amplitude of man-

dibular border movements (Fig 15-3).[17] Of particular interest was the finding that the centric relation position shifts during pain, suggesting that the occlusal changes that some patients report could be a consequence of pain rather than a cause of TMDs, as has so often been assumed.

Pain and Facial Expression

The effects of pain are not confined to the site of injury or even that region of the body. Indeed, it is usually not difficult to recognize when someone is in pain because of the changes in facial expression—the brows are lowered, the eyes become narrow, and the corners of the mouth droop (for review, see Stohler[3] and Stohler et al[19]). Other pain behaviors include guarding, gestures such as rubbing, and abnormal body postures. To produce the pain expression, the activity of several facial muscles increases. Indeed, although resting EMG activity does not increase in painful back muscles, the frontalis muscles are significantly more active in patients with back pain than in controls.[2,19] This increased facial muscle activity probably explains why some studies[20] recorded higher resting masseter and temporalis EMG activity in subjects with myofascial or neuropathic pain than in control subjects or in subjects with nonpainful disc disorders. Even when pain was unilateral, resting activity was increased bilaterally, as it is when we make a "pain face."[5] The changes in facial expression that occur as pain increases are even recognized by children and by adults of low intelligence, which is one reason why pictograms of facial expressions are used with these populations to rate pain severity (see chapter 10).

The Pain-Adaptation Model

Given the shortcomings of the vicious cycle theory and several of the other points noted above, the *pain-adaptation model* was proposed as a simple way of relating persistent pain with the associated motor signs and symptoms that were described in the previous sections and as a replacement for the vicious cycle hypothesis.[2] The model has three basic postulates; namely that *(1)* persistent pain has general effects on the motor system, including changes in facial expression and body posture and avoidance of physical work; *(2)* nociceptors in a body part (eg, skin, mucosa, teeth, connective tissue, muscle, and joint) have similar effects on the segmental motor system (Fig 15-4); and *(3)* activation of nociceptors

inhibits agonist motor neurons and facilitates antagonist motor neurons through segmental reflexes by modifying the output of central pattern generators. Since publication of the model in 1991, a large number of experiments in humans have confirmed that agonist muscle output is reduced in pain patients and by nociceptor stimulation, leading to lower MVC and reduced movement amplitude and speed.[21]

The reduction in range of motion, ability to lift heavy loads, bite hard, and move quickly in the presence of pain is traditionally characterized as dysfunction. This is correct in the sense that we are mechanically less efficient when in pain. However, in the model, these pain-related changes are viewed as adaptive because a reduced ability to move fast and contract muscles forcefully should help prevent further damage and promote healing. Even the changes in facial expression are adaptive because they tend to elicit sympathy and help for the sufferer. As pointed out in chapter 19, one of the best ways that a therapist can help suffering patients is to recognize the severity of their pain and provide the appropriate emotional support.

Summary

This chapter has described two models that were developed to explain the interrelationship between chronic pain and motor activity. The chapter also demonstrated that evidence drawn from clinical and experimental studies does not support the vicious cycle theory that was long used to explain the etiology of chronic musculoskeletal pain conditions such as TMDs. Finally, a discussion of the pain-adaptation model was presented that explains why the model was developed and summarizes its three basic postualtes: *(1)* persistent pain has general motor effects including changes in facial expression, *(2)* all nociceptors have similar effects on the segmental motor systems, and *(3)* nociceptors can inhibit agonist motor neurons and facilitate antagoinist motor neurons.

References

1. Travel J, Rinzler S, Herman M. Pain and disability of the shoulder and arm. Treatment by intramuscular infiltration with procaine hydrochloride. JAMA 1942;120:417–422.
2. Lund JP, Donga R, Widmer CG, Stohler CS. The pain-adaptation model: A discussion of the relationship between chronic musculoskeletal pain and motor activity. Can J Physiol Pharmacol 1991;69:683–694.
3. Stohler CS. Craniofacial pain and motor function: Pathogenesis, clinical correlates, and implications. Crit Rev Oral Biol Med 1999;10:504–518.
4. Dawson PE. Evaluation, Diagnosis, and Treatment of Occlusal Problems, ed 2. St Louis: Mosby, 1989.
5. Jankelson R. Neuromuscular Dental Diagnosis and Treatment. St Louis: Ishiyaku EuroAmerica, 1990.
6. Svensson P, Burgaard A, Schlosser S. Fatigue and pain in human jaw muscles during a sustained, low-intensity clenching task. Arch Oral Biol 2001;46:773–777.
7. Jensen R, Rasmussen BK, Pedersen B, Lous I, Olesen J. Cephalic muscle tenderness and pressure pain threshold in a general population. Pain 1992;48:197–203.
8. Peterson AL, Talcott GW, Kelleher WJ, Haddock CK. Site specificity of pain and tension in tension-type headaches. Headache 1995;35:89–92.
9. Sherman RA. Relationships between jaw pain and jaw muscle contraction level: Underlying factors and treatment effectiveness. J Prosthet Dent 1985;54:114–118.
10. Nilsen KB, Westgaard RH, Stovner LJ, Helde G, Ro M, Sand TH. Pain induced by low-grade stress in patients with fibromyalgia and chronic shoulder/neck pain, relation to surface electromyography. Eur J Pain 2006;10:615–627.
11. Meyenberg K, Kubik S, Palla S. Relationships of the muscles of mastication to the articular disc of the temporomandibular joint. Schweiz Monatsschr Zahnmed 1986;96:815–834.
12. Murray GM, Bhutada M, Peck CC, Phanachet I, Sae-Lee D, Whittle T. The human lateral pterygoid muscle. Arch Oral Biol 2007;52:377–380.
13. Bell WE. Temporomandibular Disorders: Classification, Diagnosis, Management, ed 3. Chicago: Year Book Medical Publishers, 1990.
14. Molin C. Vertical isometric muscle forces of the mandible. A comparative study of subjects with and without manifest mandibular pain dysfunction syndrome. Acta Odontol Scand 1972;30:485–499.
15. Arendt-Nielsen L, Graven-Nielsen T, Svarrer H, Svensson P. The influence of low back pain on muscle activity and coordination during gait: A clinical and experimental study. Pain 1996;64:231–240.
16. Stohler CS, Ashton-Miller JA, Carlson DS. The effects of pain from the mandibular joint and muscles on masticatory motor behaviour in man. Arch Oral Biol 1988;33:175–182.
17. Obrez A, Stohler CS. Jaw muscle pain and its effect on gothic arch tracings. J Prosthet Dent 1996;75:393–398.
18. Svensson P, Arendt-Nielsen L, Houe L. Sensory-motor interactions of human experimental unilateral jaw muscle pain: a quantitative analysis. Pain 1996;64:241–249.
19. Stohler CS, Zhang X, Lund JP. The effect of experimental jaw muscle pain on postural muscle activity. Pain 1996;66:215–221.
20. Bodéré C, Téa SH, Giroux-Metges MA, Woda A. Activity of masticatory muscles in subjects with different orofacial pain conditions. Pain 2005;116:33–41.
21. Farina D, Arendt-Nielsen L, Graven-Nielsen T. Experimental muscle pain decreases voluntary EMG but does not affect the muscle potential evoked by transcutaneous electrical stimulation. Clin Neurophysiol 2005;116:1558–1565.

16

Pain and Sleep Disturbances

Gilles J. Lavigne
Takafumi Kato
Pierre Mayer

Sleep is the natural process that cuts off conscious appreciation of the environment for a period of 6 to 9 hours (or longer for babies, children, and teenagers).[1] Normally, sensory stimuli that are part of the environment, such as background noise or light touch, do not interrupt sleep.[2] Rather, it is sudden or meaningful incoming information (such as an alarm clock) that usually triggers an *arousal* (brief brain, heart, and muscle activation [<10 s], without awareness) or an *awakening* (longer brain activation, with awareness of the environment).

It is important for clinicians to know that patients with orofacial pain are at risk for having poor sleep (ie, difficulty falling asleep or sleep that is interrupted by sudden onset of pain). Sleep is essential to health, and prolonged sleep deprivation increases the risk of cardiovascular and mental disorders or pain-related complaints.[3] Chronic pain patients often wake up unrefreshed[4–8] and frequently report long delays in falling asleep; insomnia is a common complaint, as is fatigue.[4] The consequences of lack of sleep or poor sleep quality include daytime sleepiness, low productivity, and increased risk of work or motor vehicle accidents.[4] This chapter will focus on the relationship between chronic pain and the mechanisms

that maintain or disrupt sleep. Tools and methodological issues relevant to this topic can be reviewed in a recent publication from our group.[9]

Normal Sleep

When passing from wakefulness to sleep, there is a gradual change from full alertness and consciousness to drowsiness and a nearly complete disengagement from the environment. At sleep onset, a surprising sudden body jerk is often experienced. This type of myoclonus, the so-called hypnic jerk, is considered normal unless it recurs frequently during sleep. Scientists divide sleep into several stages that are classified as rapid eye movement (REM) and non-rapid eye movement (NREM) sleep stages. NREM sleep stages are divided into *light sleep* (stages 1 and 2) and *deep sleep* (stages 3 and 4, also known as *slow-wave sleep* or *delta sleep*). Sleep stages 3 and 4 are believed to be the "restorative sleep"; disruption of these stages seems to be associated with a higher risk of daytime fatigue and pain.[4,7,9,10] REM sleep is also known as *active sleep* or *paradoxical sleep*. During sleep, we pass from light sleep to deep sleep to REM sleep

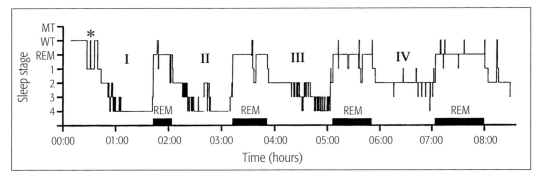

Fig 16-1a Good sleep: Data from a 23-year-old subject who had four full sleep cycles (I to IV). Only 12 sleep awakenings (thin vertical lines extending up to WT) were scored (normal < 30/night); one of the awakenings is depicted here, and in Fig 16-1b, by an asterisk. The duration of the REM periods (corresponding to the black horizontal bars) was longer and the duration of stages 3 and 4 was shorter toward the end of the sleep period. MT = movement time; WT = wake time.

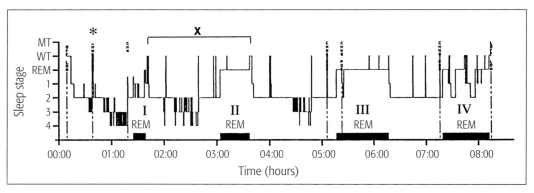

Fig 16-1b Poor sleep: Data from a 28-year-old subject who complained of unrefreshing sleep. Even though he presented four full sleep cycles (I to IV), several sleep awakenings (thin vertical lines extending up to WT) were scored (n = 27) and frequent sleep-stage shifts were noted (X). REM periods correspond to the black horizontal bars. MT = movement time; WT = wake time.

from three to six times (ultradian cycles) during the night. Each of these cycles lasts approximately 90 minutes (Fig 16-1a). In the first half of the night, stages 3 and 4 are predominant. In the second half, REM sleep dominates.

Specific criteria are used to score various sleep stages from polygraphic recordings with dedicated software (Table 16-1 and Fig 16-2). The following recordings are used: brain electric (electroenceph-

alographic [EEG]) activity, muscle (electromyo-graphic [EMG]) activity, eye movements (electro-oculogram [EOG]), heart rate (electrocardiogram [ECG]), and respiration (chest and abdominal movements and oronasal airflow).[4,9–13] Measurements of rectal temperature and salivary melatonin levels are taken to assess chronobiologic rhythms. Other measurements include esophageal acidity for gastric reflux and blood endocrine levels. Video

Table 16-1 Awake and sleep stage recognition*

Stage	Sleep time (%)	EEG/brain activity	EMG activity	EOG/eye movement	ECG/ heart rate	Arousal probability
Awake	–	Low-amplitude high-frequency β (13–30 Hz) and α (8–12 Hz) waves	High	Intense	Variable	–
NREM Light sleep Stage 1	10	Low-amplitude high-frequency and mixed-frequency of fast and desynchronized α (10–12 Hz) and θ (4–7.5 Hz) waves	High to moderate*	Slow rolling	Slower than awake	Very high
Stage 2	50	Mid-amplitude slower α (8–10 Hz) and θ (4–7.5 Hz) waves with presence of K-complexes† and EEG spindles‡	Moderate*	Slow	Slower than awake	High
NREM Deep sleep Stages 3 and 4	10–20	High-amplitude low-frequency δ (0.5–3.5 Hz) waves	Moderate to low	Absent	Slowest and regular	Low
REM/active sleep	20–25	High-frequency and mixed-frequency desynchronized pattern (absence of δ waves)	Very low/ hypotonia	Rapid and phasic	Variable	Low

* Stages with appearance of most sleep bruxism and periodic limb movements.
† K-complexes are bi-triphasic EEG waves of high amplitude (> 75 μV) lasting > 0.5 s (see C_3A_2 trace in Fig 16-2).
‡ EEG spindles are fast (12–14 Hz), sinusoidal, and fusiform waves (see toward end of C_3A_2 trace in Fig 16-2).

Fig 16-2 Sleep stage 2 in a pain-free subject. The traces represent a 20-second episode. The two upper traces are left and right ocular movements (LOC and ROC). The middle one represents the EMG activity at the chin. The lower two traces are EEG activity recorded in a central position with a reference to right earlobe (C_3A_2) and in an occipital skull position with a left earlobe reference (O_2A_1). Note the presence of a K-EEG event (large amplitude wave) in the middle of the C_3A_2 trace followed by a sleep spindle (fast and dense EEG signal) toward the end.

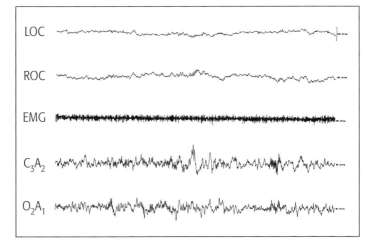

and sound recordings are also used to identify body movements that occur during sleep, including bruxism, periodic limb movement, somnambulism, snoring, talking, and REM behavior disorder (absence of body paralysis during sleep).[9]

Several neurotransmitters and peptides that have been associated with sleep (eg, serotonin [5-HT], γ-aminobutyric acid [GABA], acetylcholine [ACh], noradrenaline, cholecystokinin [CCK], opiates, prostaglandin, growth hormones, prolactin, and melatonin) are also involved in pain perception or modulation.[5,9]

Poor Sleep Quality

The assessment of sleep quality is like that of pain—highly subjective and dependent on past experience and current psychosocial status.[9] In the absence of direct measures, sleep quality assessment is frequently misinterpreted. Although sleep quality varies from individual to individual, it can be estimated from a combination of reports, including the sensation of unrefreshing sleep, not enough sleep, frequent awakenings during sleep, and the feeling of not having slept deeply. Conditions that favor good sleep quality include an environment that is safe, quiet, and comfortable. In such conditions, low-level stimuli have little or no influence on the sleep quality of a healthy person. However, a loud sound or an unexpected pain attack during sleep, such as a toothache or back pain, can generate a clear awakening response that might trigger anxiety and impede subsequent sleep. Factors that influence sleep quality include presence of pain, past pain experience, anxiety or relevance of the pain (eg, recurrence of pain in a patient whose cancer is in remission), concomitant depression, and other mood disturbances or cumulated fatigue.[4,6,9] Age may be a factor as well, since patients complain more frequently of poor sleep as they age.

Abnormal Sleep

Several variables are used to describe sleep.[4,6,9] Sleep efficiency is a measure of total sleep time over the total time in bed, from sleep onset to final awakening. It usually reaches 90% in good sleepers and is lower than 80% in poor sleepers. Reduced time in some sleep stages and frequent sleep stage shifts (from a deeper stage to a lighter one) are also indications of a sleep disturbance (see Fig 16-1b). Moreover, frequent microarousals, sleep awakenings, body movements, or sleep apnea and hypopnea episodes (50% reduction in breathing effort for >10 sec) also characterize poor sleep. Finally, the intrusion of fast (alpha) EEG waves during stages 3 and 4 is a sign of sleep lightening but is not a marker of pain during sleep.[3–6,9]

Several sleep disorders—from dyssomnias (eg, insomnia, apnea) to parasomnias (eg, enuresis, sleep walking, nightmares, sleep eating) to sleep-related movement disorders (eg, sleep bruxism, periodic limb movements, leg cramps)—and concomitant medical/psychiatric disorders (eg, fibromyalgia/widespread pain, Parkinson disease, alcoholism) are associated with an abnormal sleep structure[11] (Box 16-1).

Sleep Abnormalities in Pain Patients

Practitioners need to appreciate that patients with orofacial pain are at risk for having poor sleep.[4,5,14] Pain patients are likely to have long delays in falling asleep, frequent sleep arousals, sleep-stage shifts, and body movements during sleep.[3,4,6,9] Some may experience EEG cyclic fluctuations during sleep,[3,6,7] although these are not specific to patients with chronic pain; they are frequently seen in conjunction with other sleep-disrupting conditions.[3,4,9] Recently, a subtle form of autonomic-cardiac dysfunction was observed in both insomniacs and

Box 16-1 Examples of sleep disorders based on the International Sleep Disorders Classification[2–11]

Insomnia
(frequent in chronic pain patients)

- Delay in falling asleep or difficulty in resuming sleep if awakened during sleep hours

Sleep-related breathing disorders
(risk of cardiovascular diseases and transportation accidents)

- Sleep apnea-hypopnea syndrome (obstructive and/or central)
- Cheyne-Stokes syndrome (respiration in crescendo and decrescendo with neurologic and cardiac disease)
- Sleep-related hypoventilation/hypoxemia with sleepiness (also known as the *upper airway resistance syndrome* [UARS])
- Snoring (about 1 in 5 patients with snoring may have some form of respiratory disturbances)

Hypersomnia

- Narcolepsy
- Menstrual-related hypersomnia

Circardian rhythm sleep disorders

- Jet lag, shift work that disrupts the circadian rhythm

Parasomnias
(disorders that manifest themselves during sleep/a sleep intruder; frequent in children)

- Sleep walking
- Sleep terrors
- Sleep enuresis
- Nightmares
- REM-sleep behavior disorder/lack of muscle hypotonia during REM sleep (equated with high risk of Parkinson disease in adults)

Sleep-related movement disorders

- Sleep bruxism
- Periodic limb movement
- Leg cramps

Sleep disorders associated with other disorders

- Fibromyalgia (described also as widespread pain)
- Parkinson disease
- Sleep-related headaches (respiratory disorder needs to be excluded first)
- Sleep gastroesophageal reflux
- Sleep-related abnormal swallowing, choking, and laryngospasm

chronic pain patients with fibromyalgia. Normally, heart rate is reduced from wakefulness to light sleep, reaching its lowest level during deep sleep (stages 3 and 4), but this decrease did not occur in these patients.[9,12,13] It remains to be determined if this difference is the primary cause of unrefreshing sleep in these patients or if it is secondary to other chronic health disturbances.

Both pain and poor sleep are influenced by past experiences, personal beliefs, health status, and lifestyle, among other factors. Each case should be investigated to identify the cause of poor sleep in relation to persistent pain. Pain and poor sleep are concomitant complaints in patients suffering from conditions such as myofascial pain, rheumatoid arthritis, chronic low back pain (CLBP), and conditions with widespread pain, such as fibromyalgia.[3–8] In a comparative multicenter study,[8] patients with fibromyalgia reported 2.4 times more sleep disturbances than matched control subjects. Sleep disturbances have also been reported by 50% of patients with jaw muscle pain and by 90% of patients with fibromyalgia.[14] Some epidemiologic data suggest that a gradient (dose-response) relationship exists between jaw pain and poor sleep: whereas 20% of patients in mild pain complained of poor sleep, 59% with severe jaw pain had poor sleep.[15] An additional relationship was found between patients' reports of increased pain and complaints of poor sleep, such as taking longer to fall asleep, frequently awakening from sleep, and reduced total sleep time.[4-6] There is also some evidence of a circular relationship between sleep and pain: A day of intense pain is frequently followed by a night of poor sleep, and a night of disrupted sleep is frequently followed by a day with more intense and more variable pain.[4,5,9]

Does poor sleep cause chronic pain?

The possibility that poor sleep is a cause of pain was tested experimentally in the early 1970s. Auditory stimulation was used to deprive young healthy subjects, free of pain and sleep complaints, of the so-called restorative sleep stages (3 and 4). Interestingly, the subjects reported more muscle tenderness the following day, a possible consequence of fatigue related to sleep deprivation.[3,4,7,10] In the absence of strong evidence indicating that poor sleep is the major cause of pain, we cannot so far conclude the existence of a simple relationship between poor sleep and persistent pain. Nonetheless, sleep-related medical conditions such as insomnia, sleep respiratory disorders, and periodic limb movement need to be excluded as concomitant risk factors (see Box 16-1).

Does pain cause poor sleep?

The case for pain causing poor sleep, or vice versa, would be strengthened if it could be shown that one precedes the other. In fact, 90% of chronic pain patients reported that pain occurred before or at the onset of poor sleep.[4] While this suggests that pain has a direct influence upon sleep quality, recent experimental evidence is not supportive. Two recent studies using experimental nociceptive "brief" thermal or "long" chemical stimulation have only shown slight sleep disturbance in normal subjects.[16,17] Moreover, no major complaint of poor sleep quality was reported upon awakening.

Possible factors confounding the relationship between pain and poor sleep

It is difficult to isolate the influence of chronic health disturbances associated with persistent pain. Psychologic variables, such as a catastrophizing attitude, lifestyle and stress, fatigue, irritability, and hypervigilance toward health, are frequently noted in chronic pain patients.[3,4,7,8,9] Moreover, affective distress (eg, mood changes, anxiety, depression) has been shown to explain 25% of the variance in the interaction between pain and sleep disturbance.[4,5,9] The modifications in physiologic processes seen in insomniacs and in chronic pain (fibromyalgia) patients[7,12,13] suggest that data obtained from studies of sleep deprivation or noxious stimulation in normal subjects[3,7,9,10,16,17] should also be interpreted with caution. In the absence of persistent symptoms, a normal healthy subject may react differently to a sudden pain aggression than a patient suffering from chronic pain.

Overview of Management Strategies for Pain and Poor Sleep

In developing a management strategy, it is first important to determine whether a patient who complains primarily of poor sleep has any sleep disorders (see Box 16-1) or medical conditions that could disturb sleep. Many factors, including use of certain medications or psychostimulants, poor fitness, alcohol abuse, and poor diet, can perturb sleep. Clinicians should also be aware that antidepressant medications, such as serotonin selective reuptake inhibitors (fluoxetine, sertraline), can exacerbate motor activity such as bruxism (see Lavigne et al[4,5,18] for more information).

Next, good sleep-hygiene strategies should be reviewed, including regular sleep schedules and habits before sleep; relaxation before sleep; avoidance of coffee, excessive meals, alcohol, or smoking in the evening; and the establishment of a quiet and comfortable sleeping environment. Cognitive-behavioral techniques, relaxation, biofeedback, or autohypnosis have been suggested to be modestly effective, although further controlled studies are necessary.[4,5,19]

Medications to reduce pain in relation to sleep (eg, analgesics such as nonsteroidal anti-inflammatory drugs [NSAIDs]; see chapter 21), or those that reduce anxiety and/or muscle activity such as benzodiazepines (eg, valium, lorazepam, clonazepam) or muscle relaxants (eg, methacarbomol, cyclobenzaprine), can also be used for short periods. To improve sleep quality and continuity, hypnotic medications (eg, zolpidem, zopiclone) may be used,

again for short periods. Antidepressants (eg, amitriptyline, trazodone) have low to moderate efficacy in managing sleep and pain complaints, but their use is limited due to side effects (eg, daytime somnolence, xerostomia).

Finally, oral appliances are thought to have some efficacy in sleep bruxism and/or orofacial pain (eg, bite splints, mouth guards) or snoring/sleep apnea (eg, mandibular advancement appliances, continuous positive airway pressure), as described briefly in chapter 26; however, not all patients can tolerate them for various reasons including physical discomfort, pain, and hypersalivation.[18] Because the management of sleep breathing disorders (apneas) is a growing area of interest in dentistry, readers should increase their knowledge in this field.[11,18]

Summary

This chapter has noted that patients with orofacial pain are at risk of having poor sleep (eg, long delays in falling asleep, frequent sleep arousals, sleep-stage shifts, and body movements during sleep). There is good evidence that a day with more pain is followed by a poor night's sleep, and a night of poor sleep by more variable pain on the following day. When a chronic pain patient does report persistent problems with sleep, the following is recommended:

1. Check if the patient has good sleep hygiene (ie, regular sleep schedules and habits before sleeping; relaxation before sleeping; avoidance of coffee, excessive meals, alcohol, or smoking in the evening).
2. Determine, if the patient complains primarily of poor sleep, has any sleep disorders or medical conditions, or uses medication that could disturb sleep. It may be necessary then to refer the patient to a sleep specialist to exclude the possibility of a sleep disorder.

3. Institute short-term use of medications that may improve sleep continuity (ie, less sleep perturbation or fragmentation).
4. Consider using an oral appliance to treat sleep bruxism and/or orofacial pain (ie, bite splints, mouth guards) or snoring and/or sleep apnea (ie, mandibular advancement appliance, continuous positive airway pressure). However, recognize the limitations of such appliances.

Acknowledgments

The authors' research is supported by Canadian Institutes of Health Research and Fonds de Recherche en Santé du Quebec as well as by a Canada Research Chair in Pain, Sleep and Trauma.

References

1. Carskadon MA, Dement WC. Normal human sleep: An overview. In: Kryger MH, Roth T, Dement WC (eds). Principles and Practice of Sleep Medicine, ed 4. Philadelphia: Saunders, 2005:13–23.
2. Velluti RA. Interactions between sleep and sensory physiology. J Sleep Res 1997;6:61–77.
3. Moldofsky H. Sleep and musculoskeletal pain. In: Merskey H, Vaerøy H (eds). Progress in Fibromyalgia and Myofascial Pain. Amsterdam: Elsevier, 1993:137–148.
4. Lavigne GJ, McMillan D, Zucconi M. Pain and sleep. In: Kryger MH, Roth T, Dement WC (eds). Principles and Practice of Sleep Medicine, ed 4. Philadelphia: Saunders, 2005:1246–1255.
5. Lavigne G. Orofacial pain, sleep disturbance. In: Schmidt RF, Willis WD (eds). Encyclopedia of Pain. New York: Springer, 2007.
6. Mahowald MW, Mahowald ML, Bundlie SR, Ytterberg SR. Sleep fragmentation in rheumatoid arthritis. Arthritis Rheum 1989;32:974–983.
7. Pillemer SR, Bradley LA, Crofford LJ, Moldofsky H, Chrousos GP. The neuroscience and endocrinology of fibromyalgia. Arthritis Rheum 1997;40:1928–1939.
8. Wolfe F, Smythe HA, Yunus MB, et al. The American College of Rheumatology 1990 criteria for the classification of fibromyalgia: Report of the multicenter criteria committee. Arthritis Rheum 1990;33:160–172.
9. Lavigne G, Khoury S, Laverdure-Dupont D, Denis R, Rouleau G. Tools and methodological issues in the investigation of sleep and pain interactions. In: Lavigne G, Sessle BJ, Soja PJ, Choinière M (eds). Sleep and Pain. Seattle: IASP Press, 2007:235–266.
10. Lautenbacher S, Kundermann B, Krieg JC. Sleep deprivation and pain perception. Sleep Med Rev 2006;10: 357–369.
11. American Academy of Sleep Medicine. The International Classification of Sleep Disorders. Diagnostic and Coding Manual, ed 2. Westchester: American Academy of Sleep Medicine, 2005.
12. Bonnet MH, Arand DL. Heart rate variability in insomniacs and matched normal sleepers. Psychosom Med 1998;60:610–615.
13. Martinez-Lavin M, Hermosillo AG, Rosas M, Soto ME. Circadian studies of autonomic nervous balance in patients with fibromyalgia: A heart rate variability analysis. Arthritis Rheum 1998;41:1966–1971.
14. Dao TT, Reynolds WJ, Tenenbaum HC. Comorbidity between myofascial pain of the masticatory muscles and fibromyalgia. J Orofac Pain 1997;11:232–241.
15. Goulet JP, Lavigne GJ, Lund JP. Jaw pain prevalence among French-speaking Canadians in Québec and related symptoms of temporomandibular disorders. J Dent Res 1995;74:1738–1744.
16. Drewes AM, Nielsen KD, Arendt-Nielsen L, Birket-Smith L, Hansen LM. The effect of cutaneous and deep pain on the electroencephalogram during sleep—An experimental study. Sleep 1997;20:632–640.
17. Lavigne G, Zucconi M, Castronovo C, Manzini C, Marchettini P, Smirne S. Sleep arousal response to experimental thermal stimulation during sleep in human subjects free of pain and sleep problems. Pain 2000;84: 283–290.
18. Lavigne GJ, Manzini C, Kato T. Sleep bruxism. In: Kryger MH, Roth T, Dement WC (eds). Principles and Practice of Sleep Medicine, ed 4. Philadelphia: Saunders, 2005: 946–959.
19. Smith MT, Haythornthwaite JA. Cognitive-behavioral treatment for insomnia and pain. In: Lavigne G, Sessle BJ, Soja P, Choiniere M (eds). Sleep and Pain. Seattle: IASP Press, 2007;439–458.

Section IV

Management of Orofacial Pain: Principles and Practices

The Path to Diagnosis

Jean-Paul Goulet
Sandro Palla

Patients complaining of acute or chronic orofacial pain often first consult a general dentist, whose task is threefold: *(1)* to establish the correct diagnosis, *(2)* to determine the cause of the pain, and *(3)* to select the treatment plan. A decision to refer to an expert for further evaluation can be made at any stage, but it is mandatory in the case of chronic pain. The aim of this chapter is to describe the diagnostic process and provide a diagnostic framework for the following chapters on pain management. Chapter 27 outlines cases that illustrate this process.

Overview of the Diagnostic Process

The clinical reasoning leading to a final diagnosis follows a hypotheticodeductive process (Fig 17-1). This process includes the practitioner's memory of clinically relevant knowledge gained by formal training, as well as exposure to different clinical conditions and procedures. To develop clinical expertise, acquired knowledge and cognitive processing need to be reorganized to fit the domain of expertise. The richness of such knowledge contributes to the buildup of meaningful sets of illness scripts that are used in the deductive process to test diagnostic hypotheses by pattern recognition.[1]

Gathering all anamnestic information represents the key starting point for creating the patient's database, which then feeds the clinical reasoning process. While doing this, the clinician's working memory analyzes, weighs, compares, and reassesses incoming information so as to place it in proper perspective. The next step consists of developing a provisional or differential diagnosis from a list of all possibilities and ranking them from the most to the least probable. Clinicians' experience and knowledge of signs and symptoms, natural course, distribution, and possible mechanisms, in combination with their familiarity with the diagnostic criteria of the different orofacial pain conditions, are therefore invaluable in the making of meaningful connections with the patient's database. At this stage, the decision to seek additional clinical information or to refer the patient to a specialist usually takes place. An action plan is then developed based on a working diagnosis.

In many instances, confirming a definitive diagnosis might not be possible due to the lack of disease-specific signs, objective tests, and precise diagnostic criteria. For example, a patient may not have the "textbook" presentation. Confirming a

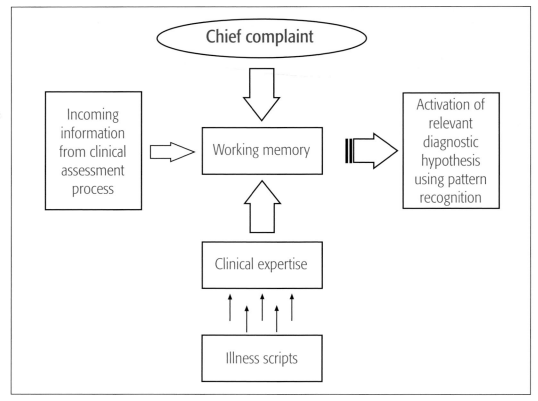

Fig 17-1 Clinical reasoning process that leads to diagnosis.

diagnosis based on the effects of treatment is also difficult given that a variety of orofacial pain conditions may respond well to the same treatment and that different treatments may be effective for the same condition (see chapters 18 and 19). When the working diagnosis remains the one with the highest probability, it is ruled as the final diagnosis unless proven otherwise.

The Clinical Assessment Process

The process of gathering evidence implies a reliance on proper strategies and procedures for data collection. As the clinician proceeds, the diagnostic space is likely to change and so will the focus of the assessment process. The assessment of the somatic, psychosocial, and behavioral aspects of the pain problem becomes invaluable when one considers that the site and source of the pain are not always the same, that tissue damage might be unnoticeable or absent, and that any state of pain has a psychologic and psychosocial impact. The clinical assessment process is usually divided into two distinct parts: (1) the appraisal of the chief complaint and the patient's medical, dental, and psychosocial status (also called the comprehensive history), and (2) the clinical examination.

It is important also to point out that the diagnostic process is different for acute and chronic pain states. For instance, it is only necessary to establish a physical/somatic diagnosis for an acute

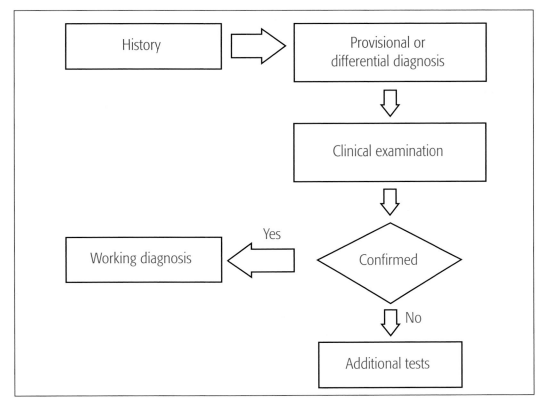

Fig 17-2 The diagnostic process.

pain condition such as a pulpitis. In cases of chronic pain, a physical as well as a psychosocial diagnosis is necessary because the pain has rarely any biologic value and is frequently accompanied by significant emotional distress and affective and cognitive disturbances that need to be addressed (see chapter 12).[2,3] In that regard, the Graded Chronic Pain Scale[4] is a good screening instrument for patients with chronic pain.

Comprehensive history

The comprehensive history constitutes the most important part of the diagnostic process. Taking the history is essential for establishing a good doctor-patient relationship, the prerequisite for successful management of the pain patient. In addition, several orofacial pain conditions lack specific signs, and their diagnosis relies on pain-related inclusion criteria that can be revealed only by the comprehensive history. The history should lead to a provisional or differential diagnosis; the clinical examination and additional tests then are needed to confirm or rule out the provisional diagnosis (Fig 17-2).

Besides appraising the patient's chief complaint, the comprehensive history helps put symptoms in the appropriate context. This is achieved through a well-organized and structured interview covering the reason the patient is seeking professional assistance, how the problem started, and how it has evolved. The clinician must inquire about localization, quality, duration, time course, triggering,

Box 17-1 Comprehensive pain description

Intensity	On a 0 to 10 scale, how does your present pain rate? For chronic pain problems, how would you rate your average, minimum, and worst pain over the past month?
Location	Is the pain intraoral or extraoral; unilateral or bilateral; localized, regional, or diffuse? Does it involve one or more branches of the trigeminal territory?
Referral patterns	Where does the pain irradiate to?
Character	What does the pain feel like (eg, throbbing, shooting, stabbing, sharp, cramping, gnawing, hot/burning, aching, heavy, tender, splitting, tiring/exhausting, sickening, fearful, punishing/cruel, unbearable)?
Duration	How long does the pain last when it occurs (eg, seconds, minutes, hours, days)?
Frequency	How often does the pain occur (eg, every day, several times a week or month, only once in a while)?
Temporal pattern	Does the pain fluctuate during the day? Is it seasonal or cyclic in pattern?
Triggering or aggravating factors	What are the effects of functional activity on pain intensity (eg, jaw opening, biting, chewing, head movements)?
Improving factors	When does the pain get better (eg, reduced functional activity, rest, relaxation, over-the-counter analgesics, heat, sleep)?
Associated signs and symptoms	Is the pain preceded or accompanied by stuffy nose, tearing, flushing, warm sensation, dizziness, vertigo, tingling, numbness, aura?

worsening or relieving factors, and accompanying symptoms (Box 17-1). A careful pain description is important since several orofacial and headache conditions are diagnosed only upon specific pain features. The classic example is trigeminal neuralgia with its normal neurologic status, pain-free intervals, and characteristic waves of paroxysmal, brief electric shock–like pain with triggering factors, (see chapter 24). Because pain is a multidimensional experience, the patients must also be asked how the pain influences their emotional behavior (see also chapters 11 and 12).

Patients focusing only on their chief complaint may underestimate the real extent of the pain involvement. This is especially true with chronic orofacial pain patients since they often suffer from different pain disorders. For instance, patients with chronic musculoskeletal orofacial pain rarely dis-

close suffering from headache or cervical pain or fibromyalgia as well. Therefore, specifically asking about pain outside the orofacial area and other pain conditions is essential for establishing a correct multiaxial diagnosis and treatment plan (see also chapter 19).

A psychosocial history is a must for patients with chronic pain. This means gathering information about any physical disability and associated disruption of lifestyle, behavior modification at the personal and social levels, beliefs regarding the cause of the pain, and coping strategies (Box 17-2). In addition to the pain duration (3 to 6 months or more), hints that the patient has a chronic pain condition are: *(1)* a vague, often changing and emotionally weighted pain description; *(2)* a tendency for the pain to expand, become persistent, and increase in intensity; *(3)* an invariably high

---

Box 17-2 Review items for assessing the impact of chronic orofacial pain

Impact of the pain problem

- Physical impairment — How does the pain interfere with orofacial function; what can the patient not do because of the pain?

- Personal disruption — What is the emotional burden caused by the pain; does the patient avoid family or other personal responsibilities or experience sleep disturbances?

- Psychosocial dysfunction — How does the pain interfere with daily activities, school, work, recreational and other social activities, and interpersonal relations (eg, family members, colleagues)?

Personal factors influencing the pain

- Mental state — How do thoughts, anger, frustration, and anxiety influence the pain?

- Stress — How do family, occupational, and social stresses influence the pain?

- Focus — What is the patient's tendency to focus on the pain problem?

- Behavior — Are certain types of behavior present that contribute to the pain problem?

---

pain intensity not influenced by functional activities; *(4)* a discrepancy between pain intensity and behavior; *(5)* high emotional and behavioral distress (Graded Chronic Pain Scale score of 3 or 4); and *(6)* a series of unsuccessful treatments.

Finally, assessing past and present illnesses, current medications, selective organ systems, recent dental treatments, and personal social history is easier when using standardized forms and questionnaires to reveal the current state of the patient.

Comprehensive physical examination

The goal of the physical evaluation is to confirm or deny the provisional or differential diagnosis by looking for specific signs and any other abnormalities (see Fig 17-2). Since signs that are uncovered must explain the symptoms (*signs plausability*), those that are fairly common in the general population, such as muscle tenderness, deviation of the mandible during opening or closing, temporomandibular joint (TMJ) sounds, and malocclusion,

should be evaluated with caution in the context of the clinical presentation.[5]

The provisional diagnosis influences the content and sequence of the clinical examination. This is therefore an inductive process where the next test/examination depends on the information gathered by the previous one and is indicated only if the additional information is likely to influence diagnosis and patient management.

Referred pain to the orofacial area from a distant source, sometimes called *heterotopic pain*, is always a possibility. In addition, comorbidity between musculoskeletal orofacial pain and other pain conditions does exist, eg, in cervical spine disorders and headache.[6,7] Therefore, other head and neck structures in addition to the oral cavity, the jaws, the masticatory muscles, and the TMJs should be part of a comprehensive physical evaluation. Whenever needed, the blood pressure, pulse rate, respiratory rate, and body temperature must be recorded. The following description summarizes these basic principles.

Extraoral examination

The head, face, ears, eyes, nose, neck, and upper extremities, including the hands, fingers, and fingernails, should be visually inspected for any gross abnormalities (eg, swelling, rashes, vesicular eruptions, lacrimation, miosis). In addition to the musculoskeletal structures of the head and neck, the lymph nodes (submandibular, submental, preauricular and postauricular, anterior and posterior cervical), major salivary glands (parotid, submandibular), paranasal sinuses (frontal, maxillary), carotid bifurcation, temporal artery, and the thyroid gland should also be palpated. The examination protocol recommended in the "Research Diagnostic Criteria for Temporomandibular Disorders"[3] should be used for the assessment of masticatory muscle and TMJ tenderness, joint noises, and the range of mandibular motion. To assess pain referral from the neck structures, palpation of the sternocleidomastoid and cervical spine muscles and assessment of the active mobility of the cervical spine are necessary. A cranial nerve screening evaluation is also indicated when signs and symptoms suggest a neurologic problem (eg, numbness or paresthesia, palsy, muscle weakness, dizziness). For both the cervical and cranial nerve examination, the goal is to document and refer the patient for a complete neurologic evaluation and appropriate management.

Intraoral examination

It is common for dental pathology to refer pain to extraoral sites. When this is suspected, a meticulous dental/periodontal examination using pulp testing, tooth percussion, biting test, and/or gingival probing is necessary to assess local causes (caries, pulp pathology, cracked tooth, periodontal pathology, occlusal trauma). In the absence of gingival inflammation, unusual pain on gingival probing may be due to allodynia, as in the case of a persistent idiopathic tooth pain (sometimes called *atypical odontalgia*).

Excessive tooth wear should prompt an inquiry about the patient's past and present parafunctional habits; occlusal changes that might have occurred just before or since the onset of the pain problem (eg, shift of the midline or development of an open bite) necessitate inquiry about joint pathology (eg, an arthritis, a neoplasia, or a disc displacement).

Careful inspection and palpation of the oral mucosa allows for assessment of the presence of soft tissue pathology. Especially important are any changes involving the posterior border of the tongue, the oropharynx, and the floor of the mouth (eg, ulcer, exophytic lesion, lump, neoplastic alterations).

Additional tests

These tests are selectively indicated whenever additional information is needed and are likely to contribute to the diagnosis and the decision regarding the patient's management (see also chapters 18 and 27).

Anesthetic blocks.
Anesthetic infiltrations and nerve blocks are helpful in identifying whether the pain is localized or referred. Qualified professionals can assess involvement of the sympathetic system (ie, sympathetically mediated pain) with anesthetic blocks of the stellate or sphenopalatine ganglion. The results of these blocks must, however, be interpreted with caution to avoid diagnostic mistakes.[8]

Imaging.
Intraoral radiographs are best to evaluate the teeth, alveolar process, and surrounding periapical bone; panoramic views are preferred for evaluating the jaws, the maxillary sinuses, and gross condylar changes. Computerized tomography is indicated for depiction of alterations to the hard tissues; magnetic resonance imaging (MRI) for showing soft tissue changes (disc form and position) and joint effusion; bone scintigraphy for uncovering metabolic changes due to neoplasias, inflammation, and

growth problems; and sialography for detecting a pathology of the salivary ducts and/or glands (eg, a stone).

Radiographic imaging is justified only if the additional information is likely to influence diagnosis and patient management. For example, ordering tomograms is not a standard care procedure to screen for condylar position since this is not related to TMJ disorders. Likewise, routine requests for MRI to "confirm a diagnosis" of a nonpainful and non-disrupting anterior disc displacement cannot be justified, since MRI normally does not provide information that would change the treatment plan.

Laboratory analysis.

Blood tests are indicated when a potential or concomitant medical problem is suspected (eg, juvenile osteoarthritis, lyme disease, psoriatic arthritis). Likewise, reports of morning headache, daytime sleepiness, or history of cessation of breathing while sleeping may suggest a sleep apnea-hypopnea syndrome that needs to be excluded by a medical consult and a sleep polygraphic study (see chapters 16 and 26). Referral to medical professionals is essential when the case is beyond the general dentist's competence to properly investigate health problems that require very specific laboratory tests and interpretation of the results for proper patient management.

Reliability of Clinical Examination Techniques and Tests

Knowing the interexaminer and between-session reliability of examination techniques is a prerequisite to sound clinical decision making (see chapter 18), but few of the routinely used procedures have been tested. Overall, the reliability of the tests used to assess mandibular mobility, muscle and TMJ tenderness, and joint sounds varies from high to acceptable among trained and calibrated examiners, and reliability is improved by recalibration.[9–11] The results of commonly used chairside clinical tests (eg, provocation tests, selective anesthesia) should be interpreted with considerable caution because their reliability either has not been tested or is questionable.

Jaw-tracking devices, electromyography, electric stimulation, sonography, vibration analysis, and thermography not only have no diagnostic validity despite many claims, but they provide a high number of false-positive indicators leading to unnecessary and often debilitating occlusal treatments.[12]

The Clinical Decision-Making Process for Orofacial Pain

The clinical decision-making process is depicted in Fig 17-3. The first question to be asked is whether the pain has a local origin and is coming from the structure where it is felt. When there is no indication of a local cause, one must check for referral from a pathologic process in a nearby structure, eg, in the maxillary sinus, ear, nose, throat, masticatory muscles, TMJ, cervical structures, major salivary glands, or major vessels. If this is not the case, one must consider referred pain from distant sources such as neuropathic pain, demyelinization disorders, neuralgias, or an ectopic manifestation of a primary headache. The latter diagnoses rely on precise inclusion criteria defined in the *International Classification of Headache Disorders*.[13]

Finally, before initiating treatment, it is necessary to establish the pain-related disability and psychosocial status for all chronic orofacial pain conditions regardless of etiology (see also chapters 11, 12, and 18). When encountering a patient with a dominant mood alteration, the clinician's role is to refer the patient to medical or psychologic experts.

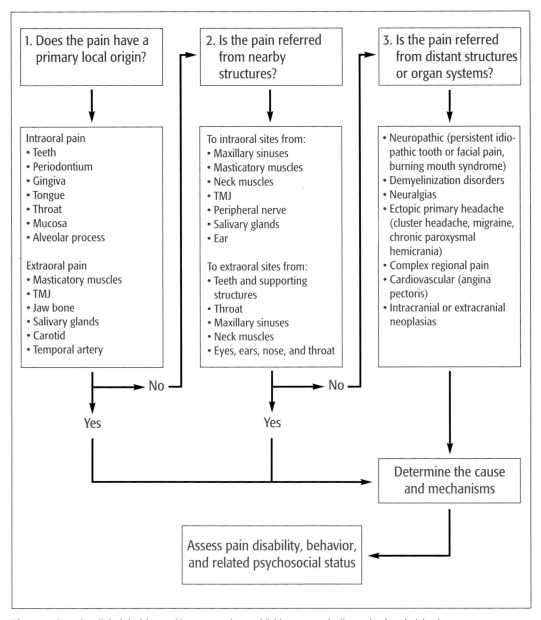

Fig 17-3 Stepwise clinical decision-making process for establishing a somatic diagnosis of orofacial pain.

Summary

This chapter has provided an overview of the intricate diagnostic process. It has emphasized the importance of a comprehensive pain history that must lead to a provisional or differential diagnosis, and thereby will set up the manner by which the physical examination process takes place.

References

1. Bordage G. Elaborated knowledge: A key to successful diagnostic thinking. Acad Med 1994;69:883–885.
2. Palla S. A need to redefine chronic pain? J Orofac Pain 2006;20:265–266.
3. Dworkin SF, LeResche L. Research diagnostic criteria for temporomandibular disorders: Review, criteria, examinations and specifications, critique. J Craniomandib Disord 1992;6:301–355.
4. Von Korff M, Ormel J, Keefe FJ, Dworkin SF. Grading the severity of chronic pain. Pain 1992;50:133–149.
5. LeResche L. Epidemiology of temporomandibular disorders: Implication for the investigation of etiologic factors. Crit Rev Oral Biol Med 1997;8:291–305.
6. Visscher CM, Lobbezoo F, de Boer W, van der Zaag J, Naeije M. Prevalence of cervical spinal pain in craniomandibular pain patients. Eur J Oral Sci 2001;109:76–80.
7. Storm C, Wanman A. Temporomandibular disorders, headaches, and cervical pain among females in a Sami population. Acta Odontol Scand 2006;64:319–325.
8. Hogan Q. Diagnostic injection. In: Turk DC, Melzack R (eds). Handbook of Pain Assessment, ed 2. New York: Guilford Press, 2001:225–247.
9. Dworkin SF, LeResche L, DeRouen T, Von Korff M. Assessing clinical signs of temporomandibular disorders: Reliability of clinical examiners. J Prosthet Dent 1990; 63:574–579.
10. Goulet JP, Clark GT, Flack VF, Changrui L. The reproducibility of muscle and joint tenderness detection methods and maximum mandibular movement measurement for the temporomandibular system. J Orofac Pain 1998;12:17–26.
11. List T, John MT, Dworkin SF, Svensson P. Recalibration improves inter-examiner reliability of TMD examination. Acta Odontol Scand 2006;64:146–152.
12. Baba K, Tsukiyama Y, Clark GT. Reliability, validity, and utility of various occlusal measurement methods and techniques. J Prosthet Dent 2000;83:83–89.
13. International Headache Society. Headache Classification Subcommittee. The International Classification of Headache Disorders, ed 2. Oxford: Blackwell, 2004.

Evidence-Based Pain Management

Jocelyne S. Feine

Health care is increasingly expensive, and health care providers, consumers, insurance companies, and governments all want to know that the services provided are efficient and cost effective. In today's society, the clinician has to be able to answer questions from patients and those who control payment plans. In some cases, clinicians must also defend their decisions before tribunals.

The fundamentals of good evidence-based health care are disarmingly simple: "doing the right thing" for patients (ie, providing appropriate care) and "doing the right thing right" (ie, providing appropriate care properly).[1] The choice is based on the best available evidence and is guided by the preference of patients who have been fully informed about the possible associated risks and benefits. Ideally, it should cost no more than an equally effective alternative service.[1]

Historically, clinical practice was opinion-based. Clinical decisions were often made by the dentist or physician after little discussion with the patient. The treatment plans were based on a mix of knowledge gained through training, subjective perception of past experiences, practice traditions, and the opinions of recognized authorities. This resulted in highly variable diagnoses and treatments for the same condition, as well as ineffective, expensive, and sometimes harmful interventions.[2] This situation is no longer acceptable to society.

The evidence-based clinical practice movement promotes the translation of new scientific evidence into clinical care. It means integrating personal clinical expertise with the best available external evidence drawn from research into the accuracy and precision of diagnostic tests; the power of prognostic markers; and the efficacy and safety of therapeutic, rehabilitative, and preventive regimens.[3] To function in this new environment, health care providers must be able to (1) formulate answerable questions that stem from clinical issues, (2) track down the best evidence to answer them, (3) evaluate the evidence, (4) apply the results of the appraisal to their clinical practice, and (5) evaluate their own future clinical performance (audit). The questions posed should be as specific as possible and include the type of patient, the clinical intervention (if treatment choice is the subject of interest), and the appropriate outcome. Once the clinical questions have been properly formulated, a search of the literature can be carried out to find the relevant publications.[4]

The Evidence

Scientific literature is now readily accessible to anyone who wishes to find the information, particularly with the rapidly changing developments in computer resources and Internet communications. A review of the literature on therapies designed to treat pain produces a wide variety of publications ranging from systematic reviews to single case reports,[4,5] which rank in value (from highest to lowest) as follows:

1. Systematic reviews
2. Randomized controlled trials (RCTs)
3. Controlled trials without randomization
4. Cohort or case-control studies
5. Descriptive studies (comparative or correlational)
6. Respected authorities, clinical experience (case reports), or expert committees

The best evidence of therapeutic efficacy will be found in properly conducted systematic reviews, particularly meta-analyses, of multiple well-designed RCTs. These are considered the gold standard for evidence because they evaluate the consistency of scientific results drawn from many RCTs carried out on different populations, often in different countries. If a systematic review or meta-analysis has not been undertaken for a relevant question, the next strongest evidence comes from at least one properly designed and executed RCT. If RCTs have not been done, the reader should look for nonrandomized trials, single-group pre-treatment and posttreatment assessments, time series, or case-control studies. The last line of evidence on which to base a clinical decision comes from case series reports and the opinions of respected authorities in the field. Reports of expert consensus committees that are scientifically unsupported are given little credibility in this hierarchy, an approach that is very different from the tradition of valuing personal opinion of the expert above all other sources of information. A review of evidence-based pain management issues details the current state of evidence-based care and concludes that the necessary evidence to support the management of various types of pain conditions is not always available.[2] For example, a systematic review on the efficacy of occlusal adjustment treatments for temporomandibular disorders (TMDs) found no evidence to support this common therapeutic approach.[6] Similarly, another systematic review concluded that there is inadequate evidence available to draw conclusions on the efficacy of splint therapy to reduce pain associated with TMDs.[7]

Assessing the evidence of RCTs

To assess the quality of a clinical trial, one must understand the basic principles of study design. Some of these principles are illustrated below using a hypothetic study designed to test whether a new analgesic will reduce the postoperative pain associated with the placement of dental implants significantly faster than the standard medication.

1. *Sample.* The group of subjects enrolled in the trial should be a good, representative sample of the general population of patients who undergo implant surgery. If these are generally older adults, then this should be the chosen population.
2. *Population size.* The population size should be large enough to satisfy statistical criteria, and a statistical test to determine the number of subjects necessary to detect real differences (and similarities) should be reported in the publication.
3. *Outcomes.* The outcomes chosen should be appropriate and valid. If the purpose of the treatment is to reduce postoperative pain and if one wishes to show that the new analgesic reduces the pain faster than the standard treatment, then the primary outcome of the study should be patients' ratings of pain measured over a period of time. Other outcomes of interest may also be used such as the use of medications and time off from work, among others.

4. *Randomization.* The treatments should be randomly allocated to patients undergoing implant surgery so that about half will receive the new analgesic and the rest of the patients will receive a standard analgesic.
5. *Blinded controls.* The study should be *blinded*, meaning neither the patients nor the clinicians should know which analgesic a patient receives. This is often accomplished by having the pharmacist prepare the medications so that they look exactly the same (eg, pills of same size, color, taste).
6. Appropriate statistical tests should be conducted to determine whether detected differences between treatments are significant and whether other factors (eg, age, sex, side effects) alter the outcome.

Box 18-1 presents an example of the use of evidence for deciding whether to use a new local anesthetic for acute pain control.

Case-control and cohort studies

If one wishes to know whether a diagnostic test will accurately distinguish between healthy and ill people, then the most appropriate study designs are cross-sectional. A *cross-sectional study* is an observational study because no intervention is undertaken. A population is selected, and individuals with and without the disease are identified using an accepted gold standard test. In the field of chronic pain, this would be the clinical examination and medical/dental history. The new diagnostic test is also used with the population and its results are compared with those of the gold standard. These studies will establish the *sensitivity* (the ability of the test to accurately detect those with the condition) and *specificity* (the ability of the test to accurately detect those without the condition) of the diagnostic test. The clinical course of a condition (prognosis or natural history) may be best described using a *cohort* or *follow-up* design, in which a population with a disorder is observed over time to determine how the illness progresses. Certain criteria must be followed for the results to be considered valid[8] and ethical.

Evaluating clinical performance

Once the clinician has sought the appropriate scientific information and has put it into practice, it is important to know whether the therapies or techniques are successful. Clinicians can assess the effectiveness of their efforts (auditing) to control both acute and chronic pain by using certain measurable factors that reflect relevant changes in the patient's condition (Box 18-2).

When treating pain in the clinic, it is also important to understand that any intervention can have a placebo effect.[9] In other words, the therapy itself may not be efficacious, yet the patient may feel that pain is reduced. This has been shown repeatedly; for example, subjects taking acetylsalicylic acid or a placebo sugar pill all reported significant pain relief.[10]

Acute pain control

Assessing the success of acute pain control is straightforward. Generally, the patient's reports of acute pain intensity and relief are appropriate indicators of changes in the condition. These can be recorded on simple scales (see chapter 10). To get a better understanding of the intensity and duration of the pain, information on the number of pills used or access to rescue medication, for example, is also gathered.

Chronic pain control

Because chronic pain has a great impact on psychologic state and quality of life (see chapter 12) and in many cases cannot be eliminated completely or permanently, most therapy is palliative and directed toward improving the ability of the patient to cope and to improve quality of life. Palliative therapies (eg, application of heat or cold to the painful area, electric stimulation, exercises, drugs, and dental appliances) are not capable of curing the condition; at best, they reduce some of the symptoms.

Although a chronic condition may manifest several features, pain is the primary reason that most patients seek care. Thus, it seems logical to measure the patient's pain perception to evaluate treatment success (see chapter 10), as described below, and also to use psychosocial scales such as the Graded Chronic Pain Scale (see chapters 11 and 12) to evaluate level of psychosocial functioning. Many dentists involved in management of chronic pain patients collaborate with psychologists

or psychiatrists who can assess the possibility of a psychosocial dysfunction.

Measuring the pain

Clinicians have traditionally assessed treatment success by asking patients whether they feel better than they did previously, thereby obtaining an estimate of the perceived degree of relief. The assumption here is that patients first recall correctly how they felt prior to treatment, then compare that memory to how they feel at present. In using these reports of relief as a basis for assessing treatment success, one assumes that the memory of the initial pain (prior to treatment) is accurate. In fact, this has been shown not to be the case for chronic pain.[11] Because ratings of relief are not highly correlated with decreases in pain levels, it is possible that these reports reflect patients' tolerance of their overall condition and/or their feelings about their condition.

Reports of relief may be a useful indicator of a patient's beliefs that he or she is benefiting from treatment. In that sense, these reports are helpful to the clinician, but it must be kept in mind that a high rating of relief is not evidence that the treatment has corrected the real cause of the problem nor reduced the intensity and duration of the pain. To know whether there has been a true change in the primary symptom of pain, it is necessary to measure the level of pain before, during, and after treatment.

Measuring care-seeking behavior

Scientists often use subsequent care-seeking behavior to measure success of treatments for chronic pain conditions in long-term clinical studies. However, few clinicians have the resources to follow patients who no longer come to the office or call to complain about their condition. Many chronic pain patients go to other health care providers when one treatment does not seem to be suc-

Box 18-2 Measurable factors for assessing changes in patient's pain condition

Acute pain	Chronic pain
• Pain reports	• Pain reports
• Reports of relief	• Reports of relief
• Use of medication*	• Use of medication*
• Response to provocation	• Response to provocation
	• Ability to perform daily tasks
	• Quality of life
	• Care-seeking behavior

*More pills or rescue medication

cessful. The patient who appears at a dental office with a bag full of splints was probably considered to be a successful case by the previous practitioner, because the patient never returned to that office.

Some pain patients, such as those with lower back pain, are unable to work as a result of their pain; a return-to-work measure is a possible criterion for success of treatment in these patients. However, the interpretation of this variable is not easy because it may have more to do with other factors, such as job availability and satisfaction, than with pain levels.[12]

Measuring the use of medication

Reports of reduced use of medication are frequently applied in chronic pain evaluation. Long-term pharmacotherapy, although easy to assess and directly applicable to conditions such as rheumatoid arthritis, is not ordinarily used to treat conditions such as TMDs because of weak evidence of efficacy.

Provocation tests

Although the manual pressure-pain threshold test is widely used in clinical practice, this technique has been shown to be highly variable.[13] While this variability can be reduced with the use of pressure algometers,[14] the results are still influenced by several factors including patient response, location of pain, magnitude of pain, rate of application of the pressure, and degree of muscle contraction.[15]

Functional measures

Some practitioners believe that patients' reports of chronic pain are unreliable because these reports are subjective and their treatment results are vulnerable to the influence of factors that have nothing to do with the condition itself. Practitioners often turn to so-called objective or functional tests, no matter how poorly these tests perform. As an example, these tests are performed routinely in patients with a temporomandibular joint (TMJ) disc displacement without reduction (see chapter 22) to assess limitations in jaw function by measuring maximum mouth opening and excursive movements of the mandible. Although these tests can give some indication as to change in condition, limited jaw function is not a consistent symptom in TMD patients. Valid measures of function for TMDs have yet to be developed; those currently in use have performed poorly in clinical studies.[16] For example, one study assessed the validity of measurements of jaw movement to distinguish between people with and without TMDs.[17] A group of young adult male and female subjects was selected, then the gold standard of examination and pain reports was used to determine if they had symptoms of TMDs. An individual who was blind to these diagnoses recorded their jaw movements with an instrument and classified them into healthy or ill groups based on the manufacturer's criteria. The results of the two classifications were compared, and it was found that the new tests identified disease in most of the group with symptoms, but also in most of the control group; ie, the test had high sensitivity but low specificity. It was concluded that the use of such tests could lead to the unnecessary treatment of healthy patients.[17] Therefore, although the clinician may wish to carry out these functional tests to have a rough record of function for medicolegal purposes, their scientific value for chronic TMDs is highly questionable.

The presence of concomitant bruxism is often noted in TMD cases, but valid diagnosis is only possible in sleep laboratories or laboratories with ambulatory systems (see chapters 16 and 26). These types of functional tests are not in common use because they are time-consuming and costly.

Some functional disability tests for patients with chronic back pain have been validated,[18] possibly because it is easier to observe pain behavior in these patients (limping, grimacing, and bracing) than to see alterations in function caused by pain. Turk and Melzack[12] have reported that the relationship between pathology, function, behavior, and pain reports is weak. Moreover, functional assessment is always influenced by the patient's psychologic state because motivation and effort are necessary in the performance of the test.[19]

Psychosocial measures

The measurement of psychologic variables, such as coping ability, distress, or depression, is unfamiliar to most dentists, although these are highly important factors in chronic pain conditions. When it appears that a patient is struggling to deal with the pain and is demonstrating distress, referral to a psychologist or psychiatrist is indicated (see chapters 11 and 12).

Measuring satisfaction with treatment

Questionnaires, surveys, and interviews can be used to measure patient satisfaction with the health care they have received. It has been suggested that patients evaluate their health care on a number of different aspects, including technical quality, personal aspects of care, accessibility, availability, continuity, acceptability and convenience of the physical setting, as well as the effectiveness of treatment.[20] However, because these are difficult to separate, a single global measure of satisfaction is often taken.

Summary

This chapter has emphasized that quality health care requires that treatment decisions be based on scientific evidence. Therefore, clinicians must be capable of understanding scientific methods and maintaining active clinical auditing within their practices. Particularly when a condition is chronic and there is little evidence that most therapies are more efficacious than placebo, it is important that a treatment be properly evaluated for its effectiveness within the environment in which it is provided. Measuring changes in pain and asking patients to rate the relief that they feel are valid methods clinicians can use to determine the effectiveness of the therapies that they provide.

References

1. Rachlis M, Kushner C. Strong Medicine: How to Save Canada's Health Care System. Toronto: Harper Collins, 1994.
2. Manchikanti L, Boswell MV, Giordano J. Evidence-based interventional pain management: Principles, problems, potential and applications. Pain Physician 2007;10:329–356.
3. Evidence-Based Medicine Working Group. Evidence-based medicine: A new approach to teaching the practice of medicine. JAMA 1992;268:2420–2425.
4. Rosenberg W, Donald A. Evidence based medicine: An approach to clinical problem-solving. BMJ 1995;310:1122–1126.
5. Wiffen PJ, Fairman FS. The Cochrane Collaboration Pain, Palliative Care and Supportive Care Collaborative Review Group. J Pain Palliat Care Pharmacother 2002;16(2):69–79.
6. Forssell H, Kalso E. Application of principles of evidence-based medicine to occlusal treatment for temporomandibular disorders: Are there lessons to be learned? J Orofac Pain 2004;18:9–22; discussion 23–32.
7. Al-Ani MZ, Davies SJ, Gray RJ, Sloan P, Glenny AM. Stabilisation splint therapy for temporomandibular pain dysfunction syndrome [comment]. Evid Based Dent 2004;5:65–66.
8. Crombie IK. The Pocket Guide to Critical Appraisal. London: BMJ Publishing, 1996.
9. Evans FJ. The placebo response in pain reduction. In: Bonica JJ (ed). Advances in Neurology, vol 4. New York: Raven Press, 1974:289–296.
10. McQuay H, Carroll D, Moore A. Variation in the placebo effect in randomised controlled trials of analgesics: All is as blind as it seems. Pain 1996;64:331–335.
11. Feine JS, Lavigne GJ, Dao TT, Morin C, Lund JP. Memories of chronic pain and perceptions of relief. Pain 1998;77:137–141.
12. Turk DC, Melzack R (eds). Handbook of Pain Assessment. New York: The Guilford Press, 1992:3–12.
13. Friedman MH, Weisberg J. Pitfalls of muscle palpation in TMJ diagnosis. J Prosthet Dent 1982;48:331.
14. Schiffman E, Fricton J, Haley D, Tylca D. A pressure algometer for myofascial pain syndrome: Reliability and validity testing. In: Dubner R, Gebhart GF, Bond MR (eds). Proceedings of the Vth World Congress on Pain. New York: Elsevier, 1988.
15. Thu Thon M, Lavigne GJ, TenBokun L, Guitard F, Goulet J-P. The effect of muscle contraction, distraction and other variables on pressure-pain threshold. In: Seventh World Congress on Pain. [Proceedings of Seventh World Congress on Pain, 22–27 Aug 1993, Paris.] Seattle: IASP Publications, 1993.
16. Widmer CG, Lund JP, Feine JS. Diagnostic validity of clinical evaluation techniques for temporomandibular disorders. J Orofac Pain 1993;7:103–104.
17. Feine JS, Hutchins MO, Lund JP. An evaluation of the criteria used to diagnose mandibular dysfunction with the mandibular kinesiograph. J Prosthet Dent 1988;60:374–380.
18. Dirks JF, Wunder J, Kinsman R, McElhinny J, Jones NF. A pain rating scale and a pain behavior checklist for clinical use: Development, norms, and the consistency score. Psychother Psychosom 1993;59:41–49.
19. Fordyce WE. Pain and suffering: A reappraisal. Am Psychol 1988;43:276–283.
20. Fitzpatrick R. Measurement of patient satisfaction. In: Hopkins A, Costain D, (eds). Measuring the Outcomes of Medical Care: Papers Based on a Conference Held in September 1989. London: Royal College of Physicians of London, King's Fund Centre for Health Services Development. 1990:19–26.

Management of Persistent Orofacial Pain

Christian S. Stohler

This chapter presents a framework for the management of persistent orofacial pain conditions. Emphasis is placed on the delivery of care. One-size-fits-all "magic-bullet" practice schemes do not take into account the wide range of case complexity (eg, the intensity and extent of pain, mood-related consequences, disability, and comorbid conditions), making it difficult for the inexperienced practitioner to choose a suitable care environment and appropriate level of care for a given patient. Experience has shown that not all patients with a particular diagnosis benefit from being managed the same way. For this reason, this chapter introduces a framework for clinical decision-making to provide a basis for subsequent chapters dealing with specific pain conditions. This outline acknowledges differences in the care needs of individual orofacial pain patients irrespective of whether the origin of their pain is musculoskeletal, neuropathic, or idiopathic.

Professional Care

Disease taxonomies that distinguish disease subsets for which a specific treatment predicts a greater benefit-risk ratio than other types of care are use-

ful. On the other hand, some disease classifications present no evidence that this benefit-risk response varies among subsets for a given intervention; these classifications imply meaningful information when in fact none exists. Any therapeutic intervention should also be based on reasonable certainty that the patient suffers from a condition for which the chosen care is likely to improve the patient's life. The guiding principles are that treatment benefits outweigh potential risks and that the costs, both monetary and biologic, are justified by the expected benefits.

Defining the Challenge

There is a great deal of subject-to-subject variation in response to treatment, and most patients experience benefits from a range of therapies, especially when treated for the first time. However, the challenge lies with a subset of patients for whom all current treatments leave much to be desired. It is the growing level of dissatisfaction among such patients that is captured in the voice of patient advocates who call for efficacious therapies, care standardization, safety assurances, and professional accountability.

Using a Case-Specific Approach

Lessons learned from the management of persistent pain teaches us key case attributes that have diagnostic and therapeutic implications include the temporal presentation of pain (persistent or not), the presence and nature of comorbid conditions, the impact on the patient's life, and the history of previous unsatisfactory treatment attempts. In this respect, it seems appropriate to make the assumption that, compared to a patient exhibiting transient pain, patients with persistent pain have greater chance of continuing to be in pain in the future. Similarly, a patient who has experienced multiple unsatisfactory treatments is more likely to encounter another treatment failure than success.

Another problem is that much comorbidity linked to orofacial pain conditions falls beyond the scope of the dental practice act in almost all jurisdictions and, therefore, requires coordination of care with another health care provider (see also chapter 12). Comorbidities include emotional consequences, such as depressive preoccupation, fear, and anxiety. Physical impairment and disability may exceed the range of services offered in a general dentistry setting. The more complex cases are better dealt with in tertiary care pain clinics, where the emphasis shifts from eradicating pain to improving activity tolerance, preventing deconditioning, and maintaining productivity.

Varying Focus in the Treatment of Pain

In contrast to acute pain and pain associated with terminal illness, *persistent pain* has an element of permanency. In fact, persistent pain implies that all treatments up to this point have not produced acceptable relief. Given the need for continued care, potential health risks due to long-term treatments need to be considered. Unnecessarily high dosages of pain medication should be avoided, and chances of adverse drug interactions increase with the number of concurrent medications consumed (see also chapter 21). When choosing treatments for persistent pain, the primary focus is safety, with secondary importance given to treatment efficacy and cost. This emphasis contrasts sharply with the management of acute pain or pain of the terminally ill, for which treatment efficacy should be the priority.

Sorting Patients According to Care Requirements

Pain severity, extent, and pain/stress-related consequences vary from patient to patient, calling for the decision as to which care intensity and environment best meet the needs of a particular patient. Whereas transient and infrequent orofacial pains represent more of a nuisance than a burden, severe and persistent pains are debilitating and cause significant life disruption. Impact on patients and their families has to be taken into account.

Both patients and health care providers benefit from the customization of therapy. Referrals should be considered based on the experience and skills of providers and the essential services that are at their disposal. The dentist can offer valuable service in combination with other health care providers, even in the most complex case, and particularly in rural settings, where access to specialty clinics is often limited. For the milder, nondebilitating forms of pain, dentists offer treatment alternatives to pharmacotherapy that are often preferred by patients.

Understanding of complex matters can be achieved through a structured approach to simplify the problem. In this approach, a system is introduced that brings order to a patient population with heterogenous care needs. Among the case attributes with both therapeutic and medicolegal implications, two criteria are critical for sorting patients according to care needs and to further define the dentist's role: *(1)* pain severity and *(2)* relevant comorbid conditions. The decision tree, displayed in

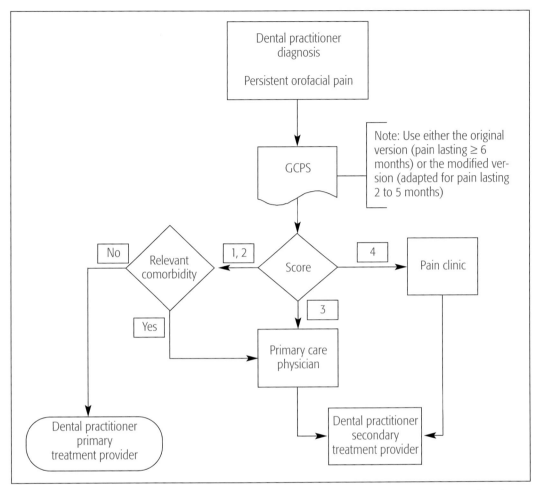

Fig 19-1 Determination of service requirements of patients with musculoskeletal and neuropathic orofacial pains based on assessments of pain severity and impact and the presence or absence of relevant comorbid conditions. Depending on the patient's response on the original[2] or modified Graded Chronic Pain Scale (GCPS), case-specific service requirements are defined. For cases scoring either Grade 1 or 2 on the GCPS, it is further suggested to consider whether the primary care physician should be consulted for comorbid conditions.

Fig 19-1, captures the most salient features and suggests the preferred care setting for case-specific reasoning: (1) dentistry as primary setting for cases of minimal complexity; (2) dentistry in collaboration with the primary medical care for cases of intermediate complexity; and (3) dentistry as a secondary resource for the most complex cases managed by specialty clinics.

The Graded Chronic Pain Scale (GCPS),[1,2] which assigns a severity grade to clinical pain lasting 6 months or more (Table 19-1), provides the framework that the inexperienced clinician needs. However, this scale does not cover the complete spectrum of cases because it requires the presence of pain for 6 months minimally. With minor modifications that allow it to acknowledge pain of 2 to 6

Table 19-1 GCPS[2] and modified von Korff scale

Question	GCPS (pain duration > 6 months)	Modified von Korff Scale (pain duration > 2 months)
1	How would you rate your facial pain on a 0 to 10 scale at the present time, that is, right now, where 0 is "no pain" and 10 is "pain as bad as could be"?	As originally proposed
2	In the past 6 months, how intense was your worst pain, rated on a 0 to 10 scale where 0 is "no pain" and 10 is "pain as bad as could be"?	In the past 2 months . . .
3	In the past 6 months, on average, how intense was your pain rated on a 0 to 10 scale where 0 is "no pain" and 10 is "pain as bad as could be"?	In the past 2 months . . .
1–3	Characteristic pain intensity = Mean (pain right now, worst pain, and average pain) x 10	As originally proposed
4	About how many days in the past 6 months have you been kept from your usual activities (work, school, or housework) because of facial pain? _____ disability days *Disability points* 0 to 6 days: 0 points 7 to 14 days: 1 point 15 to 30 days: 2 points 31+ days: 3 points	About how many days in the past 2 months . . . *Disability points* 0 to 2 days: 0 points 3 to 5 days: 1 point 6 to 10 days: 2 points 11+ days: 3 points
5	In the past 6 months, how much has facial pain interfered with your daily activities, rated on a 0 to 10 scale where 0 is "no interference" and 10 is "unable to carry on any activities"?	In the past 2 months . . .
6	In the past 6 months, how much has facial pain changed your ability to take part in recreational, social, and family activities, rated on a 0 to 10 scale where 0 is "no change" and 10 is "extreme change"?	In the past 2 months . . .
7	In the past 6 months, how much has facial pain changed your ability to work (including housework), rated on a 0 to 10 scale and where 0 is "no change" and 10 is "extreme change"?	In the past 2 months . . .
4–7	Disability score = Mean (daily activities, social activities, work activities) x 10 *Disability points* 0 to 29: 0 points 30 to 49: 1 point 50 to 69: 2 points 70+ : 3 points Disability points: Score for disability days + disability score	As originally proposed

Grade 1: characteristic pain intensity < 50, disability points < 3.
Grade 2: characteristic pain intensity > 50, disability points < 3.
Grade 3: 3 to 4 disability points regardless of characteristic pain intensity.
Grade 4: 5 to 6 disability points regardless of characteristic pain intensity.

months' duration (see Table 19-1, column 3), the instrument can identify patients not fitting the conservative definition of *chronic*, but whose care needs are greater than a general dentist can provide. This modification will assist the inexperienced clinician with the sorting of patients according to care-setting needs. Besides the assessment of pain severity and debilitating effects, the dentist must recognize the impact of coexisting illnesses. Pain in parts of the body other than the orofacial complex is not unusual. Often patients do not tell the dentist about conditions outside the orofacial complex because they may think that these are not within the dentist's scope of practice. These conditions call for coordination of care with the primary care physician.

Treatment Options Within the Scope of General Dentistry

According to 2,544 members of the American Dental Association, the most common orofacial pain treatments provided/prescribed (in descending order) are occlusal appliances, occlusal equilibration, thermal packs, medications with anti-inflammatory or muscle-relaxant properties, relaxation/stress-management training, and diet counseling.[3]

While many types of treatment are offered, there appears to be little difference in the reported levels of clinical success. Proof of efficacy and effectiveness of many interventions is limited. In general, interventions have not been studied with sufficient rigor to permit sound conclusions. Lack of randomization and double-blinding to reduce case selection and observer bias, deficiencies in case inclusion criteria and case definition, inadequate description of case withdrawals, insufficient acknowledgment of confounding medical conditions, the environment within which care was rendered, and lack of follow-up all limit the strength of the available evidence.

Occlusal therapies

Occlusal treatments to address pain include the adjustments of teeth, bite appliances, and orthodontic and fixed prosthodontic treatment with or without surgical correction to change the bite. Only dentists provide these treatments, which explains their popularity in the dental community. Occlusal treatment by means of prosthodontics or orthodontics with or without surgery and adjustment of teeth for nonrestorative indications are not warranted because its superiority over simpler approaches (eg, stabilization splints) has not been shown. However, there is also no clear evidence of efficacy over credible placebo treatment even for the popular stabilization bite splints.[4]

If long-term administration of an interocclusal appliance is considered, a full-coverage (stabilization) design with occlusal stops for all opposing teeth in the form of a flat occlusal plane has fewer undesirable effects than other designs. These appliances are typically worn at night and intermittently during the day, if required. They represent a reasonable treatment alternative to long-term pharmacologic approaches for conditions involving persistent musculoskeletal pain.[5,6] Treatment-induced changes in the occlusion are minimal, eliminating subsequent costly occlusal reconstruction. Regular patient follow-up to ensure contact of opposing teeth on the splint will minimize the risk for unwanted effects. Significant adverse effects, however, are linked to long-term use of realignment or repositioning bite appliances (eg, Pull-Forward, Gelb, Tanner, Bellavia, and Sved appliances). Resultant alterations to the dental occlusion necessitate subsequent prosthetic or orthodontic work and, in some cases, even corrective orthognathic surgery. Because no superior benefit is documented for these appliances over stabilization splints, long-term use is discouraged.

Pharmacotherapy

The general dentist employs two main classes of analgesics: (1) nonsteroidal anti-inflammatory drugs (NSAIDs) (see chapter 21) and (2) to a lesser degree, medications that are classified as antidepressants. Anticonvulsants and neuroleptics (eg, carbamazepine, pregabalin, gabapentin, and lamotrigine), part of the standard pharmacologic armamentarium of the pain specialist, are beyond the scope of the nonspecialist. Although opioids play an important role in pain control, it is not advised for general dentists to administer these unless administration is coordinated with the primary care physician or pain specialist. Side effects are not insignificant and include vomiting, nausea, drowsiness, constipation, and dependence. When it comes to the successful management of persistent pain, none of the drugs with analgesic properties are particularly effective, and drug-drug interactions are expected since polypharmacy is common among persistent pain sufferers.

NSAIDs

The most common type of medication in the world, the NSAIDs (eg, aspirin, ibuprofen, and naproxen) belong to a heterogenous class of pharmacologic agents with anti-inflammatory, antipyretic, and analgesic properties. The analgesic properties of NSAIDs are related to their ability to block the activity of cyclooxygenase (COX), the enzyme that converts arachidonic acid into prostaglandins. Although their short-term efficacy is well established, long-term efficacy and safety in the situation of persistent pain, as might be expected, is not documented. Given the widespread use of these drugs, the number of patients experiencing complications is remarkable. Twenty-one percent of adverse drug reactions reported to the Food and Drug Administration (FDA) in the United States are linked to NSAIDs, and about 20,000 hospitalizations and 2,600 deaths per year result from related compli-

cations.[7] Esophagitis, dyspepsia, gastritis, gastric erosions, and peptic ulcers leading to blood loss constitute the major complications. Hypersensitivity reactions and blockage of platelet aggregation due to the inhibited formation of thromboxane are other unwanted side effects. Postmarketing surveillance of the most recent additions to the NSAID family, the selective cyclooxygenase-2 (COX-2) inhibitors, has shown that this new class of drugs demonstrates risks that are higher than anticipated (see chapter 21).

Antidepressants

The second class of drugs, referred to as *tricyclic antidepressants,* includes medications that originally impressed because of their antidepressive properties. Even at significantly lower dosages than those administered for clinical depression, they demonstrate modest analgesic properties combined with superior safety profiles when compared with NSAIDs. Because of this, they are appealing in the long-term management of persistent pain. Favorable treatment outcome is attributed to their effect on noradrenergic and serotonergic systems in the central nervous system, which exert descending influences on trigeminal and spinal dorsal horn neurons. The additional benefit of antidepressants is thought to come from their influence on mood.

Control of unwanted side effects is a critical factor in the successful use of tricyclic antidepressants. Unwanted effects are not uncommon and include dry mouth, metallic and sour tastes, epigastric distress, constipation, dizziness, heart palpitations, sleep disturbance, tremor, sexual dysfunction, and problems with appetite. Cardiac toxicity and orthostatic hypotension represent the most serious complications. A host of clinically relevant drug-drug interactions exist, which are often attributed to the effect of other medications on the metabolism of the antidepressant by the liver. Because the potentially most serious drug-drug interactions occur with antidepressants that are classified as monoamine oxidase inhibitors (MAOIs) and selective serotonin reuptake inhibitors (SSRIs), the dental practitioner should avoid prescribing these medications.

There is a great deal of evidence on which to base the management of mental depression, but this evidence cannot be directly applied to the use of tricyclic antidepressants for pain management. There are no validated decision trees for the case-specific selection or dosing of a particular antidepressant for pain management. However, it is generally agreed that maintenance dosages for pain management are substantially lower than those required in cases of major depression. If an analgesic effect is not observed within a few days, the low initial dose should be increased unless unwanted side effects do not permit titration to a higher dose. Although side effects are often encountered with tricyclic antidepressants, they can sometimes be used to produce a favorable outcome for other existing complaints. For example, if a patient reports problems with sleep as well as pain, a practitioner could prescribe a sedating antidepressant to be taken at dinnertime, thereby turning an unwanted response into a welcome effect.

Physical treatment modalities

Although many patients appear to do better with a range of physical treatment modalities, there is little scientific proof that many of these modalities produce lasting reductions in the pain symptomatology.[8] Despite their popularity, the efficacy of most physical modalities for conditions of musculoskeletal, neuropathic, and idiopathic persistent pain is in question—no different from many other forms of treatment offered to this patient group. The effect of locally applied heat in the form of hot packs, moist heat, short wave diathermy, microwave, and ultrasound is inconsistent. Other modalities include joint manipulation to improve articular range of pain-free motion, and soft tissue mobilization, which consists of massage, stretching, and myofascial techniques. Home exercises are intended to avoid dependency and to restore a sense of control. Experimental evidence suggests that immobilization is more harmful than beneficial in arthritis, perhaps because joint loading constitutes an essential factor in regulating the articular matrix structure.[9] Aerobic exercise has positive effects on mood and inspires a sense of achievement in a patient whose life is plagued by pain and suffering.[9,10]

Summary

This chapter has presented a framework for the management of persistent orofacial pain conditions. Key case attributes that have diagnostic and therapeutic implications include the temporal presentation of pain, the nature of comorbid conditions, the impact of pain on the patient's life, and the history of previous unsatisfactory treatment attempts. When choosing treatments for persistent pain, the primary focus is safety, with secondary importance given to treatment efficacy and cost. Comorbid conditions falling beyond the scope of the dental practice act require coordination of care with other health care professionals.

References

1. Von Korff M, Dworkin SF, Le Resche L. Graded chronic pain status: An epidemiologic evaluation. Pain 1990;40:279–291.
2. Von Korff M, Ormel J, Keefe FJ, Dworkin SF. Grading the severity of chronic pain. Pain 1992;50:133–149.
3. Glass EG, Glaros AG, McGlynn FD. Myofascial pain dysfunction: Treatments used by ADA members. Cranio 1993;11:25–29.
4. Kreiner M, Betancor E, Clark GT. Occlusal stabilization appliances. Evidence of their efficacy. J Am Dent Assoc 2001;132:770–777.
5. Dao TT, Lavigne GJ, Charbonneau A, Feine JS, Lund JP. The efficacy of oral splints in the treatment of myofascial pain of the jaw muscles: A controlled clinical trial. Pain 1994;56:85–94.
6. Dao TT, Lavigne GJ. Oral splints: The crutches for temporomandibular disorders and bruxism? Crit Rev Oral Biol Med 1998;9:345–361.

7. Fries JF, Miller SR, Spitz PW, Williams CA, Hubert HB, Bloch DA. Identification of patients at risk for gastropathy associated with NSAID use. J Rheumatol Suppl 1990; 20:12–19.

8. Feine JS, Widmer CG, Lund JP. Physical therapy: A critique. Oral Surg Oral Med Oral Pathol Oral Radiol Endod 1997;83:123–127.

9. Galois L, Etienne S, Grossin L, et al. Dose-response relationship for exercise on severity of experimental arthritis in rats. Osteoarthritis Cartilage 2004;12:779–786.

10. Sculco AD, Poup DC, Fernall B, Sculco MJ. Effects of aerobic exercise on low back pain patients in treatment. Spine 2001;1:95–101.

Management of Dental Pain

G. Rex Holland

Some of the most common pain conditions are associated with the teeth. This chapter outlines the signs and symptoms of conditions expressing pain in the teeth as well as outlines principles and approaches to be used in their diagnosis and management.

Diagnostic Considerations

The successful treatment of dental pain begins with a sound diagnosis. The most common cause of pain from the mouth is inflammatory disease of the dental pulp or periodontal tissues. Diagnosis, however, may pose a challenge to the practitioner since pain may have an obscure cause or originate by referral from a distant location. *Referred pain* results from the convergence of input from a site of tissue damage and from another site (where there is no tissue damage) on the same central neurons in which central sensitization may be present (see chapter 5). Pain may be referred to one tooth from another or from a nondental or even extraoral site. The true origin is always on the same side as the site of referral.[1] Other sites from which pain may be referred to the teeth include the muscles of mastication, the ear, the sinuses, and the heart.[2–4] Thirty-seven percent of patients with myofascial

pain of the jaw muscles include pain from teeth as one of their symptoms. The management of referred pain lies in its recognition and in identification of the true cause of pain. Treating the target to which pain is referred will be ineffective.

While most pain of dental origin results from inflammatory changes, inflammation of the dental pulp and the periapical tissues is not always painful. The physiologic basis of this is unknown, although the presence of morphine receptors on pulpal nerves and the presence of opioids in the pulp, especially during inflammation, suggest that there may be local antinociceptive mechanisms[5] (see chapters 6 and 8). Many inflammatory periapical lesions following necrosis of the pulp are detected by chance on radiographs with no prior history of pain.

Relieving toothache with predictable success involves removal of the cause rather than merely addressing the symptoms. When the pain is of dental origin, the tooth (or teeth) involved must be accurately identified. Problems with localization due to referral can lead to a healthy tooth being extracted or root filled.

Table 20-1 outlines signs and symptoms that assist in the differential diagnosis of the several clinical conditions considered in this chapter.

Table 20-1   Dental pain diagnosis and management

Symptoms	Signs	Radiography	Pulp tests
Short discomfort to thermal stimulus	Exposed dentin	Normal	Normal
Stronger, longer pain to thermal stimulus	Caries Deficient restoration	Caries or poor margins	Normal
Strong and lingering pain to cold stimulus, perhaps spontaneous	Caries Deficient restoration	Caries	Lingering pain to thermal tests
Hot tooth syndrome; spontaneously very painful, tender tooth	Anesthesia difficulty	Caries	Lingering pain to thermal tests
Pain on biting loose tooth	Mesiodistal vertical fracture	Radiolucency, often J-shaped	Normal
Pain on biting	No obvious fracture Buccolingual crack detected by transillumination	Normal	Normal
Pain on biting	"High" restoration (recent endodontic treatment)	Normal	Normal
Tender buccal swelling	Tense, tender buccal swelling	Periapical radiolucency	Negative
Mildly tender buccal swelling Bad taste	Pus discharged on pressing No periodontal pocketing	Periapical radiolucency	Negative
Mildly tender buccal swelling	Periodontal pocketing Pus discharge from pocket	Periapical radiolucency	Often vital
Face/neck swollen	Tender lymph nodes Elevated body temperature Malaise	Periapical radiolucency	Negative
Soreness/swelling around erupting tooth	Partially erupted tooth	Partially erupted tooth	Normal
Pain and localized swelling in molar region	Recent extraction	Extraction socket	No tooth

Table 20-1 *(cont)*

Periapical test (percussion)	Diagnosis	Emergency treatment	Definitive treatment
Normal	Sensitive dentin	None	Occlude dentinal tubules
Normal	Reversible pulpitis	Excavate caries, temporize	Caries removal, restoration
May be slightly tender	Irreversible pulpitis	Pulpotomy Analgesics	Root canal therapy, restoration
Tender	Irreversible pulpitis with extensive sensitization	Local, regional anesthesia Intraosseous local anesthesia	Root canal therapy, restoration
Tender	Vertically fractured tooth	Reduce occlusion Temporary crown or band Analgesics	Root canal therapy, crown Likely extraction if vertical fracture extends into root
Discomfort on biting between cusps	Cracked tooth	Reduce occlusion and band or crown	Cast crown
Tender	Acute periapical periodontitis	Debride root canal Analgesics	Occlusal adjustment, root canal therapy if pulp involvement
Tender	Acute periapical abcess	Debride root canal Incise swelling Analgesics	Root canal therapy
Normal or tender	Chronic periapical abscess	Debride root canal	Root canal therapy
Normal or tender	Periodontal abscess	Debride pocket	Periodontal treatment, root canal therapy
Tender	Spreading infection	Incise, drain Antibiotics Analgesics Possible hospitalization	Root canal therapy
Normal	Pericoronitis	Irrigation of flap Analgesics	Removal of tooth if impacted
No tooth	Acute alveolar osteitis/ dry socket	Irrigation of socket Analgesics Antibiotics if systemic signs	As emergency care

Pains of Pulpal Origin

Sensitive dentin

When dentin is exposed, it is often, but not always, sensitive. Thermal, osmotic, or mechanical stimuli evoke sharp, short-lived pain. Common causes of dentin sensitivity include tooth-whitening procedures, subgingival curettage, and root planing. The principal mechanism responsible for dentin sensitivity is the movement of fluid along dentinal tubules activating nociceptors in the inner dentin or outer pulp[6] (see chapter 4). A secondary mechanism may be the direct diffusion of irritants through the dentin, although this would be opposed by the outward flow of dentinal fluid. It is unclear to what extent inflammatory changes in the underlying pulp contribute to the sensitivity.

The treatment of sensitive dentin is largely aimed at occluding dentinal tubules and preventing fluid flow. Fluoride and oxalate salts can be precipitated into dentinal tubules (see Table 20-1). Potassium ions reduce the excitability of pulpal axons, and the inclusion of potassium salts in desensitizing toothpastes may induce this effect if the ions diffuse into the pulp. Potassium salts may also be applied as a gel in trays. Strong evidence of the efficacy of potassium salts in a dentifrice is lacking. A recent Cochrane systematic review concluded that "no clear evidence is available for the support of potassium-containing toothpastes for dentine hypersensitivity."[7] Adhesive restorative materials that cover exposed dentin, such as glass-ionomer cements, can also be effective. However, they may not be retained well, and they tend to have irregular margins that provide an attractive habitat for plaque.

Reversible pulpitis

A diagnosis of reversible pulpitis is made when a tooth responds to thermal or osmotic stimuli with a sharp pain that stops when the stimulus is taken away. It is thus difficult to differentiate from sensitive dentin. If there is no exposed dentin but some etiologic factor such as caries, trauma, or a leaking restoration is present, it is likely that there are inflammatory changes in the underlying pulp. It has long been known that the relationship between clinical signs and symptoms and the pathologic condition of the pulp, at least as determined histologically, is a weak one.[8] Thus, the diagnosis of different degrees of pulpitis is arbitrary.

Treatment consists of removing caries and defective restorations and placing new restorations with intact marginal seals. Medication is not required. In preparing for restorations, great care should be taken not to add further injury to an already compromised pulp.

If removal of all the caries is likely to lead to a pulp exposure, one option is to remove most of the caries and place a dressing to seal off the remainder from the oral environment (*indirect pulp capping*). This has only a modestly positive prognosis but may be worth attempting if the alternatives, such as root canal therapy or extraction, are unattractive.

Irreversible pulpitis

The accepted wisdom is that if a tooth responds with lingering pain to thermal stimuli, the pulp is irreversibly damaged. Objective evidence for this is not strong.[8] The judicious approach is to be lenient with the interpretation of lingering pain and to err on the side of conservative treatment. Spontaneous pain from a tooth most closely correlates with significant pathologic changes in the pulp.[8]

The definitive treatment for irreversible pulpitis is root canal therapy or extraction (see Table 20-1). Symptoms are rapidly alleviated by either approach. If active treatment is not immediately available, the pain will require analgesic therapy. Long-standing nociceptive input leads to central sensitization and its two major effects, hyperalgesia and allodynia (see chapter 5). To bring about some diminution of these central changes, a combination of an anti-inflammatory drug and a centrally acting analgesic such as acetaminophen or an opioid should be used (see also chapter 21). Sometimes the pain may become self-limiting as pulpal inflammation becomes pulpal necrosis. When root canal therapy is indicated but not immediately available, partial removal of the pulp (pulpotomy) will alleviate symptoms until definitive treatment can be performed.[9] Antibiotics have no role in the treatment of pain of pulpal origin.[10]

Hot tooth syndrome

Hot tooth syndrome is an unwelcome variant of irreversible pulpitis. The affected tooth, usually a molar or premolar, is spontaneously painful and very tender. The pulp is vital and irreversibly inflamed, with the inflammation spreading from the pulp into the periapical tissues. Therefore, "hot" teeth can be difficult to anesthetize. The syndrome is best explained as a combination of peripheral and central sensitization (see chapters 5 and 7). The tooth has usually been at least uncomfortable for some time and both hyperalgesia and allodynia are present. The wise approach to this condition is to use the best pattern of local anesthesia available, combining regional anesthesia with local blocks and infiltrations, and augmenting these with intraosseous anesthesia (see Table 20-1).[11] Medication of the patient with an adequate dose of a nonsteroidal anti-inflammatory drug (NSAID), combined with a centrally acting analgesic, can be started before any clinical procedure is initiated, although the efficacy of preemptive analgesia in these circumstances has yet to be established. This condition is also an indication for the use of long-acting local anesthetics that may prolong the patient's comfort and also reduce or eliminate the nociceptive input that leads to central sensitization. Beyond this, a rapid albeit briefly uncomfortable opening of the pulp chamber is needed, followed by intrapulpal injection of local anesthetic and pulpotomy.

Barodontalgia

A sudden toothache called *barodontalgia* occurs in approximately 0.26% of high-altitude fliers.[12] This may be a result of reduced atmospheric pressure causing gas expansion within the pulp chamber that stimulates a previously inflamed pulp, although most reported cases result from pre-existing but formerly asymptomatic periapical inflammation. Deep-water divers have reported a similar experience. Incipient sinusitis can produce similar symptoms. The emergency treatment is to return to normal barometric pressure as soon as possible. Unfortunately, the discomfort can continue for several days and will only be resolved by endodontic therapy.

Cracked tooth syndrome

The term *cracked tooth syndrome* has been reserved for vital molar teeth with incomplete fractures and which are painful on clenching or when eating hard food. They may also be thermally sensitive. Cracks as opposed to vertical fractures are most commonly found in teeth with minimal restorations and run mesiodistally. The pain may be of both pulpal and periodontal origin. Once suspected, the affected tooth can usually be identified by having the patient bite on something that separates the cusps. Sometimes cracks can be revealed by transillumination of the tooth. The challenge with this condition is to effectively restore the tooth. The prognosis is usually poor as the cracks continue below a level at which restorations can be applied. The pain itself is not severe and needs no direct treatment other than that used to preserve the tooth (see Table 20-1).

Vertically fractured teeth

Teeth with complete vertical fractures may reveal no radiographic changes in the early stages. Later there will be a J-shaped radiolucency around the affected root, and a narrow pocket can be detected. The fracture line usually runs buccolingually. Pulp tests are usually negative. These teeth are almost always unrestorable.

Pain Associated with Periodontal Disease

A feature of periodontal disease that makes it characteristically insidious is that it is largely painless. If inflamed gingival tissue were painful, people with periodontal disease would present for treatment at a much earlier stage than is usual, allowing a more positive prognosis. On the other hand, gingival pain is often experienced in response to localized acute inflammation that might be associated with food impaction or trauma. This is unlikely to need more than removal of the cause. Acutely progressive oral infections involving the gingiva (eg, acute necrotizing ulcerative gingivitis) are painful, and anti-inflammatory analgesics will be needed in conjunction with definitive antimicrobial and periodontal therapy.

Periapical periodontitis

Inflammation of the supporting tissues around the apex of the tooth is often but not always painful. *Acute periapical periodontitis* can arise from trauma due to a blow, placement of a poorly designed "high" restoration, or as a sequel of root canal therapy. It most commonly occurs as an extension of pulpal inflammation and necrosis. In its early stages, periapical periodontitis is painful on biting or tapping the tooth. When pulpitis extends into the periapical tissues, it becomes easier to localize the involved tooth, which is useful for diagnosis. If the periodontitis is due to the extension of pulpitis, root canal therapy is indicated; if it is associated with a "high" restoration, occlusal adjustment may suffice. *Chronic periapical periodontitis* is usually painless, and hence resorbative inflammatory lesions around

the apices of nonvital teeth can become large before they are detected. Suppuration (pus formation) can be superimposed on both acute and chronic periapical periodontitis and can lead to an acute periapical abscess as the increase in pressure associated with pus formation leads to pain. The differentiation of abscesses resulting from pulpal necrosis and those arising from infected periapical pockets has been described. *Chronic periapical abscesses* usually drain through a sinus tract or periodontal pocket. Because there is no buildup of pressure, they are usually painless, and patients only present for treatment when a swelling is seen or recurring unpleasant taste is experienced.

In periapical disease, radiographic appearance is poorly correlated with pain symptoms. Few lesions detected radiographically are painful, but they must always be investigated and treated because a small but individually highly significant proportion of radiolucencies are associated with malignant rather than inflammatory disease. It is improper to leave any inflammatory lesion untreated, even if it is asymptomatic. Some lesions, though by no means all, will continue to expand; others may flare up into an acute abscess.

Once periodontal pockets have formed, there is an increasing possibility of an acute exacerbation of pain associated with abscess formation. Though often similar in presentation to abscesses of pulpal origin, these lateral or periodontal abscesses need to be differentiated at diagnosis because the causative factors, which must be addressed for resolution, are distinct. The tooth associated with pulpal necrosis will be nonvital, and that associated with an abscess of periodontal origin will be vital unless the periodontal pocket has extended to the apex.

Abscesses of pulpal origin should be treated definitively by cleaning and filling the root canal system (see Table 20-1). Abscesses of periodontal origin will need draining and elimination of the pocket within which the abscess formed. Abscesses of both pulpal and periodontal origin will be painful and will require the use of anti-inflammatory anal-

166

gesics. Antibiotics are indicated for both types of abscesses if systemic symptoms are present or there is evidence of pus tracking through the fascial planes. If there is visible swelling, then incision and drainage will be the most effective emergency procedure and is mandatory if the swelling is fluctuant.

Pericoronitis

The accumulation of food debris and plaque on and around the crowns of partially erupted third molars leads to infection and inflammation of the soft tissues in the area. This can be a source of pain and discomfort that may be referred to other teeth. The definitive treatment is removal of the impacted teeth once the local inflammation and infection are controlled (see Table 20-1). The immediate treatment is irrigation of the operculum overlying the tooth, use of analgesics, and (if systemic signs of infection are present) prescription of antibiotics. Again, as with all instances of pain of inflammatory/infective origin, the use of analgesics alone is inappropriate and of transitory benefit. Food impaction at other sites can also cause pain but rarely needs more than removal of the debris and irrigation followed by restorative or oral hygiene procedures to prevent recurrence.

Postendodontic treatment discomfort

Endodontic treatment is commonly followed by posttreatment discomfort (approximately 60% of cases) because the apical extrusion of debris leads to acute periapical periodontitis. This is usually mild and either needs no medication or can be controlled by over-the-counter analgesics. The discomfort resolves in a few days. Premedication of endodontic patients with NSAIDs is a common, if not universal, practice, although no clinical trial has thus far tested this approach. Rarely but significantly, the apical extrusion of debris leads to suppurative changes in the periapical tissues and an acute periapical abscess with swelling and pain.

This requires aggressive treatment that should include draining the abscess through the root canal and/or by incision and the use of NSAIDs or a combination analgesic. Antibiotics should certainly be prescribed in the event of systemic signs or spread of the infection into fascial planes.

Postextraction pain (acute alveolar osteitis, dry socket)

Pain is commonly associated with the extraction of teeth, particularly of impacted third molars, and is related to the degree of tissue damage. Because of its frequency, postextraction pain has been used as a model, for example, to test the efficacy of analgesics,[13] to develop rating scales,[14] and to determine the role of A-β fibers and central sensitization in injury-induced pain.[15]

It is hardly surprising that, following third molar extractions, local infections sometimes occur and lead to the syndrome commonly known as *dry socket*, which may involve pain that can become more than moderate. In anticipation of postoperative pain, coverage with NSAIDs is sometimes begun before an extraction. At least one clinical trial,[16] however, suggests that this method is no more effective than the use of posttreatment analgesics alone. The use of prophylactic antibiotics seems unwise on principle, although antibiotics are clearly indicated when postoperative infection gives signs of systemic involvement. As always, prevention by gentle tissue management and treatment of the cause (antimicrobial lavage of the extraction socket) are strongly advocated (see Table 20-1).

Neuralgias, Atypical Odontalgia, Phantom Tooth Pain

While classic trigeminal neuralgia is well defined, so-called atypical facial neuralgias and atypical orofacial pain are not. These conditions are outlined in chapters 1, 7, and 24, but it is to be noted here that since both can include tooth pain in their presentation, they are a source of possible misdiagnosis.[17] Differentiating factors include the severity of pain, the absence of dental lesions, and symptoms that cannot be initiated by stimulating dental tissues. Atypical odontalgia occurs predominantly in women and is often associated with emotional problems. It is often termed *phantom tooth pain* since it is usually a neuralgic condition associated with an area where there has been previous treatment, a tooth extraction, root canal therapy, or sinus surgery. It is described as a constant dull ache with occasional sharp exacerbations felt at the site of a tooth that is no longer present. While the role of local neuromas is uncertain, changes in the trigeminal brain stem sensory nuclear complex (ie, central to the site of injury) have been documented in animal models (see chapter 7).[18,19] Management of this type of pain is usually pharmacologically based, as described in chapter 24.

Summary

This chapter has outlined the signs and symptoms of several conditions affecting the teeth and has noted that in dealing with dental pain, the key principles are:

- Effective treatment can only follow accurate diagnosis.
- Always be suspicious when embarking on a pain diagnosis.
- Remember that pain is commonly referred.
- If the pain is severe and difficult to localize, a chronic pain syndrome may be present.
- Always try to reproduce the patient's symptoms.
- The best treatment is removal of the cause.
- Proceed directly with the definitive treatment whenever possible.
- Use analgesics only when indicated.
- Anti-inflammatory analgesics are usually indicated, with the addition of a centrally acting analgesic if the pain has been ongoing for some time and there is a suspicion that central sensitization may occur.
- Do not use antibiotics unless there are systemic symptoms.

References

1. Glick DH. Locating referred pulpal pains. Oral Surg Oral Med Oral Pathol 1962;15:613–623.
2. Fricton JR, Kroening R, Haley D, Siegert R. Myofascial pain syndrome of the head and neck: A review of clinical characteristics of 164 patients. Oral Surg Oral Med Oral Pathol 1985;60:615–623.
3. Diaz I, Bamberger DM. Acute sinusitis. Semin Respir Infect 1995;10:14–20.
4. Kreiner M, Okeson JP. Toothache of cardiac origin. J Orofac Pain 1999;13:201–207.
5. Mudie AS, Holland GR. Local opioids in the inflamed dental pulp. J Endod 2006;32:319–323.
6. Orchardson R, Gillam DG. Managing dentin hypersensitivity. J Am Dent Assoc 2006;137:990-998; quiz 1028–1029.
7. Keenan JV, Farman AG, Fedorowicz Z, Newton JT. A Cochrane systematic review finds no evidence to support the use of antibiotics for pain relief in irreversible pulpitis. J Endod 2006;32:87–92.
8. Seltzer S, Bender IB, Ziontz M. The dynamics of pulp inflammation: Correlations between diagnostic data and actual histologic findings in the pulp. Oral Surg Oral Med Oral Pathol 1963;16:969–977.
9. Oguntebi BR, DeSchepper EJ, Taylor TS, White CL, Pink FE. Postoperative pain incidence related to the type of emergency treatment of symptomatic pulpitis. Oral Surg Oral Med Oral Pathol 1992;73:479–483.
10. Runyon MS, Brennan MT, Batts JJ, et al. Efficacy of penicillin for dental pain without overt infection. Acad Emerg Med 2004;11:1268–1271.
11. Gallatin E, Reader A, Nist R, Beck M. Pain reduction in untreated irreversible pulpitis using an intraosseous injection of Depo-Medrol. J Endod 2000;26:633–638.
12. Robichaud R, McNally ME. Barodontalgia as a differential diagnosis: Symptoms and findings. J Can Dent Assoc 2005;71:39–42.
13. Dionne RA, Snyder J, Hargreaves KM. Analgesic efficacy of flurbiprofen in comparison with acetaminophen, acetaminophen plus codeine, and placebo after impacted third molar removal. J Oral Maxillofac Surg 1994;52:919–924; discussion 925–916.
14. Seymour RA. The use of pain scales in assessing the efficacy of analgesics in post-operative dental pain. Eur J Clin Pharmacol 1982;23:441–444.
15. Eliav E, Gracely RH. Sensory changes in the territory of the lingual and inferior alveolar nerves following lower third molar extraction. Pain 1998;77:191–199.
16. Bridgman JB, Gillgrass TG, Zacharias M. The absence of any pre-emptive analgesic effect for non-steroidal anti-inflammatory drugs. Br J Oral Maxillofac Surg 1996;34:428–431.
17. Melis M, Secci S. Diagnosis and treatment of atypical odontalgia: A review of the literature and two case reports. J Contemp Dent Pract 2007;8:81–89.
18. Torneck CD, Kwan CL, Hu JW. Inflammatory lesions of the tooth pulp induce changes in brainstem neurons of the rat trigeminal subnucleus oralis. J Dent Res 1996;75:553–561.
19. Sessle BJ. Acute and chronic craniofacial pain: Brainstem mechanisms of nociceptive transmission and neuroplasticity, and their clinical correlates. Crit Rev Oral Biol Med 2000;11:59–91.

21

Management of Inflammatory Pain

Sharon M. Gordon
Raymond A. Dionne

Many dental procedures trigger orofacial pain, necessitating that the practitioner provide pain control to improve patient postoperative comfort and to decrease anxiety about future dental treatment.[1–3] This chapter reviews strategies to manage acute orofacial inflammatory pain in particular. The use and indication of analgesics in the management of myalgia, arthralgia, mucositis, and headache are described in chapters 22, 23, and 25. Control of anxiety, although related to pain control, is beyond the scope of this chapter.

Strategies for Acute Pain Management

Pharmacologic management of dental pain is accomplished through one of three general mechanisms: blocking the nociceptive impulse along the peripheral nerve, reducing nociceptive input from the site of injury, or attenuating the perception of pain in the central nervous system (CNS). Accumulating evidence suggests that it is also possible to decrease clinical pain over the first few days postoperatively by inhibiting the development of central sensitization due to the nociceptive input that occurs during the perioperative period (see

chapter 5). These strategies are additive, often without increased adverse effects, and can be used to prevent pain rather than to manage pain after its onset.

Blocking nociceptive input

Input along trigeminal (V) nerve pathways is routinely blocked for dental procedures by administering a local anesthetic in the vicinity of the relevant nerve. The duration of local anesthetic agents such as lidocaine and mepivacaine is usually 1 to 2 hours postinjection. If the procedure has initiated the cytokine cascade leading to inflammation, the offset of local anesthesia coincides with peak release of important pain mediators such as prostaglandins and bradykinin.[4] It is not surprising, then, that anesthetic offset is accompanied by intense pain since these mediators are maximizing nociceptive input from direct effects on nerve endings. Administration of a long-acting local anesthetic such as bupivacaine or etidocaine provides a method of blocking postoperative pain for hours after painful surgical procedures. This postpones the onset of sensation until the peak levels of inflammatory mediators have subsided and analgesics are starting to exert an effect.[5–7]

Reducing nociceptive input from the periphery

Recognition of the effects of locally released mediators of pain and inflammation on the sensitization of peripheral nerve endings suggests that interfering with the release or actions of these mediators may provide therapeutic benefits. Mediators such as prostaglandin E_2 (PGE_2) sensitize nerve endings, signal pain, and potentiate the actions of other inflammatory mediators such as bradykinin. Sensitization of peripheral nociceptors is minimized in the absence of PGE_2, which attenuates pain sensations (see chapter 6 for review). Therefore, drugs that block prostaglandin synthesis or function after tissue injury are effective for reducing inflammatory pain (Fig 21-1). This information has an important practical application: pretreating patients with nonsteroidal anti-inflammatory drugs (NSAIDs) before or soon after dental surgery blocks cyclooxygenase (COX) enzymes before the initiation of tissue damage results in the synthesis of proinflammatory cytokines. A well-documented strategy for blocking pain in the immediate postoperative period is the administration of NSAIDs before pain onset (Fig 21-2).[5,9,10]

Attenuating the perception of pain in the CNS

The CNS reacts to nociceptive input with changes that lead to the development of central sensitization and hyperalgesia, both of which can prolong pain and result in pain from non-noxious stimuli. Inhibition of these processes has been demonstrated by the use of long-acting local anesthetics[6,7] and the preventive use of anti-inflammatory drugs,[9,10] which are additive as a combination for minimizing immediate postoperative pain (see Fig 21-2).[5]

Even when using preventive strategies, some patients still experience postoperative pain of moderate to severe intensity that requires the use of drugs that act in the CNS to inhibit nociceptive

transmission. For acute pain, opioid drugs are one commonly used drug class. The use of opioids for acute pain usually results in pain relief but is accompanied by a high incidence of adverse effects such as nausea, vomiting, and drowsiness. The relationship between opioid analgesia and side-effect liability is illustrated by findings of oxycodone use for postoperative dental pain. Increasing doses of oxycodone (2.5 mg, 5 mg, and 10 mg) in combination with 400 mg of ibuprofen did not result in any additive analgesia until the 10-mg dose of oxycodone.[11] The number of patients reporting side effects, however, increased linearly with increasing oxycodone dose, such that most subjects at the highest dose reported side effects including drowsiness, nausea, and vomiting. A similar relationship is seen for other opioids, such as codeine, when given alone or in combination with aspirin, acetaminophen, or NSAIDs. As a consequence, opioids should be reserved primarily for pain inadequately controlled by preventive strategies and nonopioids, or for patients who cannot tolerate aspirin-like drugs.

Drug Selection for Management of Acute Pain

Nonopioid analgesics for inflammatory pain

Nonopioid analgesics include the salicylates (aspirin and diflunisal), acetaminophen, NSAIDs (ibuprofen, ketoprofen, naproxen, and others), and COX-2 inhibitors. These drugs were formerly thought to have a peripheral mechanism of action, while opioids were thought to act at the level of the CNS. Evidence now refutes this classification scheme, with some nonopioid drugs demonstrating activity in the CNS and opioids having effects in the periphery. In general, given their low side-effect liability, efficacy for inflammatory pain, and safety with administration over a few days, nonopiods should be used preferentially for acute dental pain and as a com-

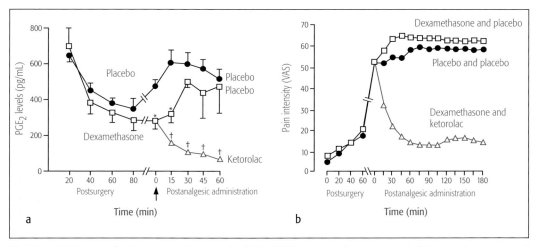

Fig 21-1 *(a)* Postoperative immunoreactive prostaglandin E_2 (PGE$_2$) concentrations at the surgical site in patients pretreated with dexamethasone or placebo, and at pain onset *(arrow)* after the administration of ketorolac or saline placebo. *(b)* Suppression of pain by the NSAID ketorolac is consistent with decreased levels of PGE$_2$. Adapted with permission from Dionne et al.[8] VAS = visual analog scale. * $P < .05$ vs placebo. † $P < .05$ vs dexamethasone and placebo.

Fig 21-2 Suppression of postoperative pain by the combination of the NSAID flurbiprofen *(dark shaded area)* and the long-acting local anesthetic etidocaine *(light shaded area)*. Their additive effect is represented by the lower line. VAS = visual analog scale.

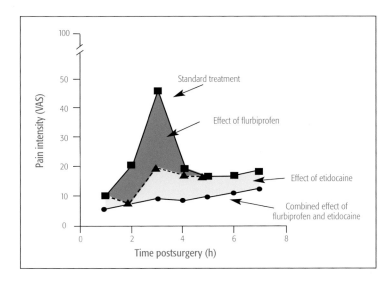

ponent of drug combinations for more severe pain. For detailed prescribing information, cautions, and contraindications, practitioners must consult the package insert or official pharmacopeia recognized by the country of practice.

Salicylates

Aspirin.

Salicylate, the active form of aspirin, is widely distributed in the body, metabolized mainly in the liver by conjugation, and excreted in the urine mostly as salicyluric acid. The efficacy of aspirin has been shown in innumerable studies; it is equipotent with acetaminophen, more effective than 30 to 60 mg codeine alone, but less efficacious than 400 mg ibuprofen. The most common side effects are epigastric distress, nausea, ulceration, and vomiting. Aspirin should not be given to patients with liver disease, hypothrombinemia, or vitamin K deficiency, nor to patients who are taking anticoagulant drugs. Allergic reactions to aspirin are uncommon but are more frequently seen in persons with asthma, nasal polyps, or a history of allergic reaction to other aspirin-like drugs (including NSAIDs). The relationship between blood levels and therapeutic effect is not direct and no fixed dose, schedule, or dosage form will provide the desired result in all patients. The usual anti-inflammatory and analgesic dose is 650 to 1,000 mg every 4 to 6 hours.

Diflunisal.

Diflunisal is a derivative of salicylic acid with a prolonged duration of action from 8 to 12 hours. Peak effect is reached in about 3 hours; as a consequence, an initial dose of 1,000 mg is recommended to attain therapeutic blood levels, followed by 500 mg every 12 hours up to a maximum of 1,500 mg per day. Diflunisal has a more prolonged duration than 650 mg aspirin, with both the 500-mg and 1,000-mg doses providing peak analgesia comparable to 600 mg acetaminophen plus 60 mg codeine, but with longer duration. Diflunisal should not be given to patients who are hypersensitive to the drug or have a history of acute asthma, urticaria, or rhinitis that is precipitated by aspirin or NSAIDs. An alternative drug should also be considered in patients with a history of ulcer disease or gastrointestinal bleeding. Diflunisal, like other salicylates, is not recommended for pregnant or nursing women, nor has its safety and effectiveness been established in children younger than 12 years.

Acetaminophen

Acetaminophen is widely used as an alternative to aspirin, NSAIDs, and selective COX-2 inhibitors for the treatment of mild to moderate pain based on its greater perceived safety in comparison to these drug classes. Acetaminophen is generally thought to be equipotent with aspirin but with fewer side effects, and it has the advantage of not inhibiting platelet aggregation. The actions of acetaminophen at the molecular level are still poorly defined despite its widespread use. Recent evidence suggests that acetaminophen inhibits COX-2 and that its analgesic effect may be partially attributed to decreased peripheral PGE_2 release in addition to its centrally mediated analgesic effects.[12]

The usual analgesic dose of acetaminophen is 650 to 1,000 mg every 6 to 8 hours. Acetaminophen may also be administered in combination with codeine, oxycodone, and hydrocodone in a variety of formulations that result in additive analgesia. Acetaminophen use is contraindicated in patients with liver damage or in conjunction with alcohol use, and attempts to improve analgesia by increasing the acetaminophen dose should be used with caution.[13,14]

NSAIDs

The NSAIDs are thought to exert their analgesic and anti-inflammatory effects partly through their common action of inhibiting synthesis of prostanoids (eg, PGE_2) following tissue injury. Their use for acute dental pain is a therapeutic improvement: NSAID use is associated with greater analgesic efficacy than is the use of single-entity agents such as aspirin or acetaminophen, but without an increase in side effects from opioid-containing combinations. NSAIDs should not be given to patients with a history of peptic ulcer disease to minimize its possible exacerbation. Furthermore, they should be used with caution in patients with a history of hypertension or heart failure. All NSAIDs inhibit the

Fig 21-3 Ibuprofen is more effective at reducing pain after dental surgery than acetaminophen (APAP) or APAP in combination with codeine (COD). * P < .05 vs placebo. VAS = visual analog scale.

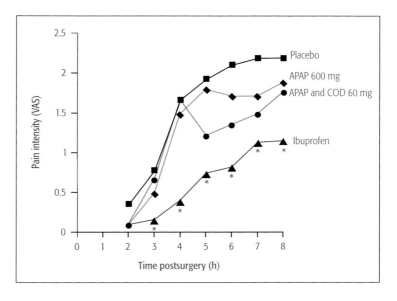

secondary aggregation of platelets and blood clotting, but to a lesser degree and duration than aspirin. They should be avoided in pregnant women and in patients predisposed to aspirin-induced asthma.

Ibuprofen.

Ibuprofen is the prototype of the NSAID class of analgesics and remains one of the most widely used NSAIDs. It has demonstrated analgesic activity over a dose range of 200 to 800 mg and has a duration of 4 to 6 hours. Ibuprofen in a dose of 400 mg has been found to be superior to 650 mg aspirin, 600 to 1,000 mg acetaminophen, combinations of aspirin or acetaminophen plus 60 mg codeine, and multiple doses of dihydrocodone[15] (Fig 21-3). Administration of doses greater than 400 mg is not likely to result in greater peak relief, but increased drug blood levels may prolong the duration of analgesia. Ibuprofen suppresses swelling over the postoperative course when edema formation associated with the inflammatory process is most prominent. The analgesic effects of ibuprofen, and presumably other NSAIDs, can be opti-mized by giving the drug prior to pain onset to suppress the onset of pain and lessen its severity.

The usual dose of ibuprofen is 400 to 600 mg every 4 to 6 hours. The proven analgesic efficacy of ibuprofen and the vast clinical experience gained through decades of clinical use make ibuprofen the drug of choice for dental pain in patients who do not have a contraindication to its use.

Other NSAIDs.

Other orally administered NSAIDs such as naproxen, ketoprofen, and flurbiprofen result in similar analgesic efficacy as ibuprofen at marketed doses. They have similar indications, contraindications, and adverse effects as ibuprofen. Ketorolac, the only NSAID available in a parenteral formulation, is particularly efficacious for dosing in the range of 30 to 60 mg, with rapid onset for the management of moderate to severe pain following a surgical procedure. Its analgesic activity is comparable to opioids such as morphine and meperidine, but with a longer duration of action and fewer side effects. The route of administration limits its use to hospitalized patients or for the initial dose prior to discharge of ambulatory patients. The efficacy of ketorolac is much less impressive when given orally; its safety profile prompted the Food and Drug Administration (FDA) in the United States to limit its recommended use to maintenance of patients already started on parenteral ketorolac.

COX-2 inhibitors

Presently, the only commercially available COX-2 inhibitor on the market in the United States is celecoxib, which has been shown to be effective for acute dental pain at doses ranging from 100 to 400 mg. If dosed at pain onset, celecoxib is less effective than 400 mg of ibuprofen for dental extraction pain.[16] Given before dental surgery, however, celecoxib is as effective as ibuprofen.[17] The 200 mg dose of celecoxib indicated for acute pain is approximately equivalent to 400 mg ibuprofen in the oral surgery pain model involving third molar extraction. The usual dose is 100 to 200 mg every 12 hours.

The incidence of epigastric ulceration as viewed by endoscopy is consistently low with celecoxib and compared with placebo. However, a large clinical trial has revealed an increased risk of myocardial infarction and stroke in patients using COX-2 inhibitors long-term, resulting in the withdrawal of two of these drugs from the US market and a warning label for celecoxib.[18] Therefore, the use of celecoxib for acute pain management should be limited to short-term use in patients not at risk for cardiovascular disease.

Opioid analgesics

Opioids have been used for centuries as analgesics and as antitussive and antidiarrheal agents, but it was belatedly realized that all opioids are qualitatively similar for producing side effects, dependence, and tolerance with repeated dosing. While the mechanism of action is not completely understood, it is assumed that exogenously administered opioids act in the brain and spinal cord to produce their pharmacologic effect by mimicking the actions of endogenous opioid ligands. The oral efficacy of most opioids is poor because of extensive metabolism in the liver following absorption, which results in little active drug reaching the site of action. While opioids also demonstrate peripheral analgesic effects and interaction with inflammatory cells in peripheral tissues,[19,20] they are generally thought to be devoid of acute anti-inflammatory effects. The incidence of side effects such as dizziness, drowsiness, nausea, and vomiting are high following opioid administration in comparison to NSAIDs, and these effects are magnified in ambulatory patients. As a consequence of these considerations, opioids are best used as adjuncts in combination with nonopioids, which actually provide the major portion of the analgesic activity.

Combination analgesics

Combinations of analgesics are frequently prescribed for the management of pain unrelieved by a full therapeutic dose of one agent alone. The rationale is to intervene in the pain process through two separate mechanisms to achieve greater analgesia. It is still considered axiomatic among clinical pharmacologists that an analgesic combination should result in a greater analgesic effect than simply increasing the dose of one of the ingredients, or should produce fewer side effects than equivalent analgesic doses of one of the ingredients. However, the vast majority of studies have demonstrated that a single-entity NSAID analgesic results in greater analgesia and fewer side effeccts than do aspirin or acetaminophen plus codeine or oxycodone combinations. Combinations of opioid and nonopioid analgesics vary by country. Practitioners should consult the package insert or the official pharmacopeia recognized by the country of practice.

Table 21-1 Hierarchy of postoperative pain management

Pain level	Procedure type	Strategy*
Prevention of pain	Surgical	Long-acting local anesthetic and NSAID prior to pain onset
Mild	Simple	Aspirin, acetaminophen, or NSAID
Moderate	Invasive	Aspirin, acetaminophen, or NSAID Add opioid if unrelieved
Severe	Surgery or trauma or unrelieved pain	Preventive measures if possible Aspirin, acetaminophen, or NSAID combined with opioid

*Choice of salicylate, NSAID, or acetaminophen is dependent on patient medical history.

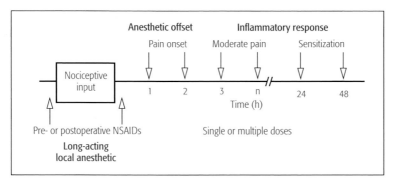

Fig 21-4 Schematic of strategies to prevent and manage acute orofacial pain in the immediate postoperative period during the offset of local anesthesia and the development of the inflammatory response. Preemptive measures administered prior to the procedure can include an NSAID, long-acting local anesthetic, or a combination of the two. An NSAID given immediately following the procedure should also decrease pain intensity. Following pain onset, the choice of drugs, doses, and dosing interval is based on side effects and the level of pain reported by the patient.

Therapeutic Recommendations to Manage Pain Related to Dental Procedures

To simultaneously minimize the perception of pain and the incidence of side effects, a flexible strategy is required to balance the analgesic needs of the individual patient and the adverse effects experienced. The generalizations made in this chapter, however, are based on the results of groups of subjects under the controlled conditions of a clinical trial. No one drug, combination of drugs, or fixed doses will work in all conditions. The challenge of pain therapy is to apply these generalizations to the individual patient to optimally balance analgesic efficacy and side-effect liability. Patients should be instructed to take doses by the clock to avoid cycles of increased pain during analgesic offset and absorption of the next dose. Patients also need to be informed of the drug risks and side effects. Table 21-1 outlines a hierarchy of pain-control strategies, and Fig 21-4 illustrates an analgesic regimen. Acute pain that is not adequately managed by these drug regimens should be re-evaluated to rule out other etiologic factors.

Summary

The analgesic strategies and drug regimens described in this chapter permit practitioners to prevent much of the acute pain that follows dental procedures. A flexible analgesic regimen can start before treatment and continue postoperatively. This flexibility allows the clinician to adjust the drugs, doses, and frequency of administration to optimize the relationship between the difficulty of the procedure, the response to the analgesic treatment, and the side effects reported by the patient.

References

1. Berggren U, Meynert G. Dental fear and avoidance: Causes, symptoms, and consequences. J Am Dent Assoc 1984;109:247–251.
2. Dionne RA, Gordon SM, McCullagh LM, Phero JC. Assessment of clinical needs for anesthesia and sedation in the general population. J Am Dent Assoc 1998;129:167–173.
3. Dionne RA, Yagiela JA, Cote CJ, et al. Balancing efficacy and safety in the use of oral sedation in dental outpatients. J Am Dent Asoc 2006;137:502–513.
4. Rozkowski MT, Swift JQ, Hargreaves KM. Effect of NSAID administration on tissue levels of immunoreactive prostaglandin E2, leukotriene B4, and (S)-flurbiprofen following extraction of impacted third molars. Pain 1997;73:339–345.
5. Dionne RA, Wirdzek PR, Fox PC, Dubner R. Suppression of postoperative pain by the combination of a non-steroidal anti-inflammatory drug, flurbiprofen, and a long-acting local anesthetic, etidocaine. J Am Dent Assoc 1984;108:598–601.
6. Gordon SM, Dionne RA, Brahim J, Jabir F, Dubner R. Blockade of peripheral neuronal barrage reduces postoperative pain. Pain 1997;70:209–215.
7. Gordon SM, Brahim JS, Dubner R, McCullagh LM, Sang C, Dionne RA. Attenuation of pain in a randomized trial by suppression of peripheral nociceptive activity in the immediate post-operative period. Anesth Analg 2002;95:1351–1357.
8. Dionne RA, Gordon SM, Rowan J, Kent A, Brahim JS. Dexamethasone suppresses peripheral prostanoid levels without analgesia in a clinical model of acute inflammation. J Oral Maxillofac Surg 2003;61:997–1003.
9. Dionne RA, Cooper SA. Evaluation of preoperative ibuprofen on postoperative pain after impaction surgery. Oral Surg Oral Med Oral Pathol 1978;45:851–856.
10. Dionne RA. Suppression of dental pain by the preoperative administration of flurbiprofen. Am J Med 1986; 80(suppl 3A):41–49.
11. Dionne RA. Additive analgesic effects of oxycodone and ibuprofen in the oral surgery model. J Oral Maxillofac Surg 1999;57:673–678.
12. Lee Y-S, Kim H, Brahim JS, Rowan J, Lee G, Dionne RA. Acetaminophen selectively suppresses peripheral prostaglandin E2 release and increases COX-2 gene expression in a clinical model of acute inflammation. Pain 2007;129:279–286.
13. Larson AM, Polson J, Fontana RJ, et al. Actaminophen-induced acute liver failure: Results of a United States multicenter, prospective study. Hepatology 2005;42:1364–1372.
14. Watkins PB, Kaplowitz N, Slattery JT, et al. Aminotransferase elevations in healthy adults receiving 4 grams of acetaminophen daily. JAMA 2006;296:87–93.
15. Dionne RA, Cooper SA. Use of ibuprofen in dentistry. In: Rainsford KD (ed). Ibuprofen: A Critical Bibliographic Review. London: Taylor & Francis, 1999:407–430.
16. Malmstrom K, Fricke JR, Kotey P, Kress B, Morrison B. A comparison of rofecoxib versus celecoxib in treating pain after dental surgery: A single-center, randomized, double-blind, placebo and active-comparator controlled, parallel group, single-dose study using the dental impaction pain model. Clin Ther 2002; 24:1549–1560.
17. Khan AA, Brahim JS, Rowan JS, Dionne RA. In vivo selectivity of a selective cyclooxygenase 2 inhibitor in the oral surgery model. Clin Pharmacol Ther 2002;72:44–49.
18. Silverstein FE, Faich G, Goldstein JL, et al. Gastrointestinal toxicity with celecoxib vs nonsteroidal anti-inflammatory drugs for osteoarthritis and rheumatoid arthritis: The CLASS Study: A randomized controlled trial. Celecoxib Long-term Arthritis Safety Study. JAMA 2000;284:1247–1255.
19. Stein C. Peripheral mechanisms of opioid analgesia. Anesth Analg 1993;76:182–191.
20. Jaber L, Swaim WD, Dionne RA. Immunohistochemical localization of mu-opioid receptors in human dental pulp. J Endod 2003;29(2):108–110.

Management of Masticatory Myalgia and Arthralgia

James R. Fricton
Eric L. Schiffman

Myalgia and *arthralgia* refer to muscle and joint pain disorders, respectively. When these disorders involve the masticatory muscles, the temporomandibular joint (TMJ), or both, they are collectively called *temporomandibular disorders* (TMDs).[1] TMD pain is typically felt in the jaw, temple, ear, and face. The hallmark of TMD pain is that it is altered by function including eating and/or by parafunction including oral habits. The most common signs include pain in the muscles and/or TMJs upon palpation, pain or limitation with jaw range of motion (ROM), irregular jaw movements, or TMJ noises. The purpose of this chapter is to present the most common disorders that can cause masticatory myalgia and arthralgia and to discuss their management.

Differential Diagnosis

Proper physical diagnosis related to the patient's pain complaint(s) and all relevant contributing factors will facilitate successful management.[1] Medical disorders and other orofacial disorders need to be considered in the differential diagnosis of TMDs. Comorbid conditions such as dental pulpitis, rheumatoid arthritis, fibromyalgia, tension-type head-

ache, and migraine headache can present with similar or overlapping pain complaints that can complicate the diagnostic process (see also chapters 19, 20, and 25).[2,3]

Masticatory myalgia is characterized as a dull persistent ache overlying the jaw and temple muscles with occasional referral to other structures such as head, neck, ear, and teeth. Symptoms can also include a restricted opening, fatigue, and stiffness. Signs include tenderness of the muscles with limited ROM. Common myalgias include *myofascial pain* (regional and referred pain associated with localized areas of tenderness called *trigger points*), *masticatory tension-type headache* (pain in the temporalis muscles area, with replication of the headache on muscle palpation or stretching), *myositis* (pain with generalized muscle tenderness), *muscle spasm* (acute pain with limited ROM), and *contracture*[4] (long-standing limited ROM).

TMJ arthralgia is characterized by joint tenderness and preauricular pain with occasional referral to the periauricular, upper neck, and temporal regions.[1] Pain is related to inflammatory and/or mechanical factors. If inflammation is significantly present, the diagnosis is arthritis, also referred to as *capsulitis* or *synovitis*. The inflammatory process may also be due to a local disorder such as disc

> **Box 22-1** Management options for TMDs
>
> Patient education and self-care
>
> Pharmacotherapy
>
> Physical medicine therapy
>
> Intraoral splints and dental treatment
>
> Cognitive-behavioral therapy
>
> TMJ surgery
>
> Complementary and alternative therapies
>
> Referral or team management

displacement or a systemic disease, including rheumatoid arthritis. Mechanically related pain may be associated with local disorders including disc displacement with reduction with intermittent locking, disc displacement without reduction with limited opening, TMJ hypermobility, or osteoarthritis (see chapter 1).[5,6] A rheumatology consultation is indicated if signs and symptoms such as swelling, warmth, redness, and involvement of other joints are present.

Management Strategies

The decision to initiate treatment for the conditions is based on the presence of pain and/or restricted jaw movement that affects use of the jaw and quality of life. The treatment goals include the following[1]:

1. Reduce or eliminate pain
2. Restore comfortable jaw function and quality of life
3. Reduce the need for future health services

There is no simple approach to be used on all patients. Patients with myalgia and arthralgia often have multiple comorbid conditions and/or contributing factors. As other chapters have noted (see chapters 17 to 19), patients have individual beliefs,

experiences, behaviors, and emotions related to their pain; each of these factors can influence treatment outcome. Cost, previous unsuccessful treatments, preferences, pain severity, and doctor-patient relationships can also influence a patient's motivation to follow recommendations. A well-designed treatment plan that is tailored to the patient's unique characteristics and focuses on treating the diagnostic condition while addressing relevant contributing factors will best achieve these goals. If any identifiable cause such as pain from third molar impaction, an uncomfortably high restoration, or recent trauma to the jaw is present, this should be managed first.

The treatment options for TMDs are also consistent with medical management of muscloskeletal disorders in other parts of the body (Box 22-1). While there is some evidence from randomized clinical trials to support the use of several of the management strategies outlined in this chapter, management of patients with TMDs still remains both an art and a science.

Patient education and self-care

Most myalgias and arthralgias can improve over time if they are allowed to heal by resting the affected muscles and joints. Consequently, initial treatment for TMDs should be reversible and directed at self-care to promote normal healing. A key to successful management involves empowering the patient through education about the problem and ensuring compliance with self-care.[7,8] Self-care is designed to rest the jaw, reduce overuse, and encourage normal function (Box 22-2).

Pharmacotherapy

Pharmacotherapy is also a useful adjunct to self-care and is reviewed in chapters 19 and 21. Analgesics, muscle relaxants, and tricyclic antidepressants have well-documented evidence of their efficacy with TMD pain.[9] Despite the advantages of medications, however, problems such as chemical dependency, adverse side effects, and conflicts with medical history can occur. Therefore, when prescribing medications, it is important to conduct routine medication reconciliation with medical consultation as needed.

Analgesics

Acute muscle and/or joint pains usually respond well to short-term use of aspirin, nonsteroidal anti-inflammatory drugs (NSAIDs), and acetaminophen. Inflammatory conditions such as arthritis suggest the need for an anti-inflammatory such as aspirin or NSAIDs. Conversely, acetaminophen is the first drug of choice for patients with mechanically related pain or gastrointestinal sensitivity to NSAIDs. However, chronic use of these medications must be approached with caution due to undesirable systemic effects.

Muscle relaxants

When myalgia is present, a muscle relaxant such as a benzodiazepine or cyclobenzaprine may be beneficial to improve muscle tension, anxiety, and sleep.[7,10] Muscle relaxants are prescribed for a few days to a few weeks and often are used before bedtime to improve sleep and nocturnal habits. If

used during waking hours, patients need to be informed of drowsiness and dizziness that could interfere with driving or use of tools. Daily use of benzodiazepines can also be associated with chemical dependency.

Tricyclic antidepressants

Research on chronic pain patients, especially those with nonrestorative sleep, indicates that tricyclic antidepressants can help relieve pain.[11] These medications can be used in chronic TMD pain for longer periods than can muscle relaxants.

Corticosteroids

Oral corticosteroids, such as a Depo-Medrol dose pack, used for 6 days can be effective for arthritis, and their effects can be prolonged with subsequent use of NSAIDs.[12] Direct injection of corticosteroids into the TMJ has short-term efficacy, but multiple injections are contraindicated.

Physical medicine therapy

A wide range of physical medicine therapies (PMTs) can be used to treat TMDs, often in combination with other treatments. Therapeutic exercises are routinely used to improve jaw relaxation, posture, ROM, and strength. Conventional physiotherapy typically includes superficial heat or cold, joint and soft tissue mobilization, or massage to reduce pain and improve ROM. Other modalities include ultrasound, phonophoresis, iontophoresis, shortwave diathermy, electric stimulation, and low-level laser therapy. Most of these PMT approaches have not been rigorously evaluated in clinical trials and have a modest, short-term palliative effect for TMDs.[13]

While exercises are recommended long-term, PMT modalities are used for a defined short-term period. If the patient reports an increase in pain or a reduction in ROM during the course of treatment, the initial diagnosis and contributing factors need

Box 22-2 Self-care approaches for masticatory myalgia and arthralgia

Apply moist heat or cold to the sore joint or muscles. Heat or ice applications used up to four times per day can reduce joint or muscle pain and relax the muscles. For heat, microwave a wet towel for approximately 1 minute or until towel is warm. Wrap this moist warm towel around a hot-water bottle or heated gel pack to keep it warm longer. Apply it to the affected area for 15 to 20 minutes. For cold, use ice wrapped in a thin cloth. An initial burning sensation is normal. Keep ice on painful area only until you first feel some numbness, but not more than 5 minutes. Use what feels best, but in general, heat is used for chronic pain conditions and cold for acute conditions.

Eat a pain-free diet. Avoid hard foods such as French bread or bagels. Avoid chewy food such as steak or candy. Cut fruits and steamed vegetables into small pieces. Do not chew gum. Advance your diet as tolerated.

Chew food on both sides of your back teeth at the same time. This will reduce strain to the muscles and joints. If biting into food with your front teeth is painful, then cut up your food with a fork and knife and chew with your back teeth.

Keep the tongue up, teeth apart, and jaw muscles relaxed. Closely monitor your jaw position during the day (waking hours) so that the jaw is maintained in a relaxed, comfortable position. This often involves placing the tongue lightly on the palate behind the maxillary anterior teeth (find this position by saying "n"), allowing the teeth to come apart while relaxing the jaw muscles.

Avoid oral habits and activities that put strain on the jaw and neck. Oral habits such as teeth clenching, teeth grinding (bruxism), teeth touching or resting together, biting cheeks or lips, tongue pushing against teeth, jaw tensing, biting objects, shoulder shrugging, and neck tensing, and other activities such as overextended yawning, prolonged dental treatments, oral sexual activities, resting your jaw on your hand, overchewing, excessive singing, or use of musical instruments can strain the jaw. Remind yourself to check regularly to see if these activities are present through reminders such as stickers or timers. If noticed, these habits should be replaced with positive habits such as tongue-up position.

Keep your head up, chin in, and shoulders down and back. Closely monitor your head position over your shoulders to maintain balanced and relaxed head, neck, and shoulder muscles without a forward head posture.

Learn and practice relaxation and abdominal breathing. This will help reduce your reactions to stressful life events and decrease tension in the jaw and neck.

Identify events that trigger the pain. Use a pain diary to review daily activities that aggravate the pain, and modify your behavior accordingly.

Get a good night's sleep. Manage your sleep environment. Reduce light and noise, and lie on a comfortable mattress. Reduce stimulating activities in late evening (including computer work and exercising). Avoid sleeping on your stomach.

Avoid caffeine. Caffeine can interfere with sleep and increase muscle tension. Caffeine or caffeine-like drugs are in coffee, tea, soda, power drinks, and chocolate. Note that some decaffeinated coffee still has half as much caffeine as regular coffee.

Use anti-inflammatory and pain-reducing medications. Short-term use of over-the-counter drugs such as ibuprofen, naproxen, acetaminophen, or aspirin (without caffeine) can reduce joint and muscle pain. If available in your country and compatible with your condition and lifestyle, consider use of a combination of analgesic and muscle relaxant in the evening.

to be reassessed, and a consultation should be considered.

Intraoral splints and dental treatment

Intraoral splints have varying levels of efficacy for both TMD arthralgia and myalgia.[1,8,14] They can prevent tooth wear in patients with bruxism and increase awareness of oral habits. A flat plane stabilization splint can be effective when worn at night, especially if pain occurs on awakening. A recent review of their basis of evidence reported mild efficacy for such approaches.[14] For TMJ arthralgia with concurrent disc displacements, a repositioning splint is also effective when used during sleep. However, not every patient finds pain relief with splints. Some patients find increased clenching or other adverse events with splints. For example, full-time use of anterior repositioning splints, partial coverage splints, or anterior bite planes such as nociception trigeminal inhibition (NTI) appliances that do not cover all the teeth can cause an open bite and are not more effective than other splints.[15,16] To ensure that adverse events are not occurring, all patients with splints require regular follow-up visits.

The evidence for occlusal dental treatment including occlusal adjustments, prosthodontic treatment, and orthodontics for TMDs is limited; thus, their use for initial treatment of TMD pain is not recommended.[14] However, an occlusal adjustment may be indicated in patients who report an uncomfortable occlusion and jaw pain from recent dental treatment.

Cognitive-behavioral therapy

Cognitive-behavioral therapies, including biofeedback and relaxation training, have been shown to be effective for TMD pain and dysfunction.[17] Such approaches can address contributing factors including emotional difficulties (eg, anxiety and depression), behaviors (eg, oral habits and sleep problems), and lifestyle problems (eg, stress). They

are often used within the context of a multidisciplinary treatment approach for chronic TMD pain.

Oral parafunctional habits include clenching, grinding, jaw bracing, finger or pen biting, lip or cheek biting, and postural habits such as telephone cradling or jaw thrust. Although many oral habits will change by making the patient aware of them, changing persistent habits requires a structured program that can be facilitated by a health care psychologist.[18] Patients should be aware that they are responsible for initiating and maintaining the program to change the behavior. Habit reversal can be accomplished by the patient gaining awareness of the habit and then knowing why and how to correct it (eg, tongue up, teeth apart, jaw muscles relaxed). When this knowledge is combined with a commitment to conscientious monitoring, most habits will change. Progress with habit reversal should be continuously monitored with the patient to maintain long-term change.

TMJ surgery

There is some evidence for efficacy of TMJ surgery in cases where persistent TMJ pain is associated with mechanically related joint disorders.[12] However, this should be considered only after nonsurgical rehabilitation care has not been successful and factors such as oral habits that contribute to surgical failure are controlled.[1,12] In general, the less invasive surgeries such as arthrocentesis (TMJ irrigation) and/or arthroscopic procedures should be considered before more invasive surgery such as disc resection (discectomy) or a disc repair procedure. Preoperative and postoperative physical and behavioral therapy will improve outcomes and reduce the risk of complications.

Complementary and alternative therapies

Specific alternative or complementary therapies such as acupuncture, chiropractic treatment, or glucosamine/chondroitin sulfate have also been reported to be useful for myalgia and arthralgia.[19,20] However, there is a lack of evidence for naturopathy, homeopathy, magnetic therapy, and other alternative treatments in the management of TMD-related pain.

Referral or team management

The general dentist can successfully manage most patients with masticatory myalgia and arthralgia by starting with patient education and self-care, followed by simple reversible treatments. However, it is important to recognize that patients with similar diagnoses could have quite different contributing factors and outcomes. In the more complex cases, addressing the problem requires the use of a team or referrals to a physical therapist, physician, and/or psychologist.

Referral to a physician is indicated when a patient presents with a concomitant medical condition. A psychologist should be consulted when significant behavioral or psychosocial issues exist (eg, abuse, stress, depression, anxiety, chemical dependency, or uncontrolled oral habits). Patients with complex orofacial pain problems often require the use of a multidisciplinary team to be successful in management, and referral to a pain clinic may be warranted, especially if the patient does not respond to initial therapy.

Summary

This chapter has noted that masticatory myalgia and temporomandibular arthralgia refer to muscle and joint pain disorders that involve the masticatory muscles, the TMJ structures, or both. Pain can range from mild and self limiting to severe and chronic. The diagnostic process must distinguish these disorders from many other disorders that can cause pain in the head. Management starts with self care and is supplemented with treatments

such as pharmacotherapy, physical therapy, splints, cognitive behavioral therapy, and, as needed, TMJ surgery. A well-designed treatment plan that is tailored to the patient's unique characteristics and focuses on treating the diagnosed conditions while addressing relevant contributing factors will best achieve the goals of relieving pain and improving function.

References

1. Okeson JP (ed). Orofacial Pain: Guidelines for Assessment, Diagnosis, and Management. Chicago: Quintessence, 1996.
2. Headache Classification Subcommittee of the International Headache Society. The International Classification of Headache Disorders: 2nd edition. Cephalalgia 2004; 24(suppl 1):9–160.
3. Fricton J. Relationship of temporomandibular disorders and fibromyalgia: Implications for diagnosis and management. Curr Pain Headache Rep 2004;8:355–363.
4. Fricton J. Myofascial pain: Clinical characteristics and diagnostic criteria. J Musculoskeletal Pain 1993;1:37–47.
5. Schiffman E, Anderson G, Fricton J, Burton K, Schellhas K. Diagnostic criteria for intraarticular T.M. disorders. Community Dent Oral Epidemiol 1989;17:252–257.
6. Dworkin SF, LeResche L. Research diagnostic criteria for temporomandibular disorders: Review, criteria, examinations and specifications, critique. J Craniomandib Disord 1992;6:301–355.
7. Herman CR, Schiffman EL, Look JO, Rindal DB. The effectiveness of adding clonazepam or cyclobenzaprine to patient education and self-care for the treatment of jaw pain upon awakening: A randomized clinical trial. J Orofac Pain 2002;16:64–70.
8. Truelove E, Huggins KH, Mancl L, Dworkin SF. The efficacy of traditional, low-cost and nonsplint therapies for temporomandibular disorder: A randomized controlled trial. J Am Dent Assoc 2006;137:1099–1107.
9. Dionne RA. Pharmacologic treatments for temporomandibular disorders. Oral Surg Oral Med Oral Pathol Oral Radiol Endod 1997;83:134–142.
10. Singer E, Dionne R. A controlled evaluation of ibuprofen and diazepam for chronic orofacial muscle pain. J Orofac Pain 1997;11:139–146.
11. Bendtsen L, Jensen R. Amitriptyline reduces myofascial tenderness in patients with chronic tension-type headache. Cephalalgia 2000;20:603–610.
12. Schiffman EL, Look JO, Hodges JS, et al. Randomized effectiveness study of four therapeutic strategies for TMJ closed lock. J Dent Res 2007;86:58–63.

13. Feine J, Lund JP. An assessment of the efficacy of physical therapy and physical modalities for the control of chronic musculoskeletal pain. Pain 1997;71:5–23.

14. Forssell H, Kalso E. Application of principles of evidence-based medicine to occlusal treatment for temporomandibular disorders: Are there lessons to be learned? J Orofac Pain 2004:18:9–22.

15. Magnusson T, Adiels AM, Nilsson HL, Helkimo M. Treatment effect on signs and symptoms of temporomandibular disorders–comparison between stabilisation splint and a new type of splint (NTI). A pilot study. Swed Dent J 2004;28:11–20.

16. Jokstad A, Mo A, Krogstad NS. Clinical comparison between two different splint designs for temporomandibular disorder therapy. Acta Odontol Scand 2005;63: 218–226.

17. Turner J, Mancl L, Aaron L. Short- and long-term efficacy of brief cognitive-behavioral therapy for patients with chronic temporomandibular disorder pain: A randomized, controlled trial. Pain 2006;121:181–194.

18. Hathaway K. Bruxism: Definition, measurement, and treatment. In: Fricton JR, Dubner R (eds). Orofacial Pain and Temporomandibular Disorders. New York: Raven Press, 1995:375–386.

19. Thie NM, Prasad NG, Major PW. Evaluation of glucosamine sulfate compared to ibuprofen for the treatment of temporomandibular joint osteoarthritis: A randomized double blind controlled 3 month clinical trial. J Rheumatol 2001;28:1347–1355.

20. Wright EF, Schiffman EL. Treatment alternatives for patients with masticatory myofascial pain. J Am Dent Assoc 1995;126:1030–1039.

Management of Mucosal Pain

Edmond Truelove

This chapter addresses the diagnosis and management of oral mucosal pain. Box 23-1 identifies the conditions commonly associated with mucosal pain. The most common mechanisms involve an initiating event (eg, infection, injury, drug toxicity, autoimmune disease) that triggers the peripheral release of mediators that cause inflammation.[1] These activate and sensitize primary afferent nociceptors, resulting in hyperalgesia and pain[2] (see also chapters 4 and 6). Conversely, some mucosal pain conditions such as burning mouth syndrome (BMS) may be associated with changes in trigeminal small-fiber afferents or changes in the central nervous system (CNS).[3,4]

Symptom management may require a primary therapy directed toward etiology, a second front targeting pain, and a third front directed at behavioral factors. It is risky to address pain management alone since the underlying condition could be serious systemic pathology.[1] Control of symptoms may lull the patient and clinician into a false sense that the condition is benign and self limiting when it is not.

Assessment and Diagnosis

If a patient complains of pain in the oral mucosa, the initial step is to identify any cause that represents a risk to local or general health. This means assessing peripheral, central, and behavioral factors that may play a role in symptom production. It is equally important to assess the impact of the mucosal pain on daily general functioning (eg, sleeping) as well as on oral functioning.[5]

History

Findings of importance in the medical history include immunosuppressive diseases, hematologic disorders, HIV, diseases of the CNS (eg, tumors, demyelinating disorders, vascular lesions, brain injury), chronic viral infections, medications, and conditions known to cause peripheral neuropathies (eg, diabetes, multiple sclerosis, antineoplastic medications). Burning in the presence of oral lesions should prompt an exploration of the patient's history of communicable diseases and medications

Box 23-1 Common painful mucosal conditions

Infections
- Herpetic stomatitis
- Varicella zoster
- Candidiasis
- Acute necrotizing gingivostomatitis

Immune/Autoimmune
- Allergic reactions (dentifrices, mouthwashes, topical medications)
- Erosive lichen planus
- Benign mucous membrane pemphigoid
- Aphthous stomatitis and aphthous lesions
- Erythema multiforme
- Graft versus host disease

Traumatic and iatrogenic injuries
- Factitial, accidental (burns: chemical, solar, thermal)
- Self-destructive (rituals, obsessive behaviors)
- Iatrogenic (chemotherapy, radiation)

Neoplasias
- Squamous cell carcinoma
- Mucoepidermoid carcinoma
- Adenocystic carcinoma
- Brain tumors

Neurologic
- Burning mouth syndrome (stomatodynia)
- Neuralgias
- Postviral neuralgias
- Posttraumatic neuropathies
- Dyskinesias and dystonias

Nutritional and metabolic
- Vitamin deficiencies (B_{12}, folate)
- Mineral deficiencies (iron)
- Diabetic neuropathy
- Malabsorption syndromes

Miscellaneous
- Xerostomia, secondary to intrinsic or extrinsic conditions
- Referred pain from esophageal or oropharyngeal malignancy
- Mucositis secondary to esophageal reflux
- Angioedema

known to cause mucositis or depress immune competence. A prior history of severe stomatitis followed by development of residual pain and burning suggests the presence of a postmucositis/stomatitis pain disorder.

Clinical findings

Most mucosal pain is associated with mucositis and oral lesions. In such cases, efforts must be directed toward diagnosis and management of the mucosal disorder. As with other painful conditions, there is great variability in pain reporting among patients; these differences may have both physiologic and behavioral origins. However, there appears to be somewhat less variation in the presentation of acute mucosal pain arising from lesions. With time and chronicity, central and behavioral factors are increasingly important.

Occasionally, the clinical examination fails to identify physical explanations for the complaint, but occult malignancy should always be considered; ie, no identifiable local pathology may be associated with BMS or with postviral or posttraumatic neuropathy. Minor evidence of inflammation or superficial tissue abrasion is sometimes seen, but this is usually secondary to parafunctional tongue activity that irritates tissue. This is often mistaken as fungal infection or nutritional deficiency, and inappropriate therapy may be prescribed. Other significant clinical findings include allodynia, hyperpathia, dysesthesia, anesthesia, edema, and increased movements of the tongue, lips, and mandible. Each of these findings suggests different underlying conditions in the absence of mucositis.

Allodynia, hyperpathia, dysesthesia, and anesthesia suggest the possibility of viral or postviral neuralgia or another neurogenic pain (see also chapters 1 and 7). After a crush injury or burn injury, the tissue can become permanently hypersensitive. The presence of any neurologic complaint should trigger a careful examination to rule out the presence of tumor or infection causing compression or inflammation of the trigeminal nerve. If the symptoms are unilateral, the presence of a peripheral or central tumor must be entertained. Anesthesia in the absence of traumatic damage points to a stroke or an occult tumor.

Edema of the lips, tongue, or oral mucosa is usually accompanied by sensations of burning or pain. Episodic edema is often the result of either a local infection or angioedema and is triggered by reactions to allergens, stressful events, thyroid disease, or hereditary disease (*familial angioedema*). Treating symptoms of mucosal burning and discomfort without addressing the angioedema places the patient at risk for airway obstruction.

Mucosal symptoms in the presence of lip or tongue hyperactivity suggest the development of orofacial tics or movement disorders such as focal dystonia (see chapter 26). In these cases, the history is important because adverse reactions to psychoactive medications (eg, neuroleptics, antidepressants) can cause dyskinesia. Nonetheless, dyskinesias and dystonias may also develop in patients with no exposure to medications known to cause orofacial movement disorders. Most patients with these disorders have no idea that abnormal movement of the tongue or other structures is occurring. Placement of a tongue blade extended onto the back of the tongue usually dramatically decreases both movement and burning.

Mucosal symptoms caused by nutritional deficiencies are often accompanied by other clinical findings including cheilitis, hyperthyroidism, anemia, and weight loss and physical signs suggesting anorexia. Diminished mental capacity and memory loss along with skin lesions suggest the presence of a nutritional or malabsorption syndrome. Full hematologic assessment including a complete blood count (CBC), differential counts, and iron and vitamin levels is warranted.

Mucosal symptoms in the absence of lesions is suggestive of metabolic, neurologic, or other physiologic pathology and should lead to consideration of five alternatives: (1) subclinical systemic or local disease, *(2)* a neuropathic disorder, *(3)* symptoms referred from other regional disorders, *(4)* symptoms as a manifestation of psychologic or behavioral problems, or *(5)* contrived symptoms for secondary gain. Indications of depression, anxiety, panic attacks, major life stressors, prior severe problems (eg, behavioral, personal, or social), or other multiple somatic complaints (eg, backaches, headaches, gastric ulcer pain, gastrointestinal pain) or nonpainful somatic complaints (eg, tinnitus, atypical smell or taste dysfunction, dizziness) gathered from the history increase the likelihood that psychologic or behavioral problems are contributing to the condition. Referral to a psychologist or psychiatrist is often necessary, but frequently patients with mucosal complaints in the absence of mucosal lesions refuse such referrals even if they are only for consultative purposes. Nevertheless, when in doubt, referral to a qualified psychologist or psychiatrist is advised.

Laboratory and special tests

For suspected infections, a diagnosis of candidiasis or bacterial infection can be confirmed by laboratory tests for identification of fungal and/or bacterial organisms. Viral agents are best detected by viral culture or fluorescent antibody testing for herpes simplex virus, varicella-zoster virus, Epstein-Barr virus, and cytomegalovirus. The advantage of fluorescent antibody testing is that the results are usually available within 24 to 48 hours. If hematology or nutritional disease is suspected, blood studies are needed, as noted previously. Tests for thyroid function and occult blood loss may also be merited.

Pain Management Therapy for Mucosal Pain

Pain and symptom management includes treatment or prevention of the underlying mucosal disorder

and palliative and supportive care. Regardless of the condition, palliative therapy may be required to increase comfort and reduce disability. Palliative treatment falls into well-understood categories (Box 23-2). CNS-modulating drugs and behavioral strategies are usually reserved for persistent pains that cannot be controlled by other therapies. However, these are also useful if the pain compromises daily function and quality of life and is associated with depressed mood. Studies have demonstrated that mucosal pain can have a significant negative effect on the quality of life.[5]

Oral hygiene procedures

Studies generally confirm that local therapies can help reduce oral pain and mucositis. Covering damaged mucosal tissues, reducing inflammation, reducing the microflora, and promoting tissue healing are important components in patient management. Good oral hygiene through use of brushing and plaque removal reduces the risk of mucositis. In cancer therapy mucositis, high-volume irrigation of the oral cavity with normal saline has been shown to provide better oral symptom control than use of astringent mouth rinses.[6] Aggressive antimicrobial therapy has not been shown to have a significant effect on pain associated with mucositis.[7] Denture hygiene and topical therapy aimed at reducing the microbial flora associated with denture stomatitis help reduce painful symptoms in edentulous tissues.

Topical agents and therapies

A number of topical agents can reduce mucosal pain if their use is tolerated by the patient.[6] The most common is topical lidocaine. Unfortunately, the duration of action is relatively short and frequent reapplication is required, increasing the risk of gastrointestinal distress. Lidocaine/prilocaine cream, a 5% eutectic mixture of 2.5% lidocaine and 2.5% prilocaine, also shows utility as a topical

> **Box 23-2** Palliative treatment
>
> Oral hygiene and management of the tissue environment
> - Covering of damaged tissue
> - Reduction in microbial flora
> - Reduction in tissue inflammation and/or irritation (from spicy food, denture fit, sharp or defective tooth restoration)
> - Promotion of tissue healing and growth
> - Promotion of salivary flow
>
> Topical agents
> - Topical lidocaine
> - Lidocaine/prilocaine cream
> - Antihistamines
> - Milk of magnesia
> - Dexamethasone
> - Morphine
> - Adhesive polymer film
> - Clonazepam
>
> Systemic agents
> - Nonsteroidal anti-inflammatory drugs
> - Opioids
> - Antidepressants
> - Benzodiazepines
>
> Management of behavioral and central factors that trigger or modify pain and disability
> - Central nociceptive processes
> - Anxiety
> - Stress
> - Depression

agent for mucosal pain, as do tetracaine and antihistamines. Recent studies have demonstrated that doxepin (a tricyclic antidepressant in liquid form) is effective in providing prolonged topical tissue anesthesia in patients suffering from cancer-related stomatitis.[8] Diphenhydramine, combined with a coating agent such as milk of magnesia, and topical steroid rinses such as dexamethasone are also used, but these agents can irritate the stomach and cause nausea. Topical morphine solution (2,000 mg morphine chlorhydrate in 1,000 mL water) dramatically reduces mucositis pain for up to 24 hours in cancer patients undergoing radiation therapy.

The use of low-energy lasers (LEL) for mucositis and related pain also has been reported to reduce mucositis scores, mucositis pain, and the need for systemic morphine, with few complications.[9,10]

Topical mucosal adhesive polymer film hydroxypropyl cellulose has also been advocated for mucosal pain associated with radiation mucositis.[11] It is usually compounded with a number of antimicrobial agents and topical anesthetics (eg, tetracaine, miconazole, ofloxacin). The use of ice chips during chemotherapy sessions also has been shown to significantly reduce severity of mucositis and mucositis pain while causing few side effects.[12]

Systemic analgesics and other medications

Systemic medications are warranted for moderate or severe pain.[13] For mild pain, nonsteroidal anti-inflammatory drugs (NSAIDs) such as ibuprofen can reduce symptoms, but as pain levels increase, management with codeine (30 to 60 mg) can be initiated. Severe trauma to the mucosa, postviral neuralgia, and extensive mucositis arising from cancer therapy indicate the need to consider more potent opioids (eg, oxycodone, hydromorphine, morphine, and sufentanil). In such circumstances, patient-controlled analgesia offers an excellent mechanism for pain control. Morphine has been found to be more effective than other analgesics and is less likely to require escalating doses than hydromorphine or sufentanil.[13] For those who can continue to take liquids, a pain cocktail consisting of 5 to 8 mg methadone and 25 mg diphenhydramine in a bland liquid (eg, milk of magnesia) every 4 or 5 hours results in significantly decreased pain and improved mood. Patients with mucositis pain that will resolve appear to be at minimum risk for developing tolerance to narcotic analgesics. The literature suggests that the employment of opioids for such pain is not problematic, it is more important to reduce pain and maintain hydration and nutrition.

Behavioral therapies

A number of behavioral approaches, including relaxation therapy, biofeedback, and hypnosis have demonstrated some value in reducing mucositis pain.[1] These management approaches have not, however, replaced topical or systemic analgesics or anesthetics as a treatment of choice. There is some evidence that behavioral treatments can reduce the amount and frequency of systemic analgesics needed to relieve mucositis pain.

Management of mucosal pain not associated with mucositis or oral lesions

Patients with BMS and mucosal pain not associated with oral lesions often require both behavioral and pharmacologic management.[5] Topical use of antihistamines (eg, diphenhydramine) reduces symptoms because of anesthetic and anti-inflammatory properties; and topical anesthetics and doxepin, as described earlier, also provide temporary relief. Some patients actually report increased pain with topical anesthetics, suggesting that symptoms are arising from neuropathic changes. Coating agents such as milk of magnesia also offer temporary soothing. Other effective methods of management include antidepressants such as amitriptyline (10 to 70 mg every 24 hours), trazodone, and amisulpride. Clonazepam (0.1 to 0.3 mg every 8 hours), which is a member of the benzodiazepine family, has additionally been reported in several studies to reduce symptoms of BMS,[6] but some patients find the side effects unpleasant and discontinue the medication. Since BMS has a high degree of psychiatric disorder comorbidity, it is wise to consider behavioral therapy as an essential component of BMS management. The use of cognitive behavioral therapy has been shown to be effective. Another novel approach in the management of BMS is use of topical capsaicin, which is thought to desensitize C-nociceptors of the oral cavity. Generally, a topical anesthetic is applied prior to each capsaicin application to reduce the burning sensation triggered by the capsaicin.[6]

Summary

Mucosal pain is a common problem that can usually be addressed by treating the associated mucositis. This chapter has emphasized that the treating clinician must take care to seek out the etiology of the mucositis and to address the pathology while controlling symptoms. Adequate topical and systemic analgesic therapies are frequently not prescribed, and patients suffer unnecessary pain and morbidity resulting in decreased quality of life. The use of an adequate amount and type of analgesic necessary to alleviate pain and to sustain oral function is important when the mucositis and pain inhibit nutritional intake. For patients with mucosal pain not associated with oral lesions, it is essential to first rule out serious systemic, CNS, and local pathology while addressing palliative therapies. Behavioral approaches to pain management are advocated in chronic mucosal pain, whether accompanied with lesions or not.

References

1. Millard DH, Mason DK (eds). World Workshop on Oral Medicine. [Proceedings of the Third World Workshop on Oral Medicine, 23-27 Aug 1998, Chicago]. Ann Arbor, MI: Univ of Michigan, 2000.
2. Miaskowski C. Biology of mucosal pain. J Natl Cancer Inst Monogr 2001;29:37–40.
3. Lauria G, Majorana A, Borgna M, et al. Trigeminal small-fiber sensory neuropathy causes burning mouth syndrome. Pain 2005;115:332–337.
4. Patton LL, Siegel MA, Benoliel R, De Laat A. Management of burning mouth syndrome: Systematic review and management recommendations. Oral Surg Oral Med Oral Pathol Oral Radiol Endod 2007;103(suppl 1): S39.e1–13.
5. Stiff PJ, Erder H, Bensinger WI, et al. Reliability and validity of a patient self-administered daily questionnaire to assess impact of oral mucositis (OM) on pain and daily functioning in patients undergoing autologous hematopoietic stem cell transplantation (HSCT). Bone Marrow Transplant 2006;37:393–401.
6. Cawley MM, Benson LM. Current trends in managing oral mucositis. Clin J Oncol Nurs 2005;9:584–592.
7. Donnelly JP, Bellm LA, Epstein JB, Sonis ST, Symonds RP. Antimicrobial therapy to prevent or treat oral mucositis. Lancet Infect Dis 2003;3:405–412 [erratum 2003;3:598].
8. Epstein JB, Epstein JD, Epstein MS, Oien H, Truelove EL. Oral doxepin rinse: The analgesic effect and duration of pain reduction in patients with oral mucositis due to cancer therapy. Anesth Analg 2006;103:465–470.
9. Cerchietti LC, Navigante SH, Bonomi MR, et al. Effect of topical morphine for mucositis-associated pain following concomitant chemoradiotherapy for head and neck carcinoma. Cancer 2002;95:2230–2236.
10. Cowen D, Tardieu C, Schubert M, et al. Low energy Helium-Neon laser in the prevention of oral mucositis in patients undergoing bone marrow transplant: Result of a double blind randomized trial. Int J Radiat Oncol Biol Phys 1997;38:697–703.
11. Oguchi M, Shikama N, Sasaki S, et al. Mucosa-adhesive water-soluble polymer film for treatment of acute radiation-induced oral mucositis. Int J Radiat Oncol Biol Phys 1998;40:1033–1037.
12. Lilleby K, Garcia P, Gooley T, et al. A prospective, randomized study of cryotherapy during administration of high-dose melphalan to decrease the severity and duration of oral mucositis in patients with multiple myeloma undergoing autologous peripheral blood stem cell transplantation. Bone Marrow Transplant 2006;37:1031–1035.
13. Coda BA, O'Sullivan B, Donaldson G, Bohl S, Chapman CR, Shen DD. Comparative efficacy of patient-controlled administration of morphine, hydromorphine, or sufentanil for the treatment of oral mucositis pain following bone marrow transplantation. Pain 1997;72:333–346.

Management of Neuropathic Pain

Eli Eliav
Mitchell B. Max

Pain caused by a lesion of the peripheral or central nervous system (CNS) is commonly termed *neuropathic pain*. This chapter will consider only lesions of peripheral nerves.

Neurogenic pain in the orofacial region, as in other areas, can result from nerve trauma, deafferentation, or amputation (eg, vascular compression, neoplasia, bone fracture, root canal therapy, maxillofacial surgery); infection (eg, postherpetic neuralgia, HIV-related neuropathies); or metabolic disturbance (eg, diabetic neuralgia). However, the latter is not frequently associated with orofacial pain.

Orofacial Neuropathic Pain Conditions

Some patients develop *posttraumatic neuropathic pain* following trauma to the face, root canal treatments, tooth extractions, or even minor procedures. The pain is of moderate to severe intensity, often burning, and usually continuous. Typically, it is unilateral; the pain may spread across dermatomes but rarely crosses the midline. A related condition, *atypical odontalgia*, is a severe throbbing

pain in the tooth without any evident major pathology. The pain is commonly continuous and burning but can also be pulsatile, episodic, and migrating. Many authors report trauma or previous dental treatment, such as tooth extraction or root canal therapy, as the initiating event for atypical odontalgia and consider this condition to be "phantom toothache." It may be misdiagnosed as dental pain, leading to unnecessary dental and surgical treatment (see also chapter 20). Repeated interventions to relieve atypical odontalgia may induce posttraumatic neuropathic pain and be a significant factor in increasing comorbidity.

Two subsets of trigeminal neuralgia are recognized: idiopathic (classic) and neuralgia secondary to other pathologies such as multiple sclerosis and CNS tumors. The pain is severe and unilateral; it is usually described as sharp, shooting, stabbing, or electric in nature and is sometimes accompanied by background pain. The pain can be spontaneous or triggered by minor stimulation of specific trigger zones.

Postherpetic neuralgia is a painful condition that follows acute herpes zoster reactivation and can remain for months or even years after the rash and blisters have healed. It occurs most often in older people and in patients who are immuno-suppressed. The pain is described as severe, sharp, throbbing, or stabbing and may be accompanied by skin allodynia.

Readers should consult *Orofacial Pain: Guidelines for Assessment, Diagnosis, and Management*[1] from the American Academy of Orofacial Pain for further information.

Apart from idiopathic trigeminal neuralgia, a unique condition with its own treatment approach (discussed in a later section), it will be assumed that drug responses in neuropathic pain are similar no matter where in the body the pain originates. This assumption is necessary because only randomized clinical trials (RCTs) provide reliable evidence about analgesic responses, and too few RCTs have been conducted in orofacial pain to consider it separately. Recent reviews have proposed useful algorithms for the treatment of neuropathic pain.[2,3]

As described in previous chapters, therapeutic strategies should include a discussion of neuropathic pain causes and prognosis, as well as behavioral advice to the patient. Psychologic support is often indicated, as is information about the use and abuse of alternative therapies. While the drug management described in this chapter is supported by scientific evidence, the use of these medications is not without risk of side effects and medical complications. It is strongly recommended that clinicians prescribe these drugs with the collaboration of a family physician, neurologist, or oral medicine specialist.

Prevention of Neuropathic Pain

Preemptive analgesia induced by anesthetic blocks during surgery can prevent pain related to primary afferent hyperactivity and central sensitization (see chapters 5 and 7). Early antiviral treatment for acute herpes zoster, particularly in elderly patients, can decrease the incidence of postherpetic neuralgia.

Treatment for Neuropathic Pain (Excluding Trigeminal Neuralgia)

The drugs most commonly used for treating neuropathic pain are shown in Table 24-1. These drugs are grouped into sections according to the strength of evidence for effectiveness and toxicity. The first section describes the opioids, antidepressants, and anticonvulsants, which are roughly equipotent, and a topical lidocaine patch, which is partly effective in postherpetic neuralgia.

The most effective doses for most of the drugs in Table 24-1 vary greatly among patients. Therefore, each drug should be titrated slowly upward until side effects become limiting or pain is reduced. Complete elimination of pain is rare. Many patients do not respond at all to many of these drugs; a reduction of pain intensity by 30% to 40% can be considered a good response. Because of limited efficacy, dose-limiting adverse effects of single-agent therapy, and recent experimental data, many clinicians use combination pharmacotherapy to treat neuropathic pain.[4]

Drugs with strong evidence of benefit

Opioid analgesics

Although it is often said that neuropathic pain is resistant to opioids, some recent studies[5,6] have suggested that opioids may in fact be more effective than any other class of treatment for some types of neuropathic pain. The main concern is that patients will become psychologically dependent on the drugs. Tramadol, a weak opioid-related drug with norepinephrine and serotonin reuptake–blocking effects that may contribute to analgesia, has rarely been reported as leading to abuse. Constipation is less severe with tramadol than with other opioids, although sedation and nausea are common. Seizures are a rare complication.

Table 24-1 Drugs commonly used to treat neuropathic pain

Drug	Dose	Side effects	Comments
Strong evidence for benefit			
Opioids:			
μ-Receptor opioid agonists: morphine, oxycodone, fentanyl, etc	Variable	Sedation, nausea	Strong evidence for efficacy in PHN
Tramadol	50–100 mg tid or qid	Sedation, nausea, rare seizures	Less constipation
Antidepressants:			
Tricyclic antidepressants: amitriptyline, nortriptyline, desipramine, imipramine	Start at 10–25 mg/day; titrate to 75–125 mg/day	Orthostatic hypotension, anticholinergic effects, risk of malignant arrhythmia or heart block in ischemic heart disease	Nortriptyline may be as effective as amitriptyline, and sedation, hypotension, anticholinergic side effects are less common
Nontricyclic antidepressants:			
duloxetine, paroxetine, citalopram	40–60 mg/day (duloxetine)	Anticholinergic effects, dry mouth, constipation, increased sweating; paroxetine may raise tricyclic antidepressant concentrations threefold to sevenfold	Duloxetine is FDA cleared in the USA for the treatment of painful diabetic neuropathy
Anticonvulsants:			
Gabapentin	1,800–3,600 mg/day	Sedation, ataxia	Efficacy similar to tricyclic antidepressants in diabetic neuropathy and PHN, but has no risk of hypotension or arrhythmia
Pregabalin	Start at 50 mg tid; titrate up to 300 mg/day	Dizziness, sedation	Good results in the treatment of PHN and diabetic neuropathy
Topical medications:			
Topical lidocaine	Local application to sensitive areas	No serious adverse effects	Partial reduction of pain in PHN, effect in peripheral neuropathy unclear
Modest evidence for benefit			
Mexiletine	600–1,200 mg/day	Sedation, nausea, risk of malignant arrhythmia in ischemic heart disease	Several RCTs suggest effective in diabetic neuropathy
Carbamazepine	600–1,800 mg/day	Sedation, ataxia, nausea, rare leukopenia	May relieve continuous or paroxysmal pains
Clonidine	0.2–0.3 mg/day	Sedation, dry mouth	Several RCTs suggest effect in diabetic neuropathy
Preliminary evidence for benefit			
NSAIDs:			
Ibuprofen	1,200–3,200 mg/day	Contraindicated in chronic renal disease	Potential effect in diabetic neuropathy
Naproxen	500–1,000 mg/day		
Dextromethorphan	60–120 mg qid	Sedation, ataxia, severe adverse effect of serotonin syndrome if combined with SSRIs or MAOIs	Two small RCTs suggest effect in diabetic neuropathy; not widely available in pure form except from pharmacies that prepare to order
Topiramate	Titrate slowly up to 50–100 mg/day	Confusion, depression, anxiety, nausea	Pain reduction in some studies of diabetic neuropathy

Abbreviations: PHN = postherpetic neuralgia; RCT = randomized clinical trial; tid = three times daily; qid = four times daily; NSAIDs = nonsteroidal anti-inflammatory drugs; SSRIs = selective serotonin reuptake inhibitors; MAOIs = monoamine oxidase inhibitors.

The classic μ-receptor opioid agonists morphine, oxycodone, fentanyl, hydrocodone, and codeine can provide greater degrees of analgesia but have a greater risk of abuse. The risk of drug abuse from prescribing opioids has not been well quantified in long-term prospective trials, but most pain experts believe that it is low in patients without a history of addiction. Many scientific societies and state statutes now support a physician's choice to prescribe opioids for chronic nonmalignant pain if the risks and benefits are discussed with the patient and the effects of treatment are carefully monitored and recorded in the chart. Guidelines for such a prescription method have been published.[7] Although rapid tolerance to opioid analgesia occurs in some animal models, and therefore higher doses may be required to maintain the analgesic effect, some patients report continued efficacy on stable doses over years.

Antidepressants

The tricyclic antidepressants (amitriptyline, nortriptyline, imipramine, desipramine, doxepin) are the most-studied drugs for neuropathic pain.[8,9] RCTs have demonstrated their efficacy in diabetic and other generalized peripheral neuropathies, atypical facial pain, postherpetic neuralgia, and postmastectomy pain. The mechanism is thought to block reuptake of norepinephrine and serotonin, transmitters released by pain-modulating systems descending from the brain stem to inhibit the spinal and trigeminal dorsal horn nociceptive neurons (see chapter 5). Blockade of these transmitters presumably allows for longer periods of inhibitory action. Tricyclic antidepressants also block sodium channels and decrease ectopic discharge from injured peripheral nerves in rat models of neuropathic pain.

The most effective tricyclic antidepressants that block reuptake of norepinephrine and serotonin are amitriptyline, nortriptyline, and imipramine (Fig 24-1). Of these, nortriptyline probably has the

most favorable side-effect profile: it produces less sedation and somewhat less orthostatic hypotension. Duloxetine, one of a new generation of nontricyclic serotonin and norepinephrine reuptake inhibitors, has been cleared by the Food and Drug Administration (FDA) in the United States for the treatment of diabetic neuropathy.[10] Antidepressants that block norepinephrine but not serotonin reuptake are less effective. Some medications from this group (the nontricyclic paroxetine and citalopram)[11] reduce neuropathic pain more than placebo, whereas others (fluoxetine, desipramine) are ineffective.

Tricyclic antidepressants may be both hazardous in patients with coronary disease, since they may provoke dangerous cardiac arrhythmias or heart blockages, and in frail elderly people, in whom orthostatic hypotension may cause syncope and serious fractures. Antidepressants are also liable to cause major drug-drug interactions. For example, paroxetine and fluoxetine block the cytochrome P450 2D6 isoenzyme that metabolizes tricyclic antidepressants; this inhibition may increase the plasma concentration of the tricyclic antidepressant as much as sevenfold.

Scant data are available on the optimal dose of tricyclic antidepressants for neuropathic pain.

Anticonvulsants

In animal models of neuropathic pain and inflammatory pain, the chemically related anticonvulsant drugs gabapentin and pregabalin blocked sensitization of spinal dorsal horn sensory neurons and behavioral signs of hyperalgesia. In an orofacial model, gabapentin reduced pain-related behavior.[12] Large clinical trials in patients with diabetic neuropathy and postherpetic neuralgia[13] demonstrated good results: 1,800 to 3,600 mg/day in divided doses reduced pain by at least 50% (beyond any placebo effects) in about 1 in 3 patients, an effect similar to that found in studies of antidepressants. Side effects are mainly dizziness and sedation, which are acceptable.[14] Metabolism is

Fig 24-1 Effectiveness of various antidepressants on symptoms of diabetic neuropathy. Medians (*vertical lines*) and 95%-confidence intervals (*boxes*) describe the differences between different antidepressants and placebo as measured by physician scoring of symptoms of pain and discomfort on a 0 to 12 scale. Data are drawn from a number of the studies by Sindrup et al.[11] As in other studies, a selective norepinephrine (NA) reuptake inhibitor was effective, and drugs that inhibit both NA and serotonin (5-HT) reuptake appeared even more effective. The results shown here differ from findings of other investigators in that the specific 5-HT reuptake inhibitors, paroxetine and citalopram, showed a statistically significant analgesic effect. TCA = tricyclic antidepressant.

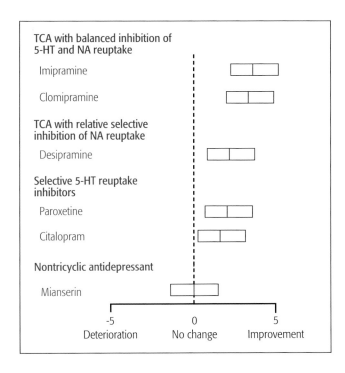

Topical drug delivery aims to induce peripheral analgesia and should be distinguished from transdermal drug delivery, which elevates the drug level systemically. Topical application of lidocaine at the thoracic level has been shown to relieve pain related to postherpetic neuralgia, although its utility for oral pain complaints is unknown. Another topical medication with only preliminary evidence of benefit includes orally applied capsaicin (Zostrix [Hi-Tech Pharmacal] 0.025% or 0.075%), which is suggested for use in orofacial neuropathic pain; however, there are no controlled studies to support its use. Capsaicin causes an unpleasant burning sensation for days before desensitization occurs. Topical application of amitriptyline with ketamine, however, was shown in an RCT to relieve peripheral neuropathic pain.[15]

Drugs with modest evidence of benefit

Mexiletine

Because the abnormal spontaneous discharge from an injured nerve is largely generated by sodium channels, sodium channel blockers may reduce neuropathic pain. Lidocaine strikingly reduces neuropathic pain when given as an intravenous infusion, but it is not available as an oral drug. Mexiletine, an oral analog, has been less impressive in RCTs, and many clinicians have noted that side effects of nausea, diarrhea, and dizziness occur before significant pain relief is achieved. Mex-

entirely renal, so dosage should be adjusted in patients with renal insufficiency. No drug-drug interactions of importance have been reported.

Topical medications

iletine may increase the risk of malignant cardiac arrhythmias in patients with cardiac disease (see Table 24-1).

Carbamazepine

Carbamazepine use for trigeminal neuralgia is discussed in a later section. A few reports suggest that patients with chronic or acute pain may benefit from its use.

Clonidine

Clonidine, an α-2 adrenergic agonist, may reduce neuropathic pain by direct inhibition of dorsal horn neurons or by reducing sympathetic efferent outflow. Several RCTs have suggested that a subgroup of patients with diabetic neuropathy may obtain modest benefit from transdermal clonidine (see Table 24-1).[16]

Drugs with preliminary evidence of benefit

Nonsteroidal anti-inflammatory drugs

Nonsteroidal anti-inflammatory drugs (NSAIDs) might potentially improve some neuropathic pain conditions (see Table 24-1) by reducing inflammation at the site of nerve injury or by direct analgesic effects in the spinal cord or brain stem.

Dextromethorphan

Extensive work in animal models has suggested that inhibitors of the *N*-methyl-D-aspartate (NMDA) glutamate receptor reduce hyperalgesia in neuropathic pain and other pain states. Small RCTs have shown reduction of diabetic neuropathy pain by the NMDA receptor antagonist dextromethorphan (see Table 24-1).[17] The required dosages averaged 400 mg/day, much higher than the upper limit of 120 mg/day suggested for the marketed antitus-

sive preparations of this drug. However, similar regimens did not relieve orofacial neuropathic pain in a small controlled trial.[18] Side effects include sedation, ataxia, and occasional psychotomimetic effects. Coadministration of dextromethorphan with selective serotonin reuptake inhibitors or monoamine oxidase inibitors may cause the potentially fatal serotonin syndrome (fever, rigidity, coma).

Topiramate

Topiramate is FDA cleared for the management of seizures and migraine (as prophylactic treatment). It has reduced pain in some studies of diabetic neuropathy.[19]

Drugs for Treatment of Trigeminal Neuralgia

The treatment of idiopathic trigeminal neuralgia (*tic douloureux*) is considered separately from other facial neuropathic pains for several reasons. First, this disorder appears to have a unique etiology, most commonly nerve compression by small blood vessels near the brain stem. In addition, RCTs have suggested that this disorder responds to a different group of drugs than do other neuropathic pain conditions. Surgical techniques are also available and include microvascular decompression, alcohol block, neurectomy, thermocoagulation, and gamma knife techniques.[20]

Commonly used drugs

Carbamazepine

Carbamazepine, an anticonvulsant and analgesic, is the mainstay of drug treatment for trigeminal neuralgia.[20] Side effects include sedation, ataxia, nausea, and anemia or decreased granulocyte count. A complete blood count should be obtained before the beginning of therapy and at 3- to 6-

month intervals thereafter. To minimize toxicity, therapy must be started at a low dosage, such as 100 mg daily, and increased 100 mg/day every 2 to 3 days to a final dosage averaging 600 to 1,200 mg/day. Sustained-release preparations may reduce side effects. Scheduling a bit more of the drug dose at night may protect against severe morning symptoms when patients brush their teeth, wash their face, and eat. After about 3 weeks of treatment, the drug often induces its own increased metabolism, requiring an increase in dosage. Carbamazepine is involved in many drug-drug metabolic interactions.

Oxcarbazepine

Oxcarbazepine is a carbamazepine derivative with fewer nervous system side effects, but dose-related hyponatremia is more common. Effective doses are usually higher; 300 mg of oxcarbazepine is equivalent to 200 mg carbamazepine.

Phenytoin

Phenytoin, another anticonvulsant, is often the second drug of choice for treating trigeminal neuralgia. Side effects are similar to those of carbamazepine, except that phenytoin is somewhat more sedating and chronic use may cause gingival hypertrophy, hirsutism, coarsening of facial features, and, rarely, pseudolymphoma. Phenytoin exhibits the unusual pattern of zero-order kinetics, ie, once metabolism is saturated, a small increase in dosage can cause a large increase in plasma concentration. Many metabolic interactions with other drugs occur.

Baclofen

The results of two RCTs show that baclofen, a muscle relaxant, is effective in treating trigeminal neuralgia. Side effects include sedation, ataxia, and nausea. A small study[21] showed that the L-isomer was more effective than the racemic mixture found in commercial preparations.

Other Drugs

An RCT has shown that the anticonvulsant lamotrigine reduces trigeminal neuralgia pain. Side effects include sedation, ataxia, an uncommon but potentially life-threatening rash, and Stevens-Johnson syndrome. Clonazepam, gabapentin, and valproic acid are also sometimes used.[20]

Summary

This chapter first briefly outlined common neuropathic orofacial pain conditions: posttraumatic neuropathic pain, atypical odontalgia, postherpetic neuralgia, and trigeminal neuralgia. Then treatment for neuropathic pain excluding trigeminal neuralgia was described. The drugs used for the management of neuropathic pain were classified as drugs with strong evidence of benefit (eg, antidepressants, opioids, anticonvulsants, and some topical medications), drugs with modest evidence of benefit (eg, mexiletine, clonidine, and carbamazepine), and drugs with preliminary evidence of benefit (eg, dextromethorphan and topiramate). Finally, the treatment for trigeminal neuralgia was outlined separately since this disorder responds to a different group of drugs than other neuropathic pain conditions.

References

1. de Leeuw R (ed). American Academy of Orofacial Pain. Orofacial Pain: Guidelines for Assessment, Diagnosis, and Management. Chicago: Quintessence, 2008.
2. Attal N, Cruccu G, Haanpaa M, et al. EFNS guidelines on pharmacological treatment of neuropathic pain. Eur J Neurol 2006;13:1153–1169.
3. Finnerup NB, Otto M, McQuay HJ, et al. Algorithm for neuropathic pain treatment: An evidence based proposal. Pain 2005;118:289–305.

4. Gilron I, Max MB. Combination pharmacotherapy for neuropathic pain: Current evidence and future directions. Expert Rev Neurother 2005;5:823–830.

5. Raja SN, Haythornthwaite JA, Pappagallo M, et al. Opioids versus antidepressants in postherpetic neuralgia: A randomized, placebo-controlled trial. Neurology 2002; 59:1015–1021.

6. Watson CP, Babul N. Efficacy of oxycodone in neuropathic pain: A randomized trial in postherpetic neuralgia. Neurology 1998;50:1837–1841.

7. Portenoy RK. Opioid therapy for chronic nonmalignant pain: A review of the critical issues. J Pain Symptom Manage 1996;11:203–217.

8. Cohen SP, Abdi S. New developments in the use of tricyclic antidepressants for the management of pain. Curr Opin Anaesthesiol 2001;14:505–511.

9. McQuay HJ, Tramer M, Nye BA, Carroll D, Wiffen PJ, Moore RA. A systematic review of antidepressants in neuropathic pain. Pain 1996;68:217–227.

10. Wernicke JF, Pritchett YL, D'Souza DN, et al. A randomized controlled trial of duloxetine in diabetic peripheral neuropathic pain. Neurology 2006;67:1411–1420.

11. Sindrup SH, Bjerre U, Dejgaard A, Brosen K, Aaes-Jorgensen T, Gram LF. The selective serotonin reuptake inhibitor citalopram relieves the symptoms of diabetic neuropathy. Clin Pharmacol Ther 1992;52:547–552.

12. Grabow TS, Dougherty PM. Gabapentin produces dose-dependent antinociception in the orofacial formalin test in the rat. Reg Anesth Pain Med 2002;27:277–283.

13. Rowbotham M, Harden N, Stacey B, Bernstein P, Magnus-Miller L. Gabapentin for the treatment of postherpetic neuralgia: A randomized controlled trial. JAMA 1998; 280:1837–1842.

14. Richter RW, Portenoy R, Sharma U, Lamoreaux L, Bockbrader H, Knapp LE. Relief of painful diabetic peripheral neuropathy with pregabalin: A randomized, placebo-controlled trial. J Pain 2005;6:253–260.

15. Lynch ME, Clark AJ, Sawynok J, Sullivan MJ. Topical 2% amitriptyline and 1% ketamine in neuropathic pain syndromes: A randomized, double-blind, placebo-controlled trial. Anesthesiology 2005;103:140–146.

16. Byas-Smith MG, Max MB, Muir J, Kingman A. Transdermal clonidine compared to placebo in painful diabetic neuropathy using a two-stage 'enriched enrollment' design. Pain 1995;60:267–274.

17. Sang CN, Booher S, Gilron I, Parada S, Max MB. Dextromethorphan and memantine in painful diabetic neuropathy and postherpetic neuralgia: Efficacy and dose-response trials. Anesthesiology 2002;96:1053–1061.

18. Gilron I, Booher SL, Rowan MS, Smoller MS, Max MB. A randomized, controlled trial of high-dose dextromethorphan in facial neuralgias. Neurology 2000;55:964–971.

19. Raskin P, Donofrio PD, Rosenthal NR, et al. Topiramate vs placebo in painful diabetic neuropathy: Analgesic and metabolic effects. Neurology 2004;63:865–873.

20. Zakrzewska JM, Lopez BC. Trigeminal neuralgia. Clin Evid 2006;(15):1827–1835.

21. Fromm GH, Terrence CF. Comparison of L-baclofen and racemic baclofen in trigeminal neuralgia. Neurology 1987;37:1725–1728.

25

Management of Orofacial Pain Related to Headache

Jeffrey P. Okeson

The complaint of headache is very commonly reported in the general population and is also a challenge in the differential diagnosis of orofacial pains (see chapter 17). Some individuals are only occasionally troubled by headaches, while others are regularly debilitated. It is very rare to find an individual who has never had a headache. Headache means different things to different people. Many people think of headache as pain felt in the temple or forehead. Others report headache in the back of their head. On occasion, a patient will report pain in the midfacial area. When this location is reported, the patient will often relate the headache to the structure where the pain is felt, such as the sinus, the jaw, or even a tooth. In this instance, the patient will often report to the dental practitioner for assistance. It is therefore important for the dentist to understand and appreciate the most common types of headaches that are encountered in practice. Failure to recognize these types of headaches may lead to a misdiagnosis and misdirected treatment (see also chapters 17 and 20).

Most headaches are expressed as a *heterotopic pain*, meaning that the location of the pain felt by the patient is not the actual origin of the nocicep-

tive input producing the pain. Therefore, when the patient is examined, the location of the headache fails to reveal any reason for the pain. In order for the headache to be successfully managed, therapy needs to be directed to the origin of the pain, which may be elusive and often arises from central mechanisms. This concept is quite different from the typical dental pains that clinicians treat (see chapter 20).

The understanding of headache classification for differential diagnosis is very complicated. The classification from the leading organization in the field, the International Headache Society (IHS), describes more than 230 types and subtypes of headaches.[1] The IHS classification attempts to separate all headaches according to etiology and involved structures. Within this classification (Box 25-1), the four primary headache types plus two of the secondary types (see nos. 11 and 13 of Box 25-1 for those dealing with facial and intraoral pain conditions) are more relevant in the differential diagnosis. The clinician also needs to consider that there are many overlapping symptoms between temporomandibular disorders (TMDs) and orofacial pain, making differential diagnosis even more difficult.[3]

Therefore, this chapter will review some of the more common headaches that may be felt in the masticatory structures but are not associated with TMDs: migraine, tension-type headache, temporal arteritis, and headache attributed to head and neck trauma. For a more thorough review of all headaches, the reader is encouraged to refer to texts specifically addressing headaches.[4,5]

Migraine

Clinical characteristics

Migraine is characterized by throbbing, often debilitating pain of moderate to severe intensity (Table 25-1). The headache is unilateral 60% of the time; it is often reported in the temple or behind the eye. Migraine can be felt in the maxillary arch, a condition referred to as *midface migraine*. This can be a diagnostic problem for the dental clinician because the pain can be felt in the teeth. The patient will often report photophobia, phonophobia, and osmophobia, and will seek a dark, quiet room. The pain is aggravated by routine physical activity and sometimes even by simple head movements.

Migraine affects approximately 16% of the population, with women affected more than men at a ratio of 3:1; about 25% of the female population is affected during their lifetime.[6] Migraine most often appears in the first 3 decades of life. When the onset is in the teenage years, it is important for the clinician to recognize this condition so that it is not mistreated. The pain episodes may occur at any time of day or night but are most frequent on arising in the morning. The pain episode commonly lasts 4 to 72 hours in adults and 2 to 4 hours in children.[7] The pain can vary greatly from mild to very intense.[8] Scalp tenderness occurs in two-thirds of patients during or after the headache.

Some migraine patients report a complex of focal neurologic symptoms that immediately precedes the headache.[8] This *aura* usually develops in 5 to 20 minutes and lasts less than 1 hour. The IHS has 2 designations for migraine: *migraine with aura* and *migraine without aura*. The former is sometimes referred to as *classic migraine*, the latter as *common migraine*. When present, the aura is commonly characterized by visual, sensory, or motor phenomena, and may even include language and brain stem disturbances. The visual symptoms are the most common symptoms and are characterized by sensations of unformed flashes of light before the eyes (*photopsia*), the partial loss of sight (*scotoma*), or a zigzag, flashing colored phenomenon that migrates across the visual field (*teichopsia*). Sensory symptoms such as paresthesia can occur.[9]

Etiology

Studies suggest that migraine patients have a genetic susceptibility to this pain condition: 50% to 60% of migraine patients have parents who also experience migraines.[10] Migraine is considered a neurovascular phenomenon since both neural and vascular structures are involved in its pathophysiology. The neural innervation of the intracranial vessels is called the *trigeminovascular system*, and current evidence suggests that there is a neurologic trigger in the brain stem that initiates a cascade of events resulting in neurogenic inflammation of the intracranial vessels that produces the headache.

Management considerations

The management of migraine with or without aura involves patient education and pharmacologic approaches (see Table 25-1).

Patient education and trigger avoidance

Patients who experience migraine headaches need to understand basic information about their pain condition. They need to know that even though the

Box 25-1 Categories of headache[2]

Part one: The primary headaches
1. Migraine
    1.1 Migraine without aura
    1.2 Migraine with aura
2. Tension-type headache
3. Cluster headache and other trigeminal autonomic cephalalgias
4. Other primary headaches

Part two: The secondary headaches
5. Headache attributed to head and/or neck trauma
6. Headache attributed to cranial or cervical vascular disorder
7. Headache attributed to nonvascular intracranial disorder
8. Headache attributed to a substance or its withdrawal
9. Headache attributed to infection
10. Headache attributed to disorder of homoeostasis
11. Headache or facial pain attributed to disorder of cranium, neck, eyes, ears, nose, sinuses, teeth, mouth or other facial or cranial structures
12. Headache attributed to psychiatric disorder

Part three: Cranial neuralgia, central and primary facial pain, and other headaches
13. Cranial neuralgias, central causes of facial pain
14. Other headaches, cranial neuralgias, central and primary facial pain

pain may be severe, it is still benign. An important aspect of education is having the patient identify any triggering factors that initiate the migraine attack (eg, exposures to certain foods, alcohol, odors, stress, or even changes in sleep patterns). The patient should be asked to maintain a headache diary to help identify factors associated with the initiation of the headache. Once these factors are identified, efforts can be made to avoid them so as to reduce the number of migraine attacks.

Pharmacologic management

Pharmacologic management of migraine is of two types: medications that are used to abort a migraine at its start and medications that are used to prevent migraine attacks. The choice of which management strategy to use is determined by the frequency of the migraine attacks. As a general rule, migraine attacks that are infrequent are managed with abortive medications so that treatment is immediately initiated during the onset of the attack. When migraine attacks occur so often that they significantly interfere with a patient's daily activities, preventive medications should be considered.[11]

Triptans are a family of medications that have been proven helpful in aborting migraines.[11] These drugs seem to stop the neurogenic inflammation in the meningeal (dural) vasculature[12] and may also act within the brain. Frequent migraines are best managed by prescribing daily medication as a preventive measure. Such medications include the β-*adrenergic agents* (β-*blockers*) such as propranolol or metoprolol,[13] or *calcium-channel blockers* such as nifedipine or verapamil.[14] The *tricyclic antidepressants* have also been useful, especially amitriptyline.[11]

Since many of the drugs have significant side effects, especially on the cardiovascular system (eg, propranolol, sumatriptan), dentists do not normally prescribe such medications unless they have advanced training in orofacial pain, oral medicine, or oral surgery. Although most of these changes are quite safe in a healthy patient, medically compromised patients or chronic pain patients who use other medications may experience significant problems that will need proper attention by appropriate health care providers.

Tension-type Headache (Temporal Headache)

Clinical characteristics

Tension-type headache is the most common headache reported in the general population (see chapter 2). The headache is described as a dull, nonpulsing tightness or pressure felt in the occipital, parietal, temporal, and frontal regions (see Table 25-1). In 90% of cases, the pain is felt bilaterally.[15] Some patients will describe the feeling of a tight "headband" compressing their head as if they were wearing a tight cap. Most tension-type headaches are of mild or moderate intensity, rarely becoming debilitating as occurs with migraine. Most tension-type headaches are episodic, lasting an average of 12 hours, although the duration can vary greatly (30 minutes to 72 hours).[16] Nausea and vomiting are rare.

Etiology

Although tension-type headache is the most common headache, its pathophysiology remains unclear. Part of the problem may be that tension-type headache, as a type of primary headache, likely has a central etiologic mechanism especially involving the limbic structures. Emotional stress, anxiety, and depression seem to present causal relationships with tension-type headaches.[17,18] However, many other disorders that result in headache present with the same clinical characteristics of tension-type headache. For example, trigger points associated with myofascial pain (see chapter 22) may result in a headache at the referred site that is often clinically described by the patient as a tension-type headache. This type of headache is secondary to the myofascial condition and therefore should not be classified as a tension-type headache. Similarly, patients with sleep bruxism may awake with headache as a secondary symptom. Also, morning headache in the temporal area is frequently associated with sleep respiratory disorders such as snoring or sleep apnea.[19,20] The headache should always be classified according to the primary disorder, which will assist in selecting the proper treatment.

Management considerations

Like many pain disorders, management of tension-type headache begins with patient education (see Table 25-1). The sufferer needs to identify those factors that aggravate the condition as well as those that might relieve it. As in the case of migraine sufferers, it is often helpful to have the patient maintain a headache diary so that factors that are not commonly considered can be recognized. The patient should be encouraged to decrease intake of caffeine (eg, coffee, tea, soft drinks) and alcohol, as well as any medications that have been chronically used for the headache. The patient should be informed that eliminating these substances may at first increase the frequency and intensity of the headaches. After 1 to 2 weeks, the withdrawal effects should subside.

Since emotional stress often plays an important role in tension-type headache, the patient should be assessed for any significant stressors; if these are identified, corrective behaviors or avoidance

Table 25-1 Clinical characteristics of the major types of headaches and management considerations

Types of headache	Symptoms	Management
Migraine	Throbbing, moderate to severe, often debilitating pain Photophobia, phonophobia, and osmophobia Duration of 4 to 72 hours	Education, trigger avoidance Abortive medication: triptans (ie, sumatriptan) Preventive medication: β-blockers or calcium-channel blockers
Tension-type	Dull, nonpulsing; tightness or pressure felt in the occipital, parietal, temporal, and frontal regions Mild or moderate intensity, rarely debilitating Photophobia, phonophobia are rare	Stress management (ie, relaxation training, biofeedback) NSAIDs Tricyclic antidepressants
Temporal arteritis	Unilateral throbbing, stabbing, burning pain felt in the temple A prominent, tortuous, very tender, and temporal artery Jaw claudication	Immediate administration of steroid Referral to rheumatologist
Headache attributed to head or neck trauma	Dull, achy pain in the temporal, frontal, orbital, and preauricular areas Pain felt in the cervical structures Headache is increased with cervical function but not by jaw function Palpation of cervical structures increases the headache	Direct therapy to the specific cervical pain disorder Referral to appropriate physician or physical therapist

should be encouraged. Stress management skills, relaxation training, and biofeedback techniques[17,18] can be very helpful therapies to manage tension-type headache, and they are frequently taught by a psychologist trained in cognitive-behavioral therapy. If a major depressive disorder or anxiety disorder is present, these conditions need to be managed by the proper health care providers.

Judicious use of mild analgesics (eg, aspirin, ibuprofen) may be needed, but the patient should be aware of the potential complications. Nonsteroidal anti-inflammatory drugs (NSAIDs) are often helpful, especially if the patient has not been using them previously. When the patient has occasion-

ally used one NSAID previously, another NSAID should be used. Often, low doses of a tricyclic antidepressant such as amitriptyline can be helpful in managing the headache and are best taken before bedtime because of their sedative effects.

When the tension-type headache is secondary to another disorder (eg, when the headache is associated with a masticatory muscle disorder), the primary disorder needs to be managed[21] (see chapter 22). Headache on awaking may be related to nocturnal bruxism or breathing disorders, and several management approaches can be used for these conditions (see chapters 16 and 26).

Temporal Arteritis

Clinical characteristics

Vascular pains originate from the vessel walls and are far less common than the neurovascular pains discussed previously. Pain originating from inflammation of a vessel wall is called *arteritis*. Dental clinicians should be familiar with temporal arteritis, which commonly presents as a severe headache in the temporal region (see Table 25-1). It is usually unilateral, affecting only one artery, but occasionally presents bilaterally. The pain is often described as throbbing or stabbing.[22] It may be felt as a superficial burning pain with a superimposed piercing quality, and the intensity may range from mild to severe. The clinician will recognize such a condition on palpation of the temporal region and will usually find a prominent, tortuous, very tender and enlarged temporal artery. While minor jaw movement will not produce pain, the patient's increased use of the jaw will increase the pain significantly (*jaw claudication*).

Etiology

The pathophysiology of cranial arteritis is unknown. It is very similar in clinical presentation to polymyalgia rheumatica, which also has an unknown etiology. Blood studies reveal an elevated erythrocyte sedimentation rate (ESR), often greater than 100 mm/hr.

The recognition of temporal arteritis is important since complete or partial loss of vision is a possible consequence, occuring in at least one-third of all cases.[23] Blindness results from the temporal arteritis producing a granulomatous inflammation of the posterior ciliary arteries that leads to an anterior ischemic optic neuropathy.[24] The inflammatory phase often appears to be self-limiting, but because of the possibility of blindness and stroke, immediate management is essential. Diagnosis is confirmed by a biopsy of the artery revealing a giant cell arteritis.

Management considerations

Since temporal arteritis is considered a semiacute inflammatory disease that can quickly threaten vision, immediate treatment is indicated (see Table 25-1). If symptoms are progressing rapidly, hospitalization may be indicated. The treatment of choice is 40 to 60 mg of prednisone daily.[22] This dosage may be tapered very quickly to a maintenance level depending on the relief of symptoms and the regulation in ESR toward a normal rate. It may be necessary to continue corticosteroids for months, though eventual discontinuance of prednisone treatment is usual in most patients. Because corticosteroids have a profound effect on immunosuppression, the clinician needs to understand the entire medical status of the patient before any medications are prescribed.

Headache Attributed to Head or Neck Trauma

Clinical characteristics

The clinician must appreciate that pain arising from cervical structures commonly presents as pain in the face and temporomandibular joint (TMJ) region. This occurs as a result of pain referral,[2] as most headaches are not felt where they originate. When pain is referred to the TMJ region, the patient will often report to the dental office for treatment. Some patients report secondary or referred pain without mention of the primary source of pain; in such a case, accurate diagnosis is more difficult. For example, the patient may come to the dental office complaining of pain in the region of the TMJ without mentioning cervical pain. The clinician must be able to identify the true source of the pain to ensure proper treatment; without this insight, treatment will likely be limited to the TMJ and will fail to resolve the primary source of the pain.

One of the most common sources of neck pain is a cervical flexion-extension injury often referred to as *whiplash*. When this type of pain persists for several weeks (which is common), it generally produces pain in the face and TMJ area. The patient may report pain with the same clinical characteristics as tension-type headache—a dull ache with a tight feeling in the back of the head is usually accompanied by a bilateral headache located in the temporal, frontal, orbital, and preauricular areas, which may be accentuated by cervical function or palpation (see Table 25-1). A key to differentiating this pain from that of tension-type headache is that jaw function does not significantly increase the pain. Further complicating the diagnosis is the possibility of minor injury to the brain associated with the trauma. This may also lead to the complaint of headache (eg, posttraumatic headache).

Etiology

There are many causes of cervical pain that may manifest as a headache. Certainly trauma is one, and a flexion-extension injury is the most common. This injury occurs when there is a sudden change in body position. In many instances the weight of the head is too great for the cervical muscles to hold the head, and under contractile force, the cervical muscles are quickly lengthened. This *eccentric contraction* causes damage to these muscles, resulting in the flexion-extension injury. Continued pain in these muscles often results in myofascial pain, which is characterized by hyperirritable bands of muscle tissue called *trigger points*—sources of deep pain resulting in the referred headache complaint. Other sources of cervical pain may be a variety of arthritic conditions or nerve root impingement disorders.

Management considerations

The management of headache attributed to head or neck trauma is directed to the specific source of the cervical pain (Table 25-1). Referring the patient to an appropriate health care provider is generally indicated. The critical issue for the dental clinician is to establish the correct diagnosis. All too often, patients with this condition are managed in the dental office with dental procedures that fail to address the source of pain. When this occurs, the pain condition becomes chronic, making it even more difficult to manage.

Summary

Headache is a very common pain complaint experienced by many patients who present in a dental office. This chapter has noted that there are many different types of headaches, some of which produce pain in the midfacial region and dental structures. When this occurs, the patient may consult with the dentist regarding treatment. It is essential for the clinician to recognize the clinical characteristics of some of the more common headaches so as not to confuse them with dental pains or TMDs, thereby avoiding inappropriate treatment.

References

1. Headache Classification Subcommittee of the International Headache Society. The International Classification of Headache Disorders: 2nd edition. Cephalalgia 2004; 24(suppl 1):9–160.
2. Okeson JP. Bell's Orofacial Pains, ed 6. Chicago: Quintessence, 2005:63–94.
3. Woda A, Pionchon P. A unified concept of idiopathic orofacial pain: Pathophysiologic features. J Orofac Pain 2000; 14:196–212.
4. Olesen J, Goodsby P, Ramadan N, Tfelt-Hansen P, Welch K (eds). The Headaches, ed 3. Philadelphia: Lippencott Williams & Wilkins, 2006.

5. Silberstein SD, Lipton RB, Dodick D (eds). Wolff's Headache and Other Head Pain, ed 8. New York: Oxford Univ Press, 2008.

6. Rasmussen BK, Jensen R, Schroll M, Olesen J. Epidemiology of headache in a general population—A prevalence study. J Clin Epidemiol 1991;44:1147–1157.

7. Classification and diagnosis criteria for headache disorders, cranial neuralgia, and facial pain. Headache Classification Committee of the International Headache Society. Cephalalgia 1988;8(suppl 7):1S–96S.

8. Stewart WF, Shechter A, Lipton RB. Migraine heterogeneity. Disability, pain intensity, and attack frequency and duration. Neurology 1994;44(6 suppl 4): 24S–39S.

9. Russell MB, Olesen J. A nosographic analysis of the migraine aura in a general population. Brain 1996;119(pt 2):355–361.

10. Walters WE, Silberstein SD, Dalessio DJ. Inheritance and epidemiology of headache. In: Dalessio DJ, Silberstein SD (eds). Wolff's Headache and Other Head Pain, ed 6. New York: Oxford Univ Press, 1993:42–58.

11. Silberstein SD. Practice parameter: Evidence-based guidelines for migraine headache (an evidence-based review): Report of the Quality Standards Subcommittee of the American Academy of Neurology. Neurology 2000;55:754–762.

12. Williamson DJ, Hargreaves RJ. Neurogenic inflammation in the context of migraine. Microsc Res Tech 2001;53: 167–178.

13. Diener HCh. Pharmacological approaches to migraine. J Neural Transm Suppl 2003;(64):35–63.

14. Adelman JU, Adelman RD. Current options for the prevention and treatment of migraine. Clin Ther 2001;23: 772–788; discussion 771.

15. Rasmussen BK, Jensen R, Olesen J. A population-based analysis of the criteria of the International Headache Society. Cephalalgia 1991;11:129–134.

16. Iversen HK, Langemark M, Andersson PG, Hansen PE, Olesen J. Clinical characteristics of migraine and tension-type headache in relation to new and old diagnostic criteria. Headache 1990;30:514–519.

17. Holte KA, Vasseljen O, Westgaard RH. Exploring perceived tension as a response to psychosocial work stress. Scand J Work Environ Health 2003;29:124–133.

18. Bertolotti G, Vidotto G, Sanavio E, Frediani F. Psychological and emotional aspects and pain. Neurol Sci 2003; 24(suppl 2):71S–75S.

19. Bailey DR. Tension headache and bruxism in the sleep disordered patient. Cranio 1990;8:174–182.

20. Ozge A, Ozge C, Kaleagasi H, Yalin OO, Unal O, Ozgur ES. Headache in patients with chronic obstructive pulmonary disease: Effects of chronic hypoxaemia. J Headache Pain 2006;7:37–43.

21. Okeson JP. Management of Temporomandibular Disorders and Occlusion, ed 6. St Louis: Mosby, 2008:377–403.

22. Redillas C, Solomon S. Recent advances in temporal arteritis. Curr Pain Headache Rep 2003;7:297–302.

23. Accetta D, Kelly JP, Tubbs RR. An elderly black woman with a painful, "swollen" face. Ann Allergy 1985;55:819–824.

24. Liozon E, Loustaud-Ratti V, Ly K, et al. Visual prognosis in extremely old patients with temporal (giant cell) arteritis. J Am Geriatr Soc 2003;51:722–723.

Management of Movement Disorders Related to Orofacial Pain

Frank Lobbezoo
Pierre Blanchet
Gilles J. Lavigne

Hypokinetic (parkinsonian) movement disorders are commonly associated with sensorimotor oropharyngeal features. In addition, four main types of *hyperkinetic* movement disorders can be distinguished: *(1)* dystonia, *(2)* dyskinesia, *(3)* stereotypies, and *(4)* bruxism. While these conditions are mainly diagnosed and managed by medical specialists, they consist of various repetitive, abnormal, involuntary movements that may affect the tongue, lips, and jaw. Orofacial pain is an under-recognized feature of several of these hypokinetic and hyperkinetic oral movement disorders. In this chapter, the management of the disorders associated with orofacial pain is presented, while their main motor and pain features, as well as their main management strategies, are summarized in Table 26-1.

Parkinson Disease

Parkinson disease (PD) is the second most common neurodegenerative disorder in humans after Alzheimer disease, affecting 1% to 2% of the population after age 50. It results from cell loss, most noticeably dopaminergic neurons, in the nervous system. Its motor features include rigidity, akinesia (paucity of movement), bradykinesia (slowness of movement), and postural instability, often associated with resting tremor. Other sensory, autonomic, and cognitive manifestations, as well as anxiety and depression, are frequent. About 40% of PD patients experience body pain. The pain is commonly related to general causes such as osteoarthritis or trauma, but it may also be related to diseases of the central nervous system (CNS), including lesions of dopamine pathways and impaired basal ganglia nociceptive processing.[1,2]

Standard medical treatment for PD includes levodopa (a catecholamine precursor), dopamine D2 agonists, and enzyme blockers that optimize levodopa pharmacokinetics. Clinicians should be aware that recurrent pain in PD patients may reflect fluctuations in drug response from one dose of levodopa to the next. Periods of low levodopa bioavailability are associated with return of motor symptoms, which may be accompanied by nonspecific oral pain or trigeminal neuralgia–like pain, the latter in absence of the usual trigger zones (see chapter 24). The pain episodes dissipate when the next dose of medication becomes effective. Other

Table 26-1 Motor features, pain features, and management of movement disorders related to orofacial pain

Movement disorder	Motor features	Pain features	Management
Hypokinetic			
Parkinson disease	Rigidity, akinesia, bradykinesia, postural instability, resting tremor	General causes (eg, osteoarthritis, trauma), central causes (eg, impaired basal ganglia nociceptive processing)	Pharmacologic
Hyperkinetic			
Dystonia	Involuntary mouth closure, opening, or deviation; blepharospasm; jerking; tremor; difficulty initiating movement	Atypical pain (eg, painful spasms, burning mouth syndrome, atypical facial pain, tension-type headache), biting injuries, temporomandibular pain	Pharmacologic (eg, botulinum toxin), occlusal splints, deep brain stimulation
Dyskinesia	Aimless, repetitive, irregular, sometimes patterned, involuntary movements of the labial, lingual, and jaw musculature	Generalized aching, orofacial pain, tongue pain, burning mouth syndrome	Pharmacologic (eg, botulinum toxin), deep brain stimulation
Stereotypies	Coordinated, repetitive, patterned movements producing grimaces, lip movements, biting, and chewing	In Gilles de la Tourette syndrome: musculoskeletal pain, neuropathic complications, self injuries	No treatment, or pharmacologic, possibly dental
Bruxism	Teeth grinding or clenching	Temporomandibular pain, tension-type headache	Occlusal splints, behavioral (counseling), pharmacologic (eg, clonazepam, clonidine)

types of oral pain (eg, burning mouth syndrome [BMS], gum or jaw discomfort) do not clearly fluctuate with the motor condition.[2] Dental status (eg, dentures, edentulism) does not appear to be of significance.

Dystonia

Orofacial *dystonia* (also known as *Meige syndrome*) is produced by excessive muscle contractions causing involuntary closure, opening or deviation of the

jaw, bruxism, and blepharospasm (prolonged eye closure). Because orofacial dystonia is confined to a restricted anatomic area, it can be considered a focal dystonia. Occasional associated signs are jerking and tremor activity as well as difficulty initiating movement. Typically, a motor act or sensory signal (*geste antagoniste*), such as food in the mouth or light touch, may reduce the intensity of the spasms. Pain is generally not a prominent feature, and although constant pain is considered atypical, dystonia may sometimes be associated with painful muscle spasms, BMS, atypical facial pain, and tension-type headache.[3,4] Oromandibular dystonia may cause painful biting injuries and temporomandibular pain.

Most adult-onset cases are of idiopathic origin. Task-specific forms of dystonia, triggered by apparently excessive repetition of motor patterns, are seen in writers, musicians, and lifetime gum-chewers, among others. Secondary causes of dystonia include focal brain lesions or drugs with dopamine receptor–blocking properties, such as antipsychotic and antiemetic/antivertigo drugs. Disruption in orofacial neuromuscular control caused by various dental procedures has been implicated as a potential trigger for oromandibular dystonia, but no correlation has been found between the severity of the injury and dystonia. Concomitant bruxism and persistent jaw pain, which have been reported in such postprocedural cases, are notoriously difficult to manage.[5]

Intramuscular injection of botulinum toxin is an excellent option for the relief of pain associated with oromandibular dystonia.[6,7] Dystonia may also benefit from a trial of anticholinergic drugs, tetrabenazine, clonazepam, or baclofen. Levodopa is generally worth trying but might exacerbate the dystonia.[3] Oral appliances such as occlusal splints may improve cases of jaw-closing dystonia.[5] Particularly disabling and refractory cases may respond to deep brain (basal ganglia) stimulation.

Dyskinesia

Oral *dyskinesia* is characterized by aimless, irregular, repetitive, sometimes patterned, involuntary movements affecting the labial, lingual, and mandibular musculature (hence the term *bucco-linguomasticatory syndrome*). It is observed as an early or delayed (*tardive*) manifestation during various drug treatments for conditions of the CNS (eg, psychosis, depression, attention deficit disorder, PD, epilepsy). Tardive dyskinesia (TD) is seen in 30% of those treated with long-term conventional anti-

psychotic drugs (eg, haloperidol), all of which are potent blockers of dopamine D2 receptors. Second-generation (*atypical*) antipsychotic drugs (eg, quetiapine) carry a lower risk. The risk of drug-related TD is five times greater in the elderly population than in younger individuals. Remission can occur, particularly if the offending drug is discontinued, but symptoms persist in most cases. Its pathophysiology is not well understood, but supersensitivity of striatal dopamine D2 receptors is the traditional explanation.

TD may be a source of generalized aching and orofacial pain. Tongue pain and BMS have been reported as a prominent manifestation.[8] This condition, known as *drug-related* tardive pain, is protracted and may be disabling. The pain may begin simultaneously with the onset of oral TD or follow it. As in dystonia, severe TD may produce complications such as painful biting injuries or temporomandibular pain.[9] The first-line approach in treating TD and associated drug-induced pain is to gradually withdraw the offending drug whenever possible. Tardive pain may benefit from the general strategies known to alleviate TD, such as treatment with the brain monoamine depletor tetrabenazine.[10] Topical oral lidocaine and analgesics are generally ineffective. In refractory cases, reintroduction of the offending agent at a higher dose, electroconvulsive therapy, and deep brain stimulation may be considered. Certain orofacial TD cases can be successfully managed with botulinum toxin.[10]

Stereotypies

Oral *stereotypies* are a form of dyskinesia characterized by repetitive, coordinated, and patterned movements that produce various grimaces and lip movements; licking, biting, and chewing motions; and bruxism. They are nonspecific and may occur in a variety of neuropsychiatric conditions including schizophrenia, autism, mental retardation, Rett syndrome, and Alzheimer disease. They resemble the tics displayed in Gilles de la Tourette syndrome (GTS), but the latter are brief, sudden, irregularly occurring, repetitive movements or utterances that most often start in childhood. Tics typically involve the craniocervical musculature, fluctuate over time, and are suppressible for a variable period of time. However, voluntary control is limited by an unpleasant, sometimes painful, growing tension that presses the individual to release the tics. Oral stereotypies occur in up to 16% of edentulous subjects.[5] Most of these subjects are aware of the presence of oral movements, which are generally mild, confined to the oral region, and never dystonic. The movements include smacking and pursing of the lips, and lateral deviation and protrusion of the tongue or jaw.

Pain is generally not reported with stereotypies but may occur in GTS patients with severe tics. In these cases, the pain is often musculoskeletal in origin but may also result from neuropathic complications or self-injuries.[11] In a survey of noninstitutionalized older adults with a high prevalence of edentulism, the subjects displaying oral stereotypies more commonly reported oral pain than controls.[12]

Stereotypies often need no treatment. The beneficial approaches used for moderate to severe tics include monoamine depletors, benzodiazepines, clonidine, antipsychotic drugs, and botulinum toxin. In edentulous patients, replacing, relining, and adjusting the dentures can reduce stereotypies.

Bruxism

Bruxism is a parafunctional activity that is characterized by clenching or grinding of the teeth. It has the highest prevalence of all the various oral movement disorders (8% to 10% in the general adult population) and may occur during sleep as well as during wakefulness.[13] The etiology of sleep and wake-time bruxism is still unknown. In the past, peripheral factors such as occlusal or orofacial structural discrepancies were thought to cause bruxism,

but we now know that they play only a minor role, if any, compared to central factors. For instance, there is evidence that sleep bruxism is part of an autonomic sleep-arousal response. In addition, bruxism appears to be modulated centrally by various neurotransmitters, which probably explains its link to smoking, alcohol, caffeine, illicit drugs, and a variety of medications. Diseases, trauma, and genetics may also be involved in the etiology of bruxism, and it has been linked to psychosocial factors such as stress.[13]

A host of dental problems have been ascribed to bruxism such as tooth wear (eg, attrition), hypertrophied masticatory muscles, and fractures/failures of restorations or dental implants.[13] It has also been linked to tension-type headache and pain associated with temporomandibular disorders (TMDs). The prevalence of bruxism in groups of undifferentiated TMD pain patients is very high. While excessive activation of the masticatory muscles sometimes leads to pain in bruxers, it is nevertheless important to note that even bruxers who have a severely worn dentition or hypertrophied muscles frequently do not have a history of myogenous TMD pain. This suggests that bruxism-related muscle pain may be a form of delayed-onset muscle soreness (see chapter 15).

Treatment of bruxism is indicated when the disorder causes any of the aforementioned problems. Unfortunately, there is a striking paucity of high-quality evidence regarding the management of bruxism. As with masticatory myalgia and arthralgia, the first line of management is patient counseling on the disorder and lifestyle instructions (eg, relaxation; see chapter 22). More specific management strategies for bruxism are described in the following sections, with emphasis on those strategies indicated by the better-designed studies.

Occlusal approaches

Two categories of occlusal management strategies commonly used for bruxism can be distinguished.

The first includes approaches such as occlusal equilibration and orthodontic treatment mainly aimed at protecting teeth from damage but also directed at managing any concomitant pain and grinding sounds. However, there is no high-quality evidence to support the use of these irreversible techniques: Most of the relevant articles are case reports and clinical guidelines.

The second category of management strategies is based on the use of occlusal appliances. Most authors recommend the use of hard acrylic resin splints. Again, the vast majority of articles on occlusal splints are case reports and guidelines, but some randomized clinical trials (RCTs) have been carried out. The efficacy of a hard occlusal splint versus a palatal control appliance (placebo splint) in the treatment of sleep bruxism was compared in two RCTs. While Dubé et al[14] concluded that both appliances reduce muscle activity associated with bruxism after 2 weeks, van der Zaag et al[15] found that neither of the appliances was effective after 4 weeks of usage. The two studies suggest either that oral appliances have only a transient effect on sleep bruxism or that there are large differences in response between subjects. Indeed, some subjects showed a decrease in bruxism activity, while others showed no change or even an increase.[15]

Behavioral approaches

In addition to patient counseling, a wide variety of behavioral approaches have been tried in the management of bruxism.[13] Most involve *biofeedback*, a technique to train bruxers to "unlearn" their behavior through feedback. While awake, patients can be trained to control their jaw muscle activity associated with wake-time bruxism through auditory or visual feedback from a surface electromyogram. For sleep bruxism, auditory, electric, vibratory, and even taste stimuli have been used for feedback. However, there is little evidence that biofeedback is an effective treatment for wake-time or sleep bruxism, especially in the long-term. Furthermore, the

negative consequences of the frequent arousals, like excessive daytime sleepiness, need further attention before this technique can be applied for the safe treatment of bruxism patients.

Other behavioral approaches that have been applied to bruxism include psychoanalysis, auto-suggestion, progressive relaxation, hypnosis, meditation, lifestyle improvement, sleep hygiene, self-monitoring or habit awareness, habit reversal (ie, teaching a bruxer a competing activity opposite to the bruxism behavior but involving the same muscles), habit retraining (ie, the replacement of a bad habit with a good one), and massed practice (ie, exaggerating the muscle activities, thereby making the habit punitive rather than rewarding). The value of these approaches, too, is questionable since they all lack a sound scientific basis. Again, most studies have been case reports, guidelines, and single cohort studies (ie, comparison of outcome variables before and after treatment).

Pharmacologic approaches

Medications for the management of bruxism have been studied increasingly over the last few years. These include botulinum toxin, anticonvulsant drugs (eg, gabapentin, tiagabine), and the selective serotonin reuptake inhibitor (SSRI) paroxetine. Unlike botulinum toxin and the anticonvulsants, SSRIs have been associated with increased bruxism activity. Unfortunately, there is only limited evidence for the efficacy of any of these drugs; most studies are case reports, so no definite conclusions can be drawn.

RCTs have only been performed for a few drugs. In a placebo-controlled sleep laboratory study, it was shown that the catecholamine precursor levodopa exerts a modest, attenuating effect on sleep bruxism.[16] However, the only other dopamine-related drug to be tested in an RCT, the dopamine D2 receptor agonist bromocriptine, did not change sleep bruxism motor activity.[17] Low doses of the tricyclic antidepressant amitriptyline were also ineffective.[18] Sleep bruxism did improve with the benzodiazepine clonazepam, although the maintenance of its therapeutic efficacy, its long-term tolerability, and its risk of addiction need further attention.[19] While propranolol, a nonselective adrenergic β-blocker, did not affect sleep bruxism, the selective α-2 agonist clonidine did reduce bruxism activity. Further safety assessments of clonidine are still required because morning hypotension was noted in about 20% of the participants.[20] Considering the collective evidence from these RCTs, it appears that although some pharmacologic approaches for bruxism seem promising, they all need further efficacy and safety assessments before being recommended for general use.

Summary

This chapter has noted that although medical specialists play a major role in the diagnosis and pharmacologic treatment of most oral movement disorders (PD, dystonia, dyskinesia, and stereotypies), some patients may also benefit from dental interventions such as a simple, protective bite-raising appliance or the replacement of ill-fitting dentures. In general, dental treatments are restricted to oral hygiene maintenance, preservation of chewing function, and acute pain management. Dentists are thus encouraged to refer any patients in whom they suspect an oral movement disorder to the appropriate medical specialists (eg, neurologists, psychiatrists).

On the other hand, dentists are primarily responsible for the management of bruxism. In the absence of a definitive treatment, bruxism can best be managed by counseling, a behavioral approach that includes addressing the patient's awareness of the movement disorder, relaxation, and lifestyle instructions; occlusal appliances mainly of the hard acrylic resin type; and pharmacologic interventions with centrally acting drugs such as benzodiazepines. However, drugs should be used only for short periods in cases with severe pain and impaired quality of life, and there is very limited evidence of the efficacy and safety of most drugs that so far have been advocated for bruxism.

References

1. Chudler EH, Dong WK. The role of the basal ganglia in nociception and pain. Pain 1995;60:3–38.
2. Sage JI. Pain in Parkinson's disease. Curr Treat Options Neurol 2004;6:191–200.
3. Jankovic J, Ford J. Blepharospasm and orofacial-cervical dystonia: Clinical and pharmacological findings in 100 patients. Ann Neurol 1983;13:402–411.
4. Galvez-Jimenez N, Lampuri C, Patino-Picirrillo R, Hargreave MJA, Hanson MR. Dystonia and headaches: Clinical features and response to botulinum toxin therapy. In: Fahn S, Hallett M, and DeLong MR (eds). Dystonia 4: Advances in Neurology, vol 94. Philadelphia: Lippincott Williams & Wilkins, 2004: 321–328.
5. Blanchet PJ, Rompre PH, Lavigne GJ, Lamarche C. Oral dyskinesia: A clinical overview. Int J Prosthodont 2005; 18:10–19.
6. Tan E-K, Jankovic J. Botulinum toxin A in patients with oromandibular dystonia: Long-term follow-up. Neurology 1999;53:2102–2107.
7. Møller E, Werdelin LM, Bakke M, Dalager T, Prytz S, Regeur L. Treatment of perioral dystonia with botulinum toxin in 4 cases of Meige's syndrome. Oral Surg Oral Med Oral Pathol Oral Radiol Endod 2003;96:544–549.
8. Ford B, Greene P, Fahn S. Oral and genital tardive pain syndromes. Neurology 1994;44:2115–2119.
9. Osborne TE, Grace EG, Schwartz MK. Severe degenerative changes of the temporomandibular joint secondary to the effects of tardive dyskinesia: A literature review and case report. Cranio 1989;7:58–62.
10. Rapaport A, Sadeh M, Stein D, et al. Botulinum toxin for the treatment of oro-facial-lingual-masticatory tardive dyskinesia. Mov Disord 2000;15:352–355.
11. Riley DE, Lang AE. Pain in Gilles de la Tourette syndrome and related tic disorders. Can J Neurol Sci 1989;16:439–441.
12. Blanchet PJ, Abdillahi O, Beauvais C, Rompré PH, Lavigne GJ. Prevalence of spontaneous oral dyskinesia in the elderly: A reappraisal. Mov Disord 2004;19:892–896.
13. Lavigne GJ, Manzini C, Kato T. Sleep bruxism. In: Kryger M, Roth T, Dement WC (eds). Principles and Practice of Sleep Medicine, ed 4. Philadelphia: Saunders, 2005; 946–959.
14. Dubé C, Rompré PH, Manzini C, Guitard F, de Grandmont P, Lavigne GJ. Quantitative polygraphic controlled study on efficacy and safety of oral splint devices in tooth-grinding subjects. J Dent Res 2004;83:398–403.

15. van der Zaag J, Lobbezoo F, Wicks DJ, Visscher CM, Hamburger HL, Naeije M. Controlled assessment of the efficacy of occlusal stabilization splints on sleep bruxism. J Orofac Pain 2005;19:151–158.

16. Lobbezoo F, Lavigne GJ, Tanguay R, Montplaisir JY. The effect of catecholamine precursor L-dopa on sleep bruxism: A controlled clinical trial. Mov Disord 1997; 12:73–78.

17. Lavigne GJ, Soucy JP, Lobbezoo F, Manzini C, Blanchet PJ, Montplaisir JY. Double-blind, crossover, placebo-controlled trial of bromocriptine in patients with sleep bruxism. Clin Neuropharmacol 2001;24:145–149.

18. Raigrodski AJ, Christensen LV, Mohamed SE, Gardiner DM. The effect of four-week administration of amitriptyline on sleep bruxism. A double-blind crossover clinical study. Cranio 2001;19:21–25.

19. Saletu A, Parapatics S, Saletu B, et al. On the pharmacotherapy of sleep bruxism: Placebo-controlled polysomnographic and psychometric studies with clonazepam. Neuropsychobiology 2005;51:214–225.

20. Huynh N, Lavigne GJ, Lanfranchi PA, Montplaisir JY, de Champlain J. The effect of 2 sympatholytic medications—propranolol and clonidine—on sleep bruxism: Experimental randomized controlled studies. Sleep 2006;29:307–316.

Illustrative Case Reports

Antoon De Laat
Sandro Palla
José Tadeu Tesseroli de Siqueira
Yoshiki Imamura

In this chapter, several cases are presented to illustrate various types of orofacial pain likely to be seen by dentists. After listening attentively to the patient's complaints and taking a careful history, the clinician should be able to establish a provisional or differential diagnosis that will then be confirmed or rejected by a clinical examination, followed by appropriate tests and images if necessary, as outlined in chapter 17.

Case 1

Patient JS, a 38-year-old woman, complains of sharp, shooting, and irradiating pain of the left maxillary region that began suddenly one morning 3 weeks ago. She cannot localize the pain to a particular tooth. Now the pain is almost continuous at a level of 3 on a visual analog scale (VAS) of 1 to 10, with 10 being the worst. The pain is exacerbated when chewing on the left side and when drinking cold water, and it worsens (level 7) in the evening when she goes to bed. Last week, the pain kept her awake one night for more than 2 hours. She is aware of daytime episodes of clenching, plus her husband says that she grinds her teeth at night. No other oral parafunctional behaviors, such as nail

biting or tongue thrust, are present. There is no history of facial or neck trauma. She does not report limitation of jaw movement or temporomandibular joint (TMJ) sounds.

Her past medical history is negative except for an appendectomy 10 years ago and sinus surgery 7 years ago due to chronic sinusitis. She has suffered from recurrent headaches, concomitant with menstrual periods and periods of stress, for several years. She takes no medication for these headaches. Her husband says she does not snore or cease breathing during sleep, and she does not complain of temporal headache on awakening, reducing the likelihood of a concomitant sleep breathing disorder.

Questions

What is your provisional or differential diagnosis? What kind of clinical examination is needed? What do you need to assess? What is the rationale?

Answers

Based on the onset, duration, and pattern of pain and exacerbating factors, dental or periodontal pathology should first be suspected. Careful intraoral and radiologic examinations will be necessary. In addition, tooth vitality testing and a local anesthesia challenge should help achieve final diagnosis. Considering the history of sinus surgery, presence of a maxillary sinusitis needs to be excluded. Here, a radiologic examination may help, but a consultation with an otorhinolaryngologist should be sought if sinusitis is suspected. Finally, in view of the history of sleep bruxism and wake-time clenching, TMJ and muscle pain needs to be excluded.

Clinical examination

Extraoral examination does not reveal any swelling, overt asymmetries, or peculiarities of the patient's face. Facial expression and mandibular movements appear normal and without pain. Intraoral examination shows an Angle Class II, division 1 occlusion and no missing teeth but several amalgam fillings. There are no obvious carious lesions and no broken fillings. Functional examination reveals no apparent premature contacts. There is abrasion or attrition of the cusps of the canines and the occlusal surfaces of the premolars and molars. There is a slight gingivitis but no loss of gingival attachment.

Tooth vitality testing with an ice-cold stick (CO_2 stick) is normal for all teeth in the second and third quadrants, but the patient displays a localized hypersensitivity of the maxillary left first premolar and second molar, as well as of the mandibular left second premolar. A provocation test, biting on a cotton roll or hard plastic stick between single pairs of teeth, provokes a sharp pain when the patient bites on the left second molars. No pain is induced upon mechanical percussion. Careful examination of the maxillary left second molar reveals no large filling or caries, but a fine crack in the buccopalatal direction is visible.

Panoramic and periapical radiographs of the maxillary left quadrant do not show any radiolucencies, carious lesions under old fillings, or periodontal problems. The fine crack is not visible on radiographs. The sinus in the vicinity of the maxillary left second molar appears normal on the panoramic radiograph. When a fine probe is forced between the two parts of the cracked tooth, a sharp pain is reported (Fig 27-1), which is eliminated by local anesthesia.

Working diagnosis

The working diagnosis is a cracked tooth, probably a result of severe and forceful wake-time bruxism of the clenching type and/or sleep clenching/grinding.

Discussion

The history and the character of the pain and its provocation by mastication, cold substances, and the probe test point to a dental etiology. There is a history of clenching habits, which could lead to some type of dental sensitivity, but this is typically less localized and tends to fluctuate over time. The past history of sinusitis and the localization of the pain in the maxillary region kept open the possibility of a maxillary sinusitis. The latter diagnosis is ruled out, however, because there is no recent history of a common cold, fever, blocked nose, or aggravation of the pain by head or bodily movements. For these reasons, the clinical examination focused on the oral cavity. If this examination had failed to show any abnormalities, a functional examination of the masticatory system (including palpation of the muscles and joints) would have been performed to check for temporomandibular disorders (TMDs) of myogenous origin and referred pain to the teeth. If no dental pathology or muscle pain had been found, the patient probably would have been referred to an otorhinolaryngologist.

The described pain is apparently caused initially by mechanical stimulation of tooth pulp nociceptors (see chapter 4). Inflammation has probably occurred gradually and has made the receptors hypersensitive to thermal and mechanical stimuli.

Fig 27-1 Cracked maxillary left second molar. A probe is forced between the two parts, which causes the patient to experience a sharp pain.

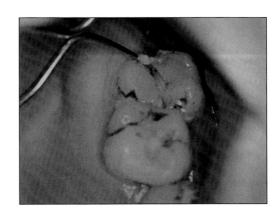

After some time, the pain starts to radiate over the region (eg, left maxilla, muscles) because of central excitatory effects (see chapters 5 and 7).

Management

Since the fracture apparently extended into the root, the tooth was extracted (see chapter 20). To prevent damage to other teeth, a bite splint was fabricated for use during periods with stress and high clenching probability (see chapters 22 and 26).

Case 2

Patient AP, a 40-year-old male, has already consulted four dentists because of pain in the left mandible that has lasted more than 6 months. The third dentist thought it was related to the mandibular left second premolar, so he removed the pulp, which temporarily eliminated the pain. However, the pain recurred, and its intensity gradually increased to the pre-endodontic treatment level. The fourth dentist extracted the tooth some months later. Since that time, the patient still feels pain sometimes located in the spot where the tooth was extracted, but most of the time it is located in the mandibular left first premolar. The pain is now constant, dull, aching, and sometimes burning; it is rated 4 to 5 on a VAS of 1 to 10. He reports no

pain during the night. Oral function (eg, chewing, talking), stress, or other factors do not exacerbate the pain. It increases slightly in the evening and when he is relaxed, watching television. Chewing gum relieves some of the pain. The patient has used several analgesics and is now taking up to six aspirin tablets per day with low to moderate relief.

His past medical history reveals that he has had a periodic left-sided headache for about 1 year. The headache periods started some time after he lost his job. He has been unemployed since then, which creates several psychosocial problems. During this period, his wife noticed more frequent tooth grinding during his sleep. More recently he has complained of chest pain, but he has not yet consulted his physician.

Questions

What will be the goal of the clinical and radiologic examination? What is your provisional or differential diagnosis?

Answers

In this particular case, the history and time course of the pain are not typical of a dental pathology, but first this should be excluded. The increase in severity of pain after the extraction, the character of the pain, and the relief brought about by chewing strongly suggest a diagnosis of atypical odontalgia. However, referred pain from the masticatory muscles or from the cervical spine is also a possibility. Consequently, careful clinical and intraoral examination, radiographic examination, and perhaps referral to specialists (eg, neurologist, pain clinic) for differential diagnosis will be needed.

Clinical examination

The patient's face looks normal in the extraoral examination, and intraorally there are no carious lesions, broken fillings, or periodontal pathology. The extraction site has healed normally but is painful to palpation by a finger or periodontal probe. Also, the mandibular left first premolar is slightly tender to percussion. All teeth are vital and react normally to cold and warm stimuli.

The mandibular movements are within normal limits and are not painful. The function and response to palpation of the TMJs are normal. The masseter muscle and the insertion of the temporalis muscle are painful to palpation, slightly more on the left side than on the right. There seem to be no neurologic signs, and in particular there are no sensory abnormalities in the area supplied by the trigeminal nerves. Movements of the head are neither limited nor painful, and palpation of the cervical muscles does not provoke pain.

Topical anesthetics applied to the gingiva in the region of the mandibular left second premolar do not decrease the pain, but a mandibular nerve block is of some benefit (50% decrease in pain). However, the pain returns to full intensity within 15 minutes, even when the region itself appears to be anesthetized.

No bone pathology is seen on the panoramic radiographs.

Working diagnosis

The working diagnosis is atypical odontalgia.

Discussion

The diagnosis of atypical odontalgia is based on the absence of dental, periodontal, or bone pathology in the painful area. In addition, the examination of the masticatory, cervical, and trigeminal areas was negative for any abnormalities, reducing the possibility of referred pain (see also chapter 20).

The time course of the pain (constant, sometimes burning, alleviated by chewing and not coincident with headache episodes) rules out an ectopic headache. The absence of other etiologic factors, the duration of the pain (more than 6 months), and the inability to provoke or exacerbate the pain, in addition to the tenderness of the area involved and the partial and only temporary relief during the mandibular block, all led to the final diagnosis. If the pain had been completely eliminated using a local anesthetic block, the diagnosis of atypical odontalgia could not have been given. Pain in the lower left mandible is sometimes related to angina pectoris. However, the fact that it was continuous, long-lasting, and not provoked by factors that typically exacerbate angina pectoris (eg, exercise, large meals, and emotional stress) eliminates this possibility. In case of doubt, consultation with the treating physician is recommended. Also, consultation with a neurologist is suggested to rule out specific lesions and other diseases (eg, irritation of the trigeminal nerve by pressure from blood vessels or tumors, demyelinating diseases).

Atypical odontalgia is considered to be of neuropathic origin. Its cause is yet unknown, although central mechanisms have been proposed (see chapters 7 and 20).

Management

Treatment of this type of orofacial pain falls out of the scope of a general dental practice. It involves the use of medications acting on the central nervous system such as tricyclic antidepressants, gabapentin or pregabalin, and *N*-methyl-D-aspartate (NMDA) receptor antagonists (see chapters 19, 20, and 24). Therefore, this patient should be referred to a neurologist or other pain specialist. Moreover, since quality of life may be perturbed, psychologic support could be helpful. If tooth grinding persists during sleep, a bite splint may help to prevent tooth damage (see chapter 26).

Since there is no identifiable lesion, surgical treatment of the extraction site or dental treatment of the neighboring teeth must be avoided; either could aggravate the pain through central sensitization (see chapters 5, 7, 8, and 24).

Case 3

Patient JS, a 15-year-old girl, complains of right pre-auricular pain and a limitation of jaw movements that began 4 days ago. The pain began suddenly when she was hit by an elbow while playing basketball. Immediately after the blow, a continuous pain was present, which gradually improved. She also has the feeling of a "full ear" and the impression of hearing difficulties since the pain occurred. In the past, she periodically had a painless click in the left and right TMJs, which worsened during jaw movements. Her past medical history is negative for any health problems except for sprained ankles.

Questions

What kind of pathology comes to mind? What steps will you take to verify this?

Answers

In contrast to the previous cases, this history suggests a traumatic etiology. Possible diagnoses are TMJ trauma leading to subcondylar or condylar fracture, inflammation, or anterior disc displacement without reduction of the right TMJ. However, the limitation of mandibular movement could also be due to myogenous pain (see chapters 14 and 15).

The clinical examination of the masticatory system should be complemented by radiographic images (initially with a panoramic radiograph, followed by computerized tomography scan or magnetic resonance imaging [MRI], if needed) of the TMJs and related structures to exclude fractures (eg, condylar neck, zygomatic arch) or TMJ disc displacement.

Clinical examination

The extraoral examination reveals no facial swelling or asymmetry. The patient can open her mouth to 35 mm with a deviation of the mandible to the right side. Maximal mouth opening can be passively increased 4 mm by the clinician. Both assisted and unassisted maximal mouth opening, as well as right lateral and protrusive movements, result in pain in front of the ear and deflection of the mandible to the right. Lateral movements are asymmetric (3 mm to the left and 10 mm to the right). Also, the mandible deflects to the right side during protrusion, which is painful. There are no sounds in the TMJ while performing these movements. Palpation of the right TMJ is painful, and pain is reproduced when the patient moves the jaw from side to side. The masseter, pterygoid, and temporalis muscles are tender to palpation on the right side. There are no signs of altered occlusion or of any dental or periodontal problems.

No bony abnormalities in the images of the TMJs are seen on a panoramic radiograph taken with the mouth open. MRI reveals an anteriorly displaced disc (Fig 27-2).

Working diagnosis

The working diagnosis is trauma to soft tissues of the TMJ and anterior disc displacement without reduction of the right TMJ, with limitation of jaw movements and myalgia and arthralgia on the right side.

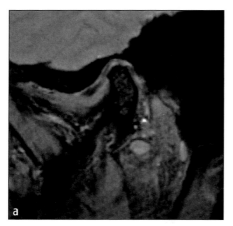 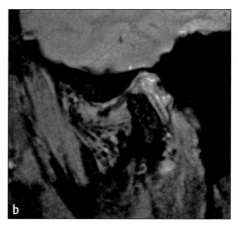

Fig 27-2 MRI of the anteriorly displaced disc (a) in maximum intercuspation and (b) at maximum opening. The disc does not reduce to its normal position during opening, thus limiting condylar translation.

Discussion

The history is highly indicative of a TMJ disorder. The clinical examination confirms right jaw muscle pain concomitant with an anteriorly dislocated disc of the right TMJ, which is also revealed by MRI. In similar cases, local TMJ trauma and resulting inflammation can also cause a limitation of mandibular movement. In these situations, the pain is of a nociceptive origin.

Management

To decrease the posttraumatic inflammation, short-term NSAIDs are indicated (see chapters 19, 21, and 22). In addition, the patient was instructed to rest the mandible as much as possible (soft diet, chewing on left side, avoiding large yawning or oral parafunctional behaviors such as nail biting and clenching). Supportive physical therapy was recommended in conjunction with the application of moist heat, massage, and, from the moment the pain decreases, progressive mobilization of the mandible with stretching exercises. After 6 weeks, the patient reported pain reduction and improved mobility.

Case 4

Patient JL, a 48-year-old woman, presents with a dull pain on both sides of the face that worsens in the evening. The pain has been present periodically for more than 6 years and gradually has increased in intensity and frequency. The last episode started after a visit with the dental hygienist for regular oral hygiene control. The pain is particularly intense during chewing and yawning. She rates the pain 4 to 5 on a VAS of 1 to 10. In general, the patient feels tired, has sleeping difficulties, and suffers periodically from gastrointestinal (GI) problems. She is not aware of any oral parafunctional habits. Because of a GI problem (gastric ulcer), she does not tolerate aspirin or other anti-inflammatory drugs. In addition, she takes medication (benazepril) to control her slightly elevated blood pressure. She also regularly takes painkillers (paracetamol with codeine) and tranquilizers (diazepam) to be able to sleep. She wakes up with tension in the neck and the shoulders. She suffers from headaches bilaterally in the occipital and temporal regions at least 10 days per month. In response to direct questions during a thorough his-

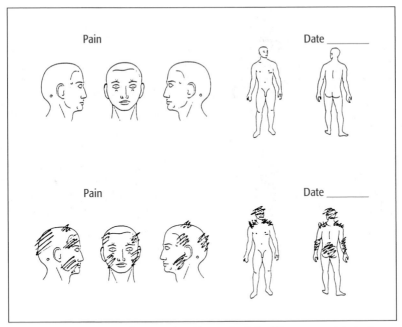

Fig 27-3 Pain drawing that illustrates the widespread pain in different parts of the body.

tory taking, she also reports pain in the shoulder, lower back, and arms, which started several years before the facial pain. The latter, however, causes her more concern. She is anxious about having a serious illness. When asked about her mood, she reports feeling depressed because of the lasting pain. She has visited many doctors and dentists without receiving a clear diagnosis or useful treatment. The most recent treatment was a new pair of partial dentures, advocated as the optimal solution for the loss of occlusal support and thus for the facial pain.

Questions

What direction should the clinical examination take? What are the possible diagnoses?

Answers

This woman has complex pain in the facial region as well as in other sites of the body. In such situations, a pain drawing may give better insight into the localization of the pain (Fig 27-3). The history is suggestive of either myofascial pain or possibly a more generalized muscle pain (eg, fibromyalgia) that includes the masticatory and cervical areas. Furthermore, the patient seems depressed, which might result from the pain but could also be contributing to the pain. Her GI problems, poor sleep, headaches, and use of anxiolytic medication are similar to common findings in patients with fibromyalgia.

Clinical examination

The patient can open her mouth to 50 mm with some slight pain. Assisted opening to 57 mm is associated with an increase in the pain. The lateral and protrusive movements of the mandible are within normal ranges. Auscultation does not reveal any joint sounds. The TMJ area is tender, and the masseter muscles are much more painful to palpation than any other masticatory muscles. Movements of the head are painful and limited. Neck and shoulder muscles are painful upon palpation, more on the left than on the right side. The neurologic screening is within normal limits. The intraoral examination reveals shortened dental arches and severe wear of the dentition. She is using maxillary and mandibular partial dentures to replace the maxillary right second premolar and first molar, the maxillary left first and second premolars and second molar, and the mandibular left first premolar and first molar, as well as the right second premolar and first molar. No evidence of dental or periodontal pathology is noted. Occlusal relationships are within normal limits.

Working diagnosis

Chronic head and neck myalgia are probably symptoms of a more generalized pain condition such as fibromyalgia, which is not a diagnosis to be made by a dentist. The patient needs to be referred to a physician and/or psychologist in addition to a physical therapist.

Discussion

In contrast to the previous cases, an interdisciplinary approach is mandatory from the start since this patient has depressed mood and a tension-type headache and suffers from pain of the masticatory system as part of a more generalized pain problem. With this type of pain it is important to ask about pain problems elsewhere in the body and other symptoms (eg, GI symptoms, poor sleep), since many patients would not report these spontaneously to a dentist.

Management

The local treatment for masticatory muscle and joint pain consisted of relaxation procedures for the masticatory muscles and supportive physical therapy. No splint was advocated since her symptoms were minor in the morning compared with the rest of the day and evening. She was also referred to a multidisciplinary pain center for her generalized symptoms, where she started a combined therapy involving (1) review of health status, sleep, hygiene, diet, and exercise; (2) medication (eg, metacarbomol, cyclobenzaprine); (3) physiotherapy and ergotherapy; and (4) cognitive behavioral therapy and psychologic support. In some cases, an antidepressant regimen (eg, low-dose amitriptyline) is used to improve sleep quality and mood disturbances if well tolerated by the patient (see chapters 16, 19 to 22, 25, and 26).

Case 5

A 58-year-old man presents with a history of very intense, threatening, shock-like pain attacks localized to the mandibular right first premolar. The pain reaches an intensity of 10 on a VAS of 1 to 10. The first consulted dentist performed a root canal treatment on the mandibular right first premolar that relieved the pain for a month. Thereafter, the attacks became more frequent and could not be alleviated by means of analgesics or anti-inflammatory drugs. The root canal treatment was redone twice, without any improvement. After approximately 2 years, the attacks increased to daily frequency, always occurred diurnally, and were triggered by routine activities such as talking, brushing teeth, chewing, or tongue movements. The patient consulted an emergency dental clinic, where a local anesthetic block was performed that only partially alleviated the pain and allowed him to perform jaw movements. This result prompted the extraction of the tooth in question. Unfortunately, 2 hours after the partial anesthetic effect was over, the pain returned, this time localized in the mandibular right lateral incisor. Consequently, this tooth was also extracted but the pain did not disappear. During the history taking, the patient denies suffering from frequent pain in other body parts.

Questions

Which kind of diagnosis comes to mind? What speaks in favor of a dental/periodontal etiology of the toothache, and what speaks against it?

Answers

Already the description of the pain (eg, its episodic, very intense, shock-like, and short-lasting character) speaks against a dental/periodontal etiology (eg, cracked tooth). This is reinforced by the lack of effectiveness of the dental therapies (root canal treatment and extractions). The most likely diagnosis is trigeminal neuralgia.

Clinical examination

Inspection and palpation of the extraoral and intraoral structures did not reveal any abnormalities of the teeth, periodontium, oral mucosa or salivary glands. The mandibular movements were unlimited and pain free. Only a mild tenderness to palpation of the masseter muscles was recorded. The palpation of the gingiva around the mandibular right first premolar triggered a pain crisis, which produced an avoidance head reaction and an expression of great suffering. The crisis lasted approximately 40 seconds, and the patient confirmed that it was the pain he normally feels. This pain could be retriggered by means of a non-noxious stimulus (eg, cotton swab).

The panoramic, periapical radiographs, and contrast medium–enhanced computerized tomograms did not reveal pathologic tissue alterations.

Working diagnosis

The working diagnosis is classical trigeminal neuralgia of the right mandibular branch (V3).

Discussion

Pain triggered by oral activities (chewing, talking, tooth brushing) does not necessarily have a dental/periodontal etiology even when the patient swears that it is a toothache. Sometimes it is referred from other sources. A precise pain description helps in making a provisional diagnosis and ruling out a dental/periodontal pathology. For instance, the pain caused by a pulpitis varies in frequency and intensity, has often a throbbing character, is triggered or exacerbated by thermal (cold/hot drinks) and mechanical (percussion, food crunching) stimuli, and may awaken the patient during the night. In addition, pulpitis pain is abolished by an anesthetic block. On the contrary, classical trigeminal neuralgia typically manifests paroxysmal, shock-like pain attacks of short duration (fractions of seconds to 2 minutes), affecting one or more trigeminal branches. This pain can be triggered by non-noxious stimuli. Furthermore, the patient is pain free between attacks; the neurologic status is normal; and the anesthetic block does not block the pain. Approximately 5% of the trigeminal neuralgias are secondary to a tumor or multiple sclerosis (in which case the condition may be referred to as *symptomatic trigeminal neuralgia*), which means that a neurologic examination is mandatory. Lastly, toothache referred from trigger points in masticatory muscles is also not paroxysmal, not shock-like, and not episodic but function-dependent and cannot be eliminated by an anesthetic block of the tooth in which the pain is felt.

The clinician's responsibilities for a patient suffering from trigeminal neuralgia are to *(1)* recognize the possible diagnosis, (2) avoid tooth extractions or root canal procedures, and (3) refer the patient to a physician or neurologist who will be responsible for excluding the presence of brain tumors or a symptomatic neuralgia and then will manage the pain.

Management

The treatment of a classical trigeminal neuralgia is pharmacologic and in cases of insufficient remission or adverse effects, neurosurgical approaches are also used. The drugs of choice are the anticonvulsants (eg, carbamazepine, oxycarbamazepine, or gabapentin and pregabalin). The dosage must be carefully titrated until the patient experiences either remission or side effects that are too severe. Patients receiving pharmacologic therapy must be permanently monitored, and in the case of carbamazepine use, a regular complete blood count is necessary (see chapter 24).

Science Transfer in Orofacial Pain: Problems and Solutions

Charles S. Greene

In this chapter, the background and current status of science transfer in the orofacial pain field will be analyzed, with special emphasis on the temporomandibular disorders (TMDs). A combination of cultural and educational barriers to the acceptance of recent developments in this field will be discussed, and some possible solutions will be proposed. The intention is to impress upon undergraduate and graduate students the need to constantly update their knowledge in this field. It is hoped that they and their teachers will benefit from learning about the problems of the past, which should enable them to face the problems of the future with open but critical minds.

General Problems in Science Transfer

It might be expected by the lay public that all practicing health care providers are ready and waiting for the latest information to arrive, while all biomedical scientists are eager to have their work applied to patients by clinicians. However, the reality is that several barriers on both sides prevent

such a smooth science-transfer process. Clinicians often allege that scientists do not appreciate the "real-life" problems facing practitioners, or that they do not care much whether their research findings can be applied to the clinical situation. As a result, many clinicians believe that the scientific community does not communicate very well with them. In addition, there is always the natural reluctance of people to make changes in the way they do things every day.

In addition, there are some special obstacles that keep health care providers from obtaining and utilizing new information. The roots of some of these problems can be traced back to a fundamental tension that exists in many health care programs, including dental schools. During those years of training, the basic science teachers frequently complain that students do not care much about the academic biomedical subjects. Instead, it seems to them that those students just want to get into the clinics, where they will quickly abandon science and replace it with clinical folklore. Unfortunately, some of the clinical faculty members may foster this behavior by downplaying the importance of science in their daily lives as "real doctors." In the end, it must be understood that many health care providers tend to resist making changes in the environment in which they work; therefore, it is important to appreciate some of the factors that might account for that resistance.

The general term that describes unwillingness or inability to adopt new ideas has been borrowed from the field of psychology: *cognitive dissonance*. This uncomfortable feeling arises from natural impulses to understand and control the world around us, so any challenge to previous beliefs has to be processed through that filter of comprehension. Of course, dental students are warned that significant scientific discoveries and changes will occur within their professional lifetime, but each major innovation in their discipline still represents another challenge to their previous understanding. The process by which individuals within a community (eg, physicians or dentists) move from their old concepts and practices to new ones has been described by Rogers as "diffusion of innovations."[1] There are four main elements in the diffusion of new ideas: *(1)* an *innovation* that is *(2) communicated* through certain channels *(3) over time (4)* among the members of a *social/professional system*. Rogers has studied this process from both ends (ie, the innovator and the recipient), and through extensive research in this field, he has identified the stages of transformation at both ends. Boxes 28-1 and 28-2 summarize these stages, and the implications for health care providers should be obvious.

Science Transfer Problems in Orofacial Pain

The field of orofacial pain has a complex history characterized by a great amount of controversy.[2,3] This is especially true for TMDs, which are a main concern for dentists. Many dentists simply want to avoid treating TMD patients because they see them as difficult to manage or because they regard the entire field as chaotic. Instead, they may try to

refer their patients to dentists who "specialize" in this field, but the referral process is usually complicated by two factors: *(1)* There are no specialists recognized by the country's licensing or accreditation bodies in this discipline, although some practitioners have spent 2 or more years in postgraduate orofacial pain training; and *(2)* the community dentists who may claim to be experts in this area often use media and Internet advertising to attract patients, but there are no standards for assessing their background or skills.

The good news on the research side of TMDs is that considerable progress has been made in their diagnosis and treatment; the bad news on the clinical side is that the profession remains divided over many diagnostic and treatment issues. Much of this division can be traced to a failure to achieve science transfer, for which both researchers and clinicians can be blamed. However, the single most important reason for this ongoing controversy can be summarized in two words: clinical success. Unlike some other fields in medicine and dentistry, the TMD field suffers from an excess of success, with well over 75% of patients with nonchronic forms of TMDs tending to respond positively to various treatments, including placebos.[4] This success has proved to be a major problem in trying to convince dental practitioners to abandon some of their outdated theories and procedures because these protocols seem to work in their hands. This might be a trivial matter if the opposing concepts were equivalent in their potential for good or harm; unfortunately, that is not the case. Instead, most of the outdated concepts of TMD etiology are based on morphologic theories, and as such they generally lead to irreversible morphology-changing treatment procedures. On the other hand, most of the current evidence-based concepts are based on a biopsychosocial medical model that generally leads to more conservative therapy. This model also places a strong emphasis on recognizing that chronic pain cannot always be cured, and therefore it calls for caring clinicians to help TMD pa-

---

Box 28-1 The innovation-decision process[1]

A new idea, practice, or technology is introduced to prospective "adopters"

Communication channels spread the message:

- Media (journals, lectures, Internet)
- Interpersonal contact (most individuals accept or reject an innovation based on peer reviews rather than relying on scientific research)
- Opinion leaders (within the social system, they promote the innovation):
  - Primary change agents are in authoritative positions
  - Secondary aides (eg, drug representatives, salespeople) try to persuade clients

Over time, five steps occur in the adoption of innovations:

- Knowledge ⟶ persuasion ⟶ decision ⟶ implementation ⟶ confirmation

---

Box 28-2 Categories of innovation adopters[1]

Venturesome people: Sophisticates that are able to understand complexities and are financially secure enough to take risks. They act as leaders and role models of innovation.

Early adopters: Persons who are more integrated in the regular culture or system and respected as being leaders. They are sought out by change agents to promote acceptance of innovation because their stamp of approval often triggers critical mass of acceptance.

Early majority: One of the largest subgroups that is slightly ahead in accepting innovation. They are very interconnected within the group, so while they do not lead the change, their acceptance tips the scales.

Late majority: A large subgroup that is slightly behind in accepting innovation. Regarded as skeptics, these people require a lot of pressure from peers before accepting innovations. They want uncertainty diminished or removed before feeling it is safe to accept.

Laggards: Often isolated people who, although they may interact with similar people, tend to be suspicious of change and also of change agents. Their resistance to innovations may be entirely rational to them because of limited resources and the need for complete certainty before giving up the old ways.

---

tients manage their pain and any associated psychosocial issues.[3]

At the clinical level, this continuing controversy has acquired some new "wrinkles." Various dental academies and institutes have established teaching programs based on the concept that the temporomandibular joint (TMJ) is the centerpiece of "ideal" dental care. As a result, not only are genuine TMD patients being placed at risk for inappropriate therapy, but even asymptomatic individuals are likely to be told that they have occult or potential TMJ problems. Therefore, they will supposedly need major dental work in order to avoid future TMJ troubles. These concepts usually include significant amounts of diagnostic testing with electronic instrumentation, complex imaging, and intricate

Box 28-3 Why we need more science transfer in orofacial pain

Dentists

May have minimal skills in differential diagnosis

- Exclude or include TMD patients incorrectly
- Have limited understanding of chronic vs acute pain
- Have limited appreciation for psychologic (Axis II) factors (see chapter 1)

May follow outdated concepts of etiology

- Overclosed vertical dimension
- Bad skeletal and dental relationships
- Malposition of mandible or condyle/fossa malrelationship
- Everything is due to stress

May not use appropriate treatments

- Fear of most prescription medications
- Limited awareness of the value of physical therapy
- Misunderstandings about oral splints—when to use them, what they can and cannot do
- Tendency to use irreversible treatments of doubtful efficacy

Physicians

Usually have little education about facial pain

- Poor understanding of TMDs
- Often refer by exclusion (especially ear, nose, and throat specialists)
- Still talking about Costen syndrome*
- Often expect dentists to "fix the bite"

*An outdated term for TMDs based on etiologic concepts of structural abnormality.

physical examination, all targeted at the TMJ and the dental occlusion, and the nearly inevitable result is that the patient is found to have "problems" that need to be addressed. For the scientific community, these entrepreneurial activities pose a different kind of challenge, because both the teaching programs and their followers have a strong financial interest in perpetuating their viewpoints. Box 28-3 summarizes many of the reasons why more science transfer in the field of orofacial pain is needed.

Enhancing Science Transfer in Orofacial Pain

To improve the science transfer situation in orofacial pain and TMDs, we need to make some assessment of what dentists and physicians in the community currently believe; this has been done at several points in the past 30 years.[5,6] These survey studies have repeatedly shown that many practitioners still believe both "facts" and opinions that

---

Box 28-4 How to enhance science transfer in orofacial pain

Individual researchers can:

- Publish more review articles to summarize the state of the art

- Do more clinical trials and publish them in popular journals

- Publish more meta-analyses of high-quality clinical studies

- Present more science transfer lectures to clinical groups, including general dental audiences (local, regional, and national), dental and medical specialty groups, and special-interest study clubs and academies

Learned societies and institutions can:

- Conduct consensus conferences (eg, National Institute of Dental and Craniofacial Research at United States National Institutes of Health)

- Empower science information committees to make public statements (eg, American Association for Dental Research)

- Develop clinical guidelines based on evidence (eg, American Academy of Orofacial Pain, American Academy of Pain Management, American Academy of Oral Medicine)

- Encourage members of expert groups to produce science transfer journal articles and lectures (eg, International Association for Dental Research–Neuroscience Group, American Academy of Orofacial Pain, American Academy of Oral Medicine)

- Present more continuing education courses on orofacial pain and TMDs

---

have already been disproved, and that those beliefs determine their day-to-day behavior as they treat patients (see Box 28-3). The presence or absence of meaningful standards and guidelines for appropriate management of TMDs by the professional community can have a powerful impact on clinician behavior—especially in a field like dentistry where every solo practitioner in a private office can do whatever seems reasonable. Box 28-4 presents some concrete suggestions to enhance the future transfer of evidence-based information and guidelines about orofacial pain to all interested clinicians.

The lack of understanding as well as the continuing controversies in orofacial pain and TMDs can probably be attributed in large part to deficiencies in undergraduate and graduate dental education. For example, a recent survey of American and Canadian dental schools[7] found that most dental schools do not have structured courses or clinical rotations dealing with the issues of orofacial pain, although TMDs may be discussed in some scattered lectures or seminars. Only a few schools had a specific curriculum for presenting the relevant basic sciences and the didactic clinical information required to prepare dental students for appropriate management of TMD patients. As a result, graduating dentists frequently are not well prepared to diagnose and treat patients with various types of nondental orofacial pain, even when those patients have some form of a TMD. Because of this deficiency, they may be attracted to various short continuing education courses or longer programs that deal with orofacial pain topics, but in doing so they may be at risk for acquiring bad information. When these clinicians do identify a TMD patient in their own practices, there is a good chance that an incorrect etiologic theory will be used to explain the problem, and as a result the treatment selected may be inappropriate. As for physicians, it is even more unlikely that their medical school education has prepared them to recognize and/or treat TMD patients. What they do learn often leads them to send patients with undiagnosed head and face pains to dentists, usually with the hope that a "bite problem" or "TMJ malalignment" will be discovered to be the basis for all symptoms.

Responsibilities of Innovators as well as Students and Practitioners

It is the position of this author that the major responsibility for science transfer in orofacial pain rests with the academic community.[8] Although it also is the responsibility of individual clinicians to keep up with current literature (and to make appropriate changes in how they practice), academics must make a more dedicated effort to transmit the latest information to them. Some efforts are already being made in this direction, but obviously more is needed (see Box 28-4). For example, the 1996 Technology Assessment Conference held by the US National Institute of Dental Research[9] and the policy statement on TMDs by the American Association for Dental Research[10] were important efforts to define the state of the art in the TMD field. To the credit of the American Academy of Orofacial Pain, they have produced (and revised three times since 1990) evidence-based guidelines for the diagnosis and management of TMDs and other orofacial pains; a new edition was published in 2008.[11]

Dental students and practitioners should understand that the obligations of science transfer also rest heavily on them. While the scientists are charged with the production and dissemination of information, the clinician audience must be prepared to receive and utilize it. This requires a positive attitude about learning new things rather than stubbornly clinging to the past, as well as the development of critical judgment in assessing new information. Most dental schools today try to teach students how to critically evaluate new information, which will always contain a mixture of valid and invalid elements. After graduation, the burden of learning and critically assessing new information shifts entirely to the clinicians as they or she embarks on a career of patient care.

Dental clinicians also need to recognize that their patients may be obtaining information and concepts from many sources. The media and the Internet are filled with a large variety of health reports that vary widely in the quality of the information they contain. Clinicians can expect to receive all sorts of questions from their patients on a variety of dental topics, and TMDs usually rank high on the list; failure to keep up with the latest developments will undermine the dentist's ability to provide the correct information that patients may need. Professional organizations, both research societies and practitioner associations, should help clinicians in providing accurate and timely information to the public about controversial dental topics. Nevertheless, the ultimate responsibility ends up in the one-to-one interaction between a patient and a dentist.

References

1. Rogers EM. Diffusion of Innovations, ed 5. New York: Free Press (Simon & Schuster), 2003.
2. Greene CS. Temporomandibular disorders: The evolution of concepts. In: Sarnat BG, Laskin DM (eds). The Temporomandibular Joint: A Biologic Basis for Clinical Practice, ed 4. Philadelphia: Saunders, 1992:298–315.
3. Greene CS. Concepts of TMD etiology: Effects on diagnosis and treatment. In: Laskin DM, Greene CS, Hylander WL (eds). Temporomandibular Disorders: An Evidence-Based Approach to Diagnosis and Treatment. Chicago: Quintessence, 2006:219–228.
4. Greene CS. Managing TMD patients: Initial therapy is the key. J Am Dent Assoc 1992;123:43–45.
5. Just JK, Perry HT, Greene CS. Treating TM disorders: A survey on diagnosis, etiology, and management. J Am Dent Assoc 1991;122:55–60.
6. Glaros AG, Glass EG, McLaughlin L. Knowledge and beliefs of dentists regarding temporomandibular disorders and chronic pain. J Orofac Pain 1994;8:216–222.
7. Klasser GD, Greene CS. Predoctoral teaching of temporomandibular disorders: A survey of U.S. and Canadian dental schools. J Am Dent Assoc 2007;138:231–237.
8. Baum BJ. Can biomedical science be made relevant in dental education? A North American perspective. Eur J Dent Educ 2003;7:49–55; discussion 56–59.
9. National Institutes of Health Technology Assessment Conference on Management of Temporomandibular Disorders. Bethesda, Maryland, April 29–May 1, 1996. Proceedings. Oral Surg Oral Med Oral Pathol Oral Radiol Endod 1997;83:49–183.
10. American Association for Dental Research. Policy Statement on Temporomandibular Disorders (TMD). AADR Reports 1996;18(4).
11. American Academy of Orofacial Pain. de Leeuw R (ed). Orofacial Pain: Guidelines for Assessment, Diagnosis, and Management. Chicago: Quintessence, 2008.

Index